Women in Jamaica

PATTERNS OF REPRODUCTION AND FAMILY
by George W. Roberts and Sonja A. Sinclair

Introduction by Vera Rubin

ICA

The findings of a major research project sponsored by the American Association for the Advancement of Science, administered by the Research Institute for the Study of Man and conducted by the Census Research Programme of the University of the West Indies, Jamaica, this Study provides the basis for a deep understanding of the position of women in Jamaica, with special reference to their reproductive performance and family relationships. Bringing together both published and newly-acquired data, it covers many significant aspects of the lifestyles of West Indian women.

The formation of family unions, the extent and character of changes in the family structure, the three types of unions (married, common law and visiting), the periods of time spent in each, as well as their relative stability, have all been delineated in the course of this investigation.

Also included in this work are many social and biological aspects of reproduction and childcare in the society, such as pregnancy wastage, infant mortality, breastfeeding, support of children, family planning, menstrual patterns and knowledge of reproduction and menstruation.

This work of Roberts and Sinclair is a critically important sociological document for a proper understanding not only of the role of women in the Jamaican family, but of the greatly varied relationships within families throughout the West Indies.

Women in Jamaica: Patterns of Reproduction and Family is a volume in the series entitled THE CARIBBEAN—Historical and Cultural Perspectives, edited by Robert A. Hill, presently at the University of California at Los Angeles.

WOMEN IN JAMAICA

Patterns of Reproduction
and Family

by

George W. Roberts and Sonja A. Sinclair

With an Introduction by Vera Rubin

GEORGE W. ROBERTS, a graduate of London University, is Professor of Demography and Director of the Census Research Programme of the University of the West Indies, Kingston, Jamaica. His publications include **The Population of Jamaica**, **Study of External Migration Affecting Jamaica 1955-1957**, **Recent Population Movements in Jamaica** and **Fertility and Mating in Four West Indian Populations.** In addition, he has written many papers on the demography of the West Indies.

SONJA A. SINCLAIR, a graduate of Pittsburgh University and a registered nurse, is Demographer at the Census Research Programme of the University of the West Indies, Kingston, Jamaica. Her publications include **Recent Population Movements in Jamaica** (co-author) and **Fertility in Jamaica, with Special Reference to St. Ann.**

kto press

A U.S. Division of Kraus-Thomson Organization Ltd.
Millwood, New York

Library of Congress Cataloging in Publication Data
Roberts, George W.
 Women in Jamaica.
 Includes bibliographical references.
 1. Women—Jamaica. 2. Family—Jamaica. 3. Fertility, Human
—Jamaica. 4. Women—Health and hygiene—Jamaica. I. Sinclair,
Sonja A., joint author. II. Title.
HQ1518.R6   301.41′2′097292   76–56911

ISBN 0–527–75870–1

First Printing 1978
Printed in the United States of America

TABLE OF CONTENTS

LIST OF TABLES

LIST OF FIGURES

Preface

This work has been undertaken in order to attain further understanding of the family in Jamaica, mainly in the context of union formation and reproduction. An appreciable amount of information is already available on fertility and mating forms in the region. This, deriving both from censuses and special surveys, conducted in Trinidad, Barbados, Jamaica and elsewhere, brings out many significant aspects of the West Indian family. The processes of formation of unions, the extent and character of changes from one type to another in the course of the family cycle, the periods of time spent in the three types of union, the relative stability of each—these have all been delineated in the course of recent investigations.

Likewise, a fairly coherent picture of fertility levels and differentials has become available, again deriving from censuses and surveys. This brings out unquestionably the differentials in terms of union status, educational attainment, religious persuasion, and other variables. Also available is a picture of the extent to which childlessness has dominated levels of fertility in the region until quite recently. Equally well depicted are the trends in fertility over the present century and some of the factors that have been responsible for these movements.

The introduction of contraceptive practices in several West Indian countries, beginning with the interesting and successful programme launched by Barbados in 1955, has led to more careful assessment of trends in fertility and to analyses aimed at determining whether these plans for fertility control are achieving their objectives.

In a review of the situation in 1974 with Dr. Vera Rubin, Director of the Research Institute for the Study of Man, the conclusion reached was that it was time to conduct an investigation which would go beyond the available quantitative material, and, relying on information of an attitudinal and qualitative nature, explore further many issues relating to reproduction and mating in the society. To some extent this necessitated obtaining additional information on these patterns. But the emphasis had to be on material needed to interpret these manifest forms. In particular, questions to be explored should center around topics such as the social and biological factors which influence mating behaviour and reproduction, knowledge of the reproductive processes, the effect of infant mortality on the family and on reproduction.

Preparatory work on the survey commenced towards the end of 1974 and by the beginning of 1975 it was possible to select the areas to be included in the study, to recruit interviewers and to get all the operations under way.

The project was supported by the Cultural Factors in Population Programme sponsored by the American Association for the Advancement of Science under grant from the United States Agency for International Development (Contract No. AID/CM/tha-C-73-25) and administered under subcontract by the Research Institute for the Study of Man. The Census Research Programme, responsible for the conduct of this project, has been during the period of its execution supported by a grant from the United Nations Fund for Population Activities.

The present work represents an extensive revision and expansion of the original study, with greater emphasis on characteristics of the prevailing family forms.

We should like to express our deep thanks to Dr. Vera Rubin for making this study possible. Her long interest in the Caribbean and her active promotion of and participation in many lines of research into the lives of its peoples are widely recognised. Her encouragement, unfailing interest and guidance, particularly in the final months of preparation, helped in large measure to ensure the timely completion of this monograph.

Professor Lambros Comitas, Associate Director of the Research Institute for the Study of Man, willingly gave his advice and assistance at several stages of the project for which we remain grateful.

We have benefited from discussions with Dr. Paul Glick, Professor David Glass and Professor Asher Tropp, all of whom read and made useful comments on particular areas of the manuscript.

We were fortunate in being afforded the opportunity of discussing the findings with members of the Advisory Board of the American Association for the Advancement of Science, as a result of which this work is considerably improved. To Dr. Margaret Mead we are deeply indebted for directing attention to many areas of this study calling for revision and conceptual clarification. Drs. Ward Goodenough, Solomon Katz, David Mutchler, Moni Nag, Priscilla Rhining and Irene Tinker also made valuable comments, as a result of which the work has been materially improved.

Members of the staff of the Research Institute for the Study of Man have assisted in bringing this work to a satisfactory conclusion and we wish to record our appreciation, particularly to June Anderson, Yvonne Darby and Florence Rivera.

The small staff of the Census Research Programme involved in this project have worked long and arduously. Special credit is due to Elaine Brooks, who from the inception of the project has been engaged in all of its operations. She carried out the demanding task of transcribing, in a very short period, the material from the tapes and supervising the checking of questionnaires. Another part of the project for which she is responsible is the preparation of most of the case studies included in the monograph. To her thanks are due also for carrying out the heavy task of checking and organising the manuscript for publication. Other members of the staff, Carol Daley, Cicilyn Davis and Dorrel Lewis, carried out considerable work in preparing the tabulations used in this study and in getting together all the remaining types of information needed for the analysis. We express to these four our deep appreciation and sincere thanks as without their conscientious efforts it would have been impossible to bring the work to completion in the scheduled time.

We are indebted to Mrs. Sumner Gerard for the preparation of additional case studies.

To the 18 field interviewers we owe a particular debt. Without their hard and dedicated work this study would not have been possible. Not only have they done very good field interviewing, but they have after the completion of these operations been in consultation with us on several problems which have arisen and which have called for clarification. Sheila Weatherly and Dorothy Monteith have proved especially helpful in this respect.

For fruitful discussions on several aspects of religion and the family, we are indebted to Rev. A. McKenzie and to Rev G. McKenzie.

We are grateful to Mary Manning Carley who has provided editorial assistance of the highest quality, thus removing many errors. Grateful acknowledgments are made to Kathleen Miles for her careful and rapid typing of the manuscript and to Auville Case for assistance in the preparation of the Figures.

To Marion Sader, Editor at Kraus-Thomson, we express our deep appreciation for the valuable assistance rendered in the preparation of the manuscript and for her readiness at all times to deal with the various problems that arose in the publication.

Finally to the women who willingly gave information about themselves and their beliefs we express our thanks and hope that this work will make their attitudes and problems more widely known and thus help to improve the condition of the lives of women of Jamaica and that of their families.

The authors assume full responsibility for errors and shortcomings that remain.

Census Research Program
University of the West Indies
Kingston, Jamaica
December 1976

GEORGE W. ROBERTS
SONJA A. SINCLAIR

Introduction

Understanding of the complex social organization of the multicultural stratified societies of the Caribbean requires a sound demographic baseline; for over twenty years social science researchers as well as government planners have drawn on the demographic works of Professor George W. Roberts for such a base. Consequently, when the Research Institute for the Study of Man undertook a cross-cultural project to examine sociocultural factors in fertility,* the possibility of carrying out a comparative study in Jamaica was explored with Professor Roberts of the University of the West Indies and his research staff, of which Sonja Sinclair had become a member. Since Professor Roberts and his staff had recently completed an extensive island-wide survey that raised numerous sociocultural questions, considerable interest was shown in carrying out more intensive research. The project was launched toward the end of 1974 under the direction of Professor Roberts and Sonja Sinclair.

Females are the demographic center of this research universe; the present study reflects the world of Jamaican women and throws significant new light on West Indian family forms. The so-called "West Indian Family" has been described by social scientists as characterized by "unstable unions" with high rates of "illegitimacy", "marginal parenthood", and households headed by women with "visiting" males in husband/father roles. In fact, there is a range of forms of mating unions including legal marriage; however, their incidence varies with age group and socioeconomic status. Movements from one type of union to another do not necessarily follow a standard domestic developmental cycle.

The diversity of these mating forms has generated a broad range of

*The Jamaica study is part of a series of seven research projects, organized by RISM, funded by the American Association for the Advancement of Science and USAID, to study social and cultural factors in fertility in several countries.

theories. Major theoretical explanations include the premise of African origins and continuities; historical roots in slavery and/or the plantation system; failure of the church to promote legal marriage; pluralism; cultural ecological factors; the economic marginality of males; "imbalance" in the sex ratio due to male migration; and a predicated "culture of motherhood," transmitted transgenerationally, that reinforces fertility behavior regardless of marital status. Social scientists have debated these issues that are a seemingly endless source of contentious fascination.

The conventional wisdom about the West Indian mating system that has also been engendered, generally reflects moral judgments, with some degree of relativistic benevolence. At issue is the form of mating that has been dubbed the "visiting union," where males are the "visiting" partners, and central relationships are formed around women in the mothering role. Both visiting and common-law unions are recognized census categories throughout the West Indies, along with the standard typologies of married, single, widowed, and divorced.

The prevalence of the visiting union is a distinctive feature of social organization in Jamaica as in other Caribbean societies; the subject has been the focus of census research and regional community studies in the search for causality as well as correlations. While there are vast areas of disagreement over primary causes, it is evident that multiple factors are involved in the perpetuation of the visiting union as an institution in the Caribbean. However, between the broad overview of national census statistics and the existential limitations of community studies, the quality of the visiting union has not always been grasped. Numerous questions arise—among others whether these unions are "promiscuous" (as the moralists say); whether they are "unstable" (as the structuralists say); whether they are responsible for high fertility rates (as the family planners say); whether the male partners are irresponsible in their husbanding/fathering roles; whether the children are deprived of father figures; and whether the women are involuntary partners in a non-choice situation.

Women in Jamaica: Patterns of Reproduction and Family is a remarkable study because the answers to these questions, and a number of others, are generated by a straightforward survey—a survey, however, with a difference. In addition to being semistructured, with tape-recorded responses that permitted content analysis, the questionnaire was designed on the basis of extensive previous survey and census research data. Results were analyzed in the framework of biomedical as well as demographic and sociocultural dimensions. The authors comment on "the willingness of the great majority of respondents to enter into eager discussion." They have, consequently, among other analytic contributions, been able to delineate the multidimensional quality of the visiting union, although this type of mating has been "the most challenging to analyze," and to establish a significant subtype, correlated with teen-age fertility, and perhaps with psychocultural factors in fertility.

It is of considerable interest that emergent forms of mating in North America appear to approximate the controversial visiting union. The free and more egalitarian sexuality sought by middle-class women's movements in North America apparently exists among working-class Jamaican women, as a matter of course. In addition, the study indicates that there is apparently a conscious desire on the part of the women to maintain the visiting union status until they are ready to enter a marital union, or re-enter a "single" state. Women appear to be opting for "freedom" in the visiting union; unlike their North American counterparts, however, they need not be isolated from functioning kinship networks, or give up child-bearing. When the time comes they may choose to marry. They are involved all along in family structures that may supersede actual household composition and provide the psychological as well as socioeconomic support of family networks, including visiting males. This substantive finding throws light on the current triangular theoretical controversy concerning the relative importance of household composition vis-a-vis familial networks. In any event, it appears that the visiting union may not be a "marginal adaptation," any more than "illegitimacy" is a "marginal adaptation." Both institutions are structured and socially recognized, as well as enduring ways of life, with moral strengths, and little intraclass stigma.

Equal rights for women through equal pay for equal work, availability of medical and social services, education about human biology as well as adult education—these are problems yet to be resolved in a hard-pressed society where "marginality" is not a question of gender. Whatever the origins of the institution of the visiting union, human interactions have long been structured as compassionate adaptive strategies by both men and women, and undoubtedly will continue to exist until new forms of social organization are invented.

This fascinating study illuminates many aspects of the "dynamic nature of the mating process" and introduces new data on "the challenging issues posed by visiting unions" that will prove to be an enduring and extensive research source. Clearly, the study also has challenging implications for social planners; some of these that are spelled out in the conclusions are not beyond realization, given the commitment of the society to the enhancement of the status of women.

February 1977

VERA RUBIN
Director
Research Institute
for the Study of Man

Chapter 1
Family Unions: Historical and Religious Perspectives

The whole subject of existing mating patterns in Jamaica, and indeed among all New World negro societies, is an extremely complex one and has been approached in different ways by social scientists, particularly in discussions of the "origins" of these patterns. Two schools of thought are usually identified in writings on the "origins" of family forms among New World societies of African descent. One, whose main exponent is Herskovits, argues that many of the familial institutions of these people have their roots in survivals from Africa.[1] The other, headed by Frazier, inclines to the view that prevailing forms of negro family in these societies can be traced to the pervasive influence of slavery.[2] Both of these approaches have figured in varying degrees in writings of West Indian scholars on the subject. We are not here concerned with the relative merits of either of these positions; indeed we acknowledge the merits that attach to each.

The fairly extensive literature on the West Indian family deals with a variety of its historical and functional features. Our concern here is to raise a somewhat different issue, one resting basically on the role of religious institutions in establishing prevailing family forms. However, the association between religion and the family does not constitute the focus of this study. The aim of the present chapter is to draw attention to an aspect of the subject to which sufficient attention has not, in our view, so far been paid.

It is our hypothesis that mating forms now characterising Jamaican and other Caribbean societies can be meaningfully approached when they are viewed in the context of the religious institutions and ceremonials involved in their establishment and functioning. An attempt will be made to show that a consideration of four ceremonials of the church, each of which assists in defining the position of the individual within the family and within the wider community, contributes to the understanding of the family within a society which clings closely to Christianity. These four ceremonials are baptism, confirmation, marriage and burial. The first of these is in fact much more than

1

a mere ceremonial, being a fundamental sacrament, an important element in the individual's entry into the church. A further aspect of the hypothesis is that, unlike other elements of the society, family forms have not undergone any material change since emancipation. Possibly the best approach in an investigation of the type proposed here would be to carry out a statistical analysis of baptisms, burials, confirmations and marriages over a long period of time. This would entail access to the church registers for the production of comprehensive tabulations of the data on these events. Until such time as an investigation of this nature can be conducted, the only relevant statistical sources which can be tapped relate to marriage. In fact for much of the substantive material concerning the role of religious rites in the society, the views of a few knowledgeable church leaders have had to be relied on. These include Anglican, Baptist and United Church ministers.

This chapter discusses first the principal aspects of prevailing mating patterns and some data on fertility levels shown by each type. With this necessary background, it will be possible to proceed to the main themes which consider changes in the society and relate existing mating forms to features of Christian religion. The latter is not by any means an attempt to put forward a kind of religious determinism of the family. It merely emphasises the relevance of the religious setting in any analysis of the West Indian family, especially where such analysis involves the question of its "origins."

Types of Family Forms and Their Relative Significance

Discussions of family forms in Jamaica, and indeed of the Caribbean at large, now center generally around a typology adopted mainly for demographic analysis, that is one in which exposure to the risk of childbearing figures prominently.[3] It is not, however, confined to demographic study, being used by many sociologists in place of more elaborate classifications which could be used.[4] The typology involved is a threefold one in terms of married, common-law and visiting. These are all defined in terms of couples who are in some form of steady sexual relationship, although, as will be shown in Chapter 4, a family union involves much more than sexual relations. Moreover the identification of the union is solely with reference to the female partner. In a sense, the characteristics of one of the three types —the visiting—tend to make this approach inevitable, as will presently be seen. But this reference to one member of the union is an acknowledged limitation of this simple typology.

Two features form the basis of this classification. The first is the presence or absence of legal sanction attaching to the union; the second is whether or not the couples share a common household. Thus a union which is legally sanctioned, that is established before an accredited marriage officer, and in which the partners share a common household constitutes a formal marriage. Where the partners live together in the same household but the union does not have any legal sanction, then the union is designated common-law. A union between a couple in which there is no legal sanction and in which the partners do not share a common household is termed visiting. It is relatively simple, in terms of this typology, to identify all females of married and common-law unions which have been broken by the death of the male partner or by some form of separation. Women of such broken unions are, in censuses, classified as previously living with husband or common-law partner. In the context of a census, however, it is not easy to extend this classification of broken unions to visiting types. No such problems, however, should be encountered in the case of a properly ordered survey, which could easily accommodate all types of unions and all forms of broken unions. While in general the approach in this study follows the above threefold classification of types of union, there may be, as will be seen in the course of this study, grounds for recognising as a subcategory of the visiting, a so-called "casual" type. This is characterised by the break-up of the union following the termination of the first pregnancy and, often, by the failure of the woman to contract another relationship until after the lapse of some time. This will be discussed in detail in Chapter 4.

It is important to note that no religious sacrament or rite figures in the establishment of the threefold classification outlined here, although most writers agree that one of the types identified—married—is fully sanctioned by the church.

It is now necessary to show the distribution of the female population of Jamaica in terms of these union categories at two recent censuses; this material is given in Table 1.1 and Figure 1.1. This table shows that most unions contracted during the early years of the childbearing span are of the

Table 1.1 Proportion distribution (%) of females by type of union, Jamaica, 1960 and 1970

Age group	Married		Common-law		Visiting*		No longer living with partner	
	1960	1970	1960	1970	1960	1970	1960	1970
15–19	1.2	1.3	7.9	10.3	89.2	86.8	1.7	1.6
20–24	10.9	11.5	29.6	28.8	52.5	54.8	7.0	5.0
25–29	25.8	26.1	34.3	36.4	29.9	30.2	10.0	7.4
30–34	36.2	39.4	30.2	32.0	21.2	19.7	12.4	8.8
35–39	41.9	47.5	25.9	27.3	17.7	14.9	14.6	10.3
40–44	45.4	51.2	20.2	21.2	16.1	13.3	18.2	14.3

Source: Censuses of Jamaica, 1960 and 1970.

*In 1960 this is termed Never Lived with Partner; in 1970 it combines Never lived with partner and Visiting.

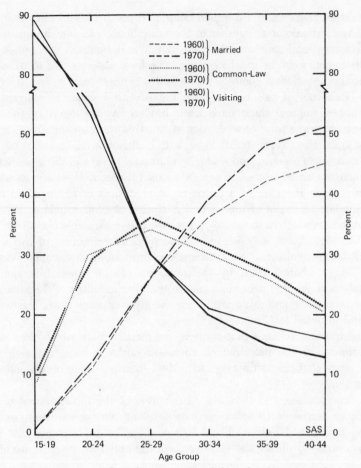

Figure 1.1 Proportion distribution (%) of females by type of union and age, Jamaica, 1960 and 1970

visiting type, while the second most frequent type occurring in this early period is the common-law and the least frequent is the married. Further up the age scale, however, important changes appear. The frequency of the married type rises steadily throughout the age span of reproduction; so that at age 45 the proportion so classified stands at 45% in 1960 and 51% in 1970. The proportion of women returned as common-law increases with the age of the woman also, but attains a maximum in the late 20s and then declines. The high proportion of visiting unions at young ages declines steadily throughout the childbearing span, so that, whereas within the age interval 15 to 19 the proportion within this type stands at 89% in 1960 and 87% in 1970, it falls, at the end of the childbearing span, to only 16% and 13% respectively. Thus the major feature revealed is one of shifts from visiting to married and, to a lesser extent, from common-law to married. In short, there is a general convergence to the married type with increasing age, and a corresponding withdrawal from the other two. It appears that the proportion of women married in 1970 is at all ages somewhat higher than in 1960.

One of the most interesting aspects of these three family forms turns on their relative levels of fertility. These differentials can be depicted in a variety of measures derived from modern censuses and from surveys. For the present purpose it suffices to consider three measures derived from the 1970 Census, which bring out some significant aspects of the underlying differentials. These are the proportion of women of various ages who are mothers, the number of children ever born to these mothers, as well as a measure combining the preceding two, that is the number of children ever born per woman. These three measures are given in Table 1.2 for women of Jamaica within the age span 15 to 54.[5] Within the period of childbearing, that is up to age 44, the first measure, the proportion of women who are mothers, shows a slight advantage for the common-law over the married up to about age 30, after which the married group has the higher proportion. Both of these considerably exceed the corresponding proportions for the visiting unions at all ages. The proportion of women who are mothers reaches a maximum of about 93% for the married and common-law types, whereas the highest value for the visiting type is only 71%. The low position of the visiting type may, however, be to some extent due to the difficulty of identifying women in this type of union at a census, and the possible overstatement of the numbers so classified.

The second measure, the number of children ever born per mother, affords a better comparison of the relative positions of the three union types, as these rates rest on more satisfactorily defined numbers at risk—that is all women

Table 1.2 Three measures of fertility among women in married, common-law and visiting unions, Jamaica, 1970

Age group	Mothers/Women			Children/Mothers			Children/Women		
	Married	Common-law	Visiting	Married	Common-law	Visiting	Married	Common-law	Visiting
15–19	.691	.737	.236	1.492	1.554	1.277	1.028	1.145	0.302
20–24	.820	.900	.510	2.304	2.587	3.003	1.890	2.328	1.533
25–29	.898	.938	.669	3.492	3.928	3.018	3.134	3.683	2.018
30–34	.931	.932	.704	4.650	5.032	3.794	4.327	4.687	2.672
35–39	.927	.921	.696	5.480	5.592	4.207	5.081	5.149	2.926
40–44	.904	.882	.642	5.862	5.598	4.069	5.301	4.935	2.613
45–54	.882	.842	.570	5.475	5.154	3.442	4.828	4.340	1.963

Source: Sonja A. Sinclair, "Fertility," in G. W. Roberts et al., *Recent Population Movements in Jamaica*, Census Research Programme, University of the West Indies, C.I.C.R.E.D. Series, Paris, 1974.

who have already borne children. While the generally low level of the visiting women is again in evidence, the differentials are not so prominent as in the case of the first measure. It should be noted that up to the age interval 35 to 39 the highest values are shown by the common-law women, whereas towards the end of the childbearing span highest values are those for married women. A combination of the two rates discussed above, in terms of the measure of children ever born per woman, puts the common-law above the married through most of the childbearing span, that is up to ages 35 to 39, while at all ages up to 44 the visiting type is clearly in the lowest position.

In terms of measures of completed fertility, the advantage lies definitely with the married, while the levels of the visiting type are very much lower than those of the other two. Thus children ever born per woman in the age interval 45 to 54 for visiting unions (just under 2) is less than half the corresponding values for the other two union types.

These important differentials have been the subject of many discussions aimed at assessing the factors underlying them. Arguments in terms of relative levels of exposure, of movement from one type to another, of the number of partners with whom the women are involved have been advanced by demographers studying these differentials.[6] In Chapter 4 some of these will be considered.

Change in the Society

As a background to the discussion of change it is necessary to recall briefly a few aspects of the West Indian family. Prevailing mating forms in Jamaica have some elements of their origins in conditions obtaining during slavery and the immediate post-emancipation period. But one important aspect which presumably could be expected to introduce a new phase into the situation was that marriage, which was virtually unknown among slaves, became a recognised institution with the passing of the marriage laws of the 1840s. This, in theory at least, made the institution readily accessible to the society at large. However, this development did not bring family forms close to the European pattern on which West Indian marriage laws were modelled. For marriage, in the majority of cases, still does not precede childbearing, but tends to take place after an appreciable size of family has been attained. This order of the institution within the family cycle gives rise to two characteristics of the Jamaican society. The first is the prevalence of unions of the type already defined as common-law and visiting. The second, following from the first, is the high level of rates of so-called illegitimacy.

One factor being emphasised in this chapter is that this lack of fundamental change in familial forms since emancipation contrasts with changes in other parts of the society. There is evidence that appreciable changes have taken place in Jamaica since slavery and these tend towards European forms. On all fronts—political, economic and social—considerable change has been recorded. The period between 1838 and 1865, in the words of Lord Olivier, "transformed an amorphous aggregate of 320,000 negro slaves, reputed to be irreclaimable savages, into the organic and self-respecting citizenry of a British community."[7] Dealing first with political development, we note that the first efforts to alter the political system came about a generation after emancipation. The society was no longer content with a political system that dated back to slavery. And although the disturbances of 1865 led to no more than direct colonial rule, the profound searching into the social and economic conditions of the island, undertaken in attempts to ascertain why these disturbances erupted, resulted in a much greater awareness of the deplorable conditions of the society. The process of what scholars call decolonisation has been up to World War II slow, and occasionally violent.[8] But rapid progress has been witnessed in the past 30 years. In 1944 adult suffrage was secured, while full independence came in 1962. The electorate has demonstrated much political sophistication in the period since 1944, putting out of office governments which failed to make good the promises of social and economic advance made before they assumed power.[9]

Economically as well there have been, especially within the past 50 years, appreciable advances in terms of overall production, although the masses of the society remain, in a sense, in a state of poverty. Income per head now exceeds $630 (Jamaican), which puts the island high up on the scale of Third World countries. Educationally the society has shown considerable progress since the days of slavery, when any schooling was considered a danger to the plantation system. The present level of literacy (that is the proportion with schooling) is in excess of 85%, which again represents a comparatively high place on the scale of Third World countries. Urbanisation may also be taken as indicative of social and economic advance during the period since slavery. The steady increase in the proportion of the island's population located within its main urban center, Kingston-St. Andrew, illustrates the degree of urban development. There is at present nearly 40% of the total population within all urban centers of the island, which means that depopulation of rural areas is proceeding apace. The nineteenth-century movement from the plantations to villages and small settlements outside of the complete control of the planter class led to the establishment of a viable peasantry and, concomitantly, some diversification of agriculture, as their departure from the sugar plantations left them free to exploit crops other than sugar. In addition there have been dramatic improvements in health throughout the society, as is illustrated in the growing control over a wide range of diseases and the attainment of a level of mortality not far removed from that of Europe.

Indeed, despite the element of truth of the assertion that the society still bears the marks of plantation slavery, much has happened to remove major cultural imprints of the slave regime. Before proceeding further with the analysis of this hypothesis, it is necessary to consider another demographic feature of the island, which affects many aspects of its social and economic life.

It is difficult to overstate the significance of external migration as a factor of social development in Caribbean countries. In the nineteenth century there were two distinct streams, in both of which Jamaica participated. The first was the introduction of indenture labour for work on the sugar plantations. In the case of Jamaica this did not play as important a role in demographic and social change as it did in the colonies of the Eastern Caribbean, but its role here should not be underplayed. The influx of Indians, though small in comparison with the numbers entering Eastern Caribbean countries, may have had some impact. With more certainty it can be stated that the outward movement to areas within the Caribbean and beyond, which extended over the period 1888 to 1921, must have exposed the island to many forms of social change. Movements to Central America and Cuba brought the inhabitants into contact with Latin American cultures, while the movement to the United States brought them into contact with a rapidly developing industrial society. As these migrations did not involve travel of a very extended nature, it was possible for emigrants to return to Jamaica from time to time, bringing with them customs they acquired from abroad. Yet despite these increasing contacts with other societies and their effects on certain aspects of life within Jamaica, there is no evidence that they had any influence on the family structure of the population.

One consequence of external migration during the period 1888 to 1921 was a marked disturbance in the sex ratio of the population, which followed from the highly sex-selective nature of the movement. The much greater proportion of males than females involved resulted in a great preponderance in the island of females over males in the age range 15 to 44. It has been contended that this was a factor involved in establishing prevailing family forms.[10] This however is untenable, for as will be argued here, these features of mating patterns long antedated the period of heavy sex-selective emigration. In any event, during the formative years of slavery, when possibly the roots of existing forms may have been established, the imbalance between the sexes was of an entirely different nature. In place of a preponderance of females, this sex was greatly outnumbered by males, because the major demand was for male slaves, and this is what the slave trade provided.

There have been therefore marked social and economic changes in the island during the post-slavery era. But it is contended here that there is no evidence of any change in mating forms over this period. One writer did in fact claim that, "Marriages are happily beginning to be very common and it is thought a disgrace to live otherwise than in honourable marriage life."[11] An observant writer remarked on the prevalence of two features which we have already emphasised as aspects of the Jamaican family: "Marriage is more common, but none marry until they have lived some time together; and the man generally lives with two or three women before he marries and leaves them with children and he seldom does anything to maintain them."[12]

Statistically, two sets of complementary data available since 1878 can be relied on to support this. The first of these is the series of marriage rates. These have remained almost unchanged since the introduction of vital registration, at between 3 and 4 per 1,000. The only important departure from this level occurred in 1907, and this can be attributed to an act of God, the destruction of Kingston by earthquake and fire in that year. During the year 1906–7, the number of marriages celebrated amounted to 5,500, and 1,228 of these took place within one month of the disaster. In the following year the number rose to 6,200, giving a marriage rate of 7.7, the highest ever recorded in the island. In keeping with our hypothesis, we may consider this dramatic rush to marriage as a collective effort on the part of the society to seek closer conformity with formal religion at a time of natural disaster. But apart from this short-lived upturn in the marriage rate and a slight decline during the period of world-wide economic depression of the early 1930s, marriage rates have not moved very much.[13]

The second series, the rates of illegitimacy, also have shown no real change over the period covered by vital registration. As in the case of the marriage rates the only departures were in the years 1906–7 and 1907–8 during which a concomitant decline was observed in illegitimacy rates.[14] These rates have been, by European standards, extremely high, that is in the high 60s and low 70s. This was the phenomenon which attracted most attention and comment in the early reports of the first Registrar General of Jamaica, S. P. Smeeton. He protested strongly against what he called "this Hydra-headed evil" and even for a time had the names of fathers entered in the registers—although this contravened the law—in the hope of reducing this high level of illegitimacy.[15] But there has been no change in this level, which remains the strongest evidence in support of our argument that no fundamental change in family forms has taken place since emancipation.

The Religious Aspect

As was stated at the commencement of this chapter, there are four ceremonials of Christianity which impinge on the formation and development of the family and it is instructive to consider the role these have played in the development of the West Indian family. In dealing with the four ceremonials of relevance—baptism, confirmation, marriage and burial—it is necessary to see how these fit into the original tenets of Christianity. The sacraments originally acknowledged by the Roman Catholic Church were Baptism,

Confirmation, the Eucharist, Repentance, Ordination, Marriage and Healing the Sick. Of these, it would seem, three bear special relevance to the formation and maintenance of the family—baptism, marriage and confirmation—while burial ceremonies are significant to any people expecting some form of existence after death. In this context, marriage signifies the initiation of a sexual union. Holy matrimony was raised to the level of a sacrament because it was "assigned a divine origin and made an indissoluble union typifying the union of Christ with his church as his mystical body."[16] The distinction between baptism and confirmation came somewhat late in the history of the Christian church, not in fact until baptism came to be applied almost exclusively to infants. The association of these two with the family lies in the fact that they relate to another aspect of the family cycle, additions to the family through births. Here it must be noted that of the ceremonials under discussion, only baptism is accepted as a true sacrament of the Protestant church. Marriage is merely a religious rite.

Before discussing the religious background of the slave regime, the question of the extent to which they were converted to Christianity by the missionaries should be raised. Accounts on this are not altogether consistent. According to Edward Brathwaite, "The evidence of the available missionary diaries suggests, on the whole, a stubborn and remarkable resistance to Christian teaching—at least as far as the Moravians were concerned."[17] But in contrast to this assessment of the position in Jamaica, there are accounts, referring especially to the Eastern Caribbean, which attest to the conversion of slaves to Christianity.

From the previous discussion of ceremonials and rites of Christianity, it would be expected that conversion to this religion would basically ensure that the slaves accept the sacrament of baptism, not necessarily that they practise the rite of marriage; and throughout the history of the region, it seems, this has been the case. There are numerous accounts indicating that during slavery it was the spread of baptism that the church originally sought. Thus one of the early missionaries, the Rev. John Smith, stressed very heavily his efforts to baptise the slaves, and was always anxious to detail the numbers he baptised, whether of infants or adults. Smith states his general policy of baptism as follows: "When they apply, I ask them whether they have a note from their master; if they answer, No, I tell them they must bring one, and then I will talk about baptising them. If, on the contrary, they have a note from their master, I examine them as to their views of the ordinance, etc. On these occasions, I generally begin by asking them how many wives they have. Then I question them in Dr. Watt's catechism. If they give satisfactory answers to these questions, profess to believe in Christ, and to be sorry for their sins, I do not refuse them."[18]

The obverse of the foregoing process—that is the acceptance of baptism by the slaves themselves—is equally important to our argument. According to

Herskovits, baptism had close parallels to African religious practice, a factor which made for its ready acceptance during slavery.[19] Moreover the view was widespread among slaves that once they were baptised they complied fully with the requirements of the church. This is forcefully expressed by a slave in the United States, as quoted by Genovese. This slave, on being charged with immoral conduct, maintained that baptism left him free to do anything: "Look yeah, massa ... don't de Scriptur say, 'Dem who believes an' is baptise shall be save'? ... 'Dem as believes and is baptise, shall be save'; want to know dat ... I *done* believe and I *done* baptise, and I *shall be save suah* ...."[20] Just as relevant to the present discussion is the attitude of the slave owners towards baptism of their slaves. The general reserve they maintained to any form of change among slaves should be stressed. They were averse to education of slaves as this would enable them to read the Bible and possibly to interpret the scriptures to support their claim to freedom. They opposed widespread conversion to Christianity for the same reason. Nevertheless there are accounts of their agreement that baptism be extended to some slaves. For instance, Smith quotes instances of slave owners sending their slaves to him to be baptised.[21]

When we turn to consider marriage, we have in the first place to show that no special attention was paid by the church to the spread of marriage among slaves or, after emancipation, among the freed population. Certain slave codes in the region made provision for marriage among slaves, but there was no complementary action on the part of the church to ensure that families were established in this way. Marriage among slaves was not unknown, as registrations of marriages among converted slaves appear in the early registration volumes in these territories. The promotion of marriage among slaves formed part of the ameliorating laws passed during the 1820s, but it is questionable whether the church made any arrangements for carrying out these expensive rites. According to Wallbridge, there was, in Guyana, a law prohibiting marriage among slaves.[22] He merely notes this. There is no discussion of its broad implications for a slave society or for their family life. Nor is there any indication as to how the church viewed such a prohibition.

An important set of legislation was proposed by the British government in 1838 to help prepare for the transition from slavery to freedom, and one of these dealt with marriage. The Order in Council dealing with this subject recognised the existence of marriages *de facto* among slaves and carried provision for their formal recognition after freedom.[23] Its preamble states: " ... since the abolition of slavery ... marriage laws ... have been found inappropriate to the altered condition thereof and inadequate to the increased desire for lawful matrimony therein." A uniform procedure of marriage by publication of banns was to be established, the cost of the ceremony to be four shillings. Records of such marriages were to be kept by the Island Secretary. The legislation also aimed at settling the legality of

certain "marriages contracted and solemnized previous to the abolition of
slavery ... between slaves ... and since the abolition of slavery between
apprentices and other persons ... by members of the Christian religion other
than clergy of the United Church of England and Ireland." Such marriages
were declared to be "good, valid and effective ...." The most realistic part of
the proposed legislation aimed at giving legal sanction to the unions formed
among slaves before emancipation. "And whereas in consequence of imperfect instruction in the Christian religion, and from other causes, many
marriages *de facto* have taken place between persons one or both of whom
were in the condition of slavery, but which marriages *de facto* have never
been sanctioned by any public ceremony or formally registered ... and it is
expedient that provisions should be made for enabling such persons to confer
upon their children the benefit of children born in lawful wedlock ... it is
further ordered that it shall be lawful for all persons having contracts of
marriage as last aforesaid at any time within one year after coming into
operation of this order, duly to solemnise the marriage ceremony before any
clergyman of the Established Church or in any other manner authorised by
this order; and every person so recognising a previous marriage *de facto* shall
at the same time make and sign the following declaration ... ." In the
declaration the parties affirmed that they on a given date and in a given place
"inter-married with each other and ... had issue of the said marriage."

Of interest here is the fact that the framers of this law traced the failure to
have marriage *de facto* publicly sanctioned or formally registered to
"imperfect instruction in the Christian religion." Moreover these seemingly
realistic measures called for full acceptance and cooperation of the church for
their success, and in any case seemed more applicable to a highly literate
society than to one just emerging from slavery. Possibly because they were
not acceptable to the church as a whole, the measures of the law dealing with
marriages *de facto* were eventually removed from the island's marriage law.
In any event these early measures contained many defects and it was not until
their administration was brought under the Registrar General that the system
became effective.

It is not easy to detail the part played by burial in the society during slavery
and the post-emancipation years. Probably the popularity of burial societies
today has its roots in the realisation that a proper disposal of the corpse, with
full Christian ceremonial, was an essential element of Christianity. Whether
the church places as much emphasis on burial rites as on baptism is difficult
to say, although as it was not a sacrament it probably was not accorded equal
status with baptism. It would seem however that the populace insisted on the
performance of the appropriate Christian rites at burial.

That from the post-emancipation period up to 1878 the only source of
information on births, marriages and deaths is to be found in the religious
records appears clear. As Smeeton remarks, the information on births and
deaths for this period was contained in church records of baptisms and

burials, while, due to the failure of the clergy to comply fully with the requirements of the early marriage law of forwarding the records to the Island Secretary, the only sure source of data on marriages was also the church records.[24]

While in the case of Jamaica civil registration came to provide the basis for performance of the Christian rites associated with baptism, burial and marriage in 1878, Barbados offers an example of a much longer period of ecclesiastical recording of vital events. Here an effective system of recording these events on a purely religious basis had long been developed and continued until the early 1920s before it was replaced by a system of civil registration.

Official Investigations

It is of interest to note that over the years several Committees of Investigation have examined the question of illegitimacy and prevailing family forms. Some have found it necessary to take these into consideration although they were not the main focus of attention. At least two were expressly set up to consider these issues, and it is useful to examine briefly some of their findings. The first Committee was set up in 1904 to enquire into the workings of the marriage and registration law.[25] It considered many aspects of illegitimacy, devoted much attention to the historical factors that seemed responsible for the emergence of the forms of family prevailing in the island. The factors that militated against the practice of marriage were touched on, and it was noted that the belief that an elaborate and expensive ceremony was required probably made it impossible for a large proportion of the population to practise formal marriage, on the grounds of its excessive cost. On the question of the reduction of the high level of illegitimacy, the report states, "it is not legislation that is required so much as the cultivation of a higher moral tone and a better public opinion among all and especially the lower classes." Despite the prominence accorded the moral tone of the society, this report does not consider that the church has any part to play in redressing the position or in any way stimulating marriage.

Much more relevant to the present discussion is the report of another Committee set up in 1936 to consider the same issues dealt with in the Committee of 1904. It enquired into the prevalence of concubinage and the high rate of illegitimacy and their effects on the moral, social and economic progress of the people. Probably because it reported during the war years (1941), its findings and recommendations have never received the attention they deserved.[26]

This Committee, headed by the Bishop of Jamaica, and numbering among its members such distinguished persons as Edith Clarke, May Farquharson, and Dr. W. E. McCulloch, stated that the problem of illegitimacy and concubinage was "one of the most complex and difficult to solve," and had "a detrimental effect upon the spiritual and moral life of the Island, and have undermined the self-respect and dignity of manhood and womanhood, and have hindered the development of homelife." Of interest is the fact that of the several causes of these phenomena the Committee listed, none was of a religious nature.

Many recommendations for dealing with the situation were made, touching on education in schools, birth control, bastardy and other matters. It urged that "without a widespread understanding of the consequences of parental irresponsibility, it is unlikely that any serious effort will be made by the community to create public opinion against parental irresponsibility and its consequences, promiscuity, illegitimacy and over-population." It returned to the device long advocated by Smeeton, and which for a time he followed. This consisted of having the name of the father entered in the birth register. One of its very interesting recommendations was that legal sanction should be accorded to "cases of permanent concubinage by some form of common-law marriage." Recommendations with religious associations are worth noting. In the first place, "The Churches and social agencies might be asked to form groups of workers to influence public opinion against illegitimacy and parental irresponsibility and supply these groups with suitable publications for this purpose." Also, "The Churches and religious bodies might be specially asked to try to correct the misunderstanding by some people of such texts as 'Increase and multiply'—'The Lord will provide'—and 'Take no thought for the morrow'—the practical effect of which misunderstanding has undoubtedly been to decrease the sense of forethought and of personal responsibility."

The Modern Position

It is now necessary to examine the modern situation with regard to the four rites which have been identified as playing a part in the functioning West Indian family. At the outset the degree to which Christianity permeates the society has to be emphasised. Most of the censuses taken in Jamaica have sought information on the religious affiliation of each individual. The tabulation of material on religion has traditionally proved to be a formidable task as the island is rich in its variety of religious denominations and sects. The following classification summarises the position at 1970:

Anglican	21%
Baptist	20%
Church of God	13%
Roman Catholic	8%
Other	26%
No religion	12%

It should be noted that the fundamentalist religions are very strongly represented in the classification "Other," which in fact includes more than fifty denominations and sects. Non-Christian religions are not strongly represented; for instance the proportions returned as Moslem and Hindu are negligible. It is nevertheless acknowledged that a wide range of superstition among the population forms an important complement to their religious practice.

The practice of baptism or blessing of infants remains a very important part of the Christian religion in Jamaica. It is not possible to ascertain the proportion of births which are involved in this sacrament. But information received from religious leaders in many denominations indicates that only small proportions of infants are not baptised. Mothers, it is reported, feel that it bodes ill for their infants if they are not baptised at an early age. Associated with baptism is the practice of naming godparents. This is another aspect of church doctrine which is closely adhered to. How far back this practice goes in the island's history is not clear; it is difficult to assess its prevalence during the nineteenth century or during the period of slavery, although its wide-spread nature at present suggests that it must have been in the past a frequent accompaniment to baptism. Informants from the churches also state that the general rule is to choose godparents who are of a higher socio-economic status than that of the child's parents. It has also been suggested that there is a general preference to have children baptised in the "established" churches, such as Anglican, Methodist and Roman Catholic.[27]

One aspect of baptism raised from time to time is whether it should be extended to illegitimate infants. For instance it has been urged that withholding this sacrament from such infants may reduce the high levels of illegitimacy. One factor which militates against such a course of action is that certain denominations do not withhold this sacrament on grounds of illegitimacy, although the tendency has been to ensure that it does not take place on Sundays. However it would seem that at present no denomination refuses this sacrament. The significance of baptism as a sacrament affecting the family is emphasised by the fact that the church will not, in general, bury an unbaptised person.

Confirmation is another important rite which is still strongly maintained. This usually takes place between the ages of 11 and 18. At this stage the child is reconfirming the promise made on his behalf by his godparents at his baptism and is therefore reaffirming his faith and beliefs in the teaching of the church. Again it is not possible to give estimates of numbers going through this ceremony. Our religious informants state that it is much less common than baptism, but that a substantial proportion of the population with some religious affiliation is confirmed. From our standpoint, the significance of this rite is that it is necessary if the person is to partake of the sacrament of communion.

When we turn to the rite of marriage, we note that, as in the past, it continues to mark the initiation of a family union in a small proportion of cases, probably less than one-third. Both the low level of marriage rates and the prevalence of unions of the types designated common-law and visiting attest to this. If statistical evidence that the proportion of infants baptised is very high compared with the proportion of family unions initiated by formal marriage could be established, then this would be in keeping with our hypothesis that, as marriage is not a sacrament of the church, its frequency will be less than that of baptism. That marriage is a rite and consequently does not play as significant a part in the people's religious life as does baptism is confirmed by religious leaders.

At the same time there is evidence that marriage is regarded as a norm towards which most couples aspire, and which in fact more than half attain by the end of the childbearing period. By the latter age also only about 14% of the unions are of the visiting type. A further important line of evidence relevant here is that whenever marriage is performed it tends to be solemnised in the church. This goes back to the days of slavery when such laws as were passed making provision for marriage among slaves envisaged that the clergy would be responsible for its performance. And up to the early 1960s the proportion of marriages performed before non-religious marriage officers was less than 15%. Religious leaders also stress that, in general, persons marrying tend to do so through the church.

There may be some acknowledgment of the significance of marriage in the family and in the religious life of the society. For it would seem that when a woman bears her first child in a visiting or common-law union, this tends to dissuade her from attending church. In fact the only formal participation in church activity in which she is involved is the baptism of her subsequent children. Usually when later in life she marries, then she resumes her close involvement in formal religious activity.

However there are undoubtedly other aspects to be taken into account. For instance it would seem from recent survey findings that in their younger years women choose to remain primarily in visiting unions because they derive certain advantages from conditions inherent in unions of this type, not least of which is "freedom." This is discussed more fully in Chapter 4.

Conclusion

We have attempted to show the role of the Christian rites most closely linked to the functioning family. Baptism, long the acknowledged means of conversion to Christianity, is the most widely practised of all the rites and we have ascribed this to the fact that of the four it is the only true sacrament of the church. The fact that babies are brought for baptism at an early age in conjunction with, in many cases, the mother's voluntary withdrawal from church attendance indicates a distinct understanding for, but a disregard of, the aspects of life which are not in accord with their desires. Confirmation in the Anglican church, and its corresponding rite in the other religions, also plays a dominant role in the religious life of the society, strengthening the person's bond to the Christian faith. Likewise burial has come to be regarded as a necessary element to the Christian and elaborate steps are taken, by means of such institutions as burial societies, to make sure that proper financial provision is made for this rite.

Probably nothing said with regard to the foregoing demarcates the position of Jamaica from other Christian societies. But in the case of marriage the situation is different. Two factors seem to separate Jamaica, and indeed all West Indian societies, from both European and African customs. In the first place the institution is much less frequently practised than is the case in Europe or Africa. In the second place it is not performed in the same order within the family. By contrast with its European counterpart, this institution comes, in a large proportion of the society, after several baptisms. In fact in many cases it has no part to play in the formation or continuation of a union. Marriage represents the rite on which the people have put their own interpretation. Conceivably this signifies that certain advantages accrue to the society as a consequence of other forms of families, although it is not easy to determine these. In fact from accounts obtained at surveys, the impression is gained that their assessment of the situation has led to a conscious desire on the part of the females to perpetuate visiting and to a lesser extent common-law unions.

It has already been acknowledged that social scientists advance several interpretations of the West Indian family. In particular both the argument centering around survivals from African customs and that linking family forms to slave conditions are accepted as being important in any interpretation of the West Indian situation. Likewise the position of Oscar Lewis remains relevant.[28] His penetrating writings, resting largely on conditions in Puerto Rico and Central America, do have relevance to the situations we are discussing. And without claiming for the "culture of poverty" all that he does, it is easy to accept that poverty may play a role in establishing the forms designated here—common-law and visiting. But if, for the sake of argument, we accept Lewis' thesis, does this mean that we have to equate slavery with the "culture of poverty"? Very few scholars will be prepared to push the meaning of this concept to the extent that it becomes equivalent to plantation slavery. In any event it has been our argument that sufficient economic advance has been made since emancipation to at least expect some shifts in mating patterns. The fact that these have not appeared suggests strongly that economic conditions have had little to do with their formation.

Our contention that an examination of certain elements of Christianity helps to throw some light on the West Indian mating situation calls for much more substantiation than we have been able to produce so far. In particular a statistical examination of the trends of numbers of infants baptised and the ages at which the ceremony takes place should shed much more light on the relation between this sacrament and births. Our argument that marriage has been interpreted essentially as a religious rite, even in modern times, is supported by the opinions of leaders of the church with whom we have discussed the matter. And the position of the latter here is illuminating. They acknowledge that failure to initiate a family union by formal marriage is not in accord with the practice of Christianity. But it is difficult to find many outspoken comments condemning the practice or action which conceivably could be taken to arrest it. For instance the possibility of refusing the sacrament of baptism to children born to unmarried parents has on occasion been put forward in this context, but has found no widespread support.[29] One seemingly firm conclusion is that the prevailing forms of mating may be perfectly in accord with most elements of the society.

Notes

1. M. J. and F. S. Herskovits, *Trinidad Village* (New York: Alfred A. Knopf, 1947); M. J. Herskovits, *The Myth of the Negro Past* (New York, 1966). For comprehensive discussions of the modern West Indian family see in particular M. G. Smith, *Kinship and Community in Carriacou* (Seattle: University of Washington Press, 1962); and R. T. Smith, *The Negro Family in British Guiana* (London: Routledge & Kegan Paul and I.S.E.R., 1956); and "Culture and Social Structure in the Caribbean: Some Recent Work on Family and Kinship Studies," *Comparative Studies in Society and History* 6, no. 1 (October 1963).
2. E. Franklin Frazier, *The Negro Family in the United States*, rev. & abr. edition (Chicago: University of Chicago Press, 1966).
3. G. W. Roberts and Lloyd Braithwaite, "A Gross Mating Table for a West Indian Population," *Population Studies* 14, no. 3 (January 1961).
4. Edith Clarke, *My Mother who Fathered Me*, 2nd ed. (London: George Allen & Unwin, 1966).
5. This discussion is based on Sonja A. Sinclair, "Fertility," in G. W. Roberts et al., *Recent Population Movements in Jamaica* (Paris: Census Research Programme, University of the West Indies, C.I.C.R.E.D. Series, 1974).
6. G. W. Roberts, *Fertility and Mating in Four West Indian Populations* (Kingston: I.S.E.R., University of the West Indies, 1975); G. E. Ebanks, P. M. George and C. E. Nobbe, "Fertility and Number of Unions in Barbados," *Population Studies* 28, no. 3 (November 1974).
7. Lord Olivier, *Jamaica: The Blessed Island* (London, 1936).
8. For a discussion of aspects of decolonisation see T. Munroe, *The Politics of Constitutional Decolonization in Jamaica, 1944–1962* (Kingston: I.S.E.R., University of the West Indies, 1972).

9. Modern political behaviour is discussed in Carl Stone, *Class, Race and Political Behaviour in Urban Jamaica, 1973: Electoral Behaviour and Public Opinion in Jamaica, 1974* (Kingston: I.S.E.R., University of the West Indies, 1974).

10. A. Marino, "Family Fertility and Sex Ratios in the British Caribbean," *Population Studies* 24, no. 2 (July 1970).

11. *Extracts from the Journal of John Chandler whilst Travelling in Jamaica* (London, 1840), p. 14.

12. Robert Paterson, *Remarks on the Present State of Cultivation in Jamaica: the Habits of the Peasantry* (Edinburgh, 1843), p. 14.

13. G. W. Roberts, "Growth of the Population" in G. W. Roberts et al., *Recent Population Movements in Jamaica*, p. 7.

14. Kalman Tekse, *Population and Vital Statistics. Jamaica. 1832–1964* (Kingston: Department of Statistics, 1974).

15. S. P. Smeeton, *First Annual Report of the Registrar General's Department* (Kingston, 1879), p. 3.

16. Encyclopaedia Britannica article, "Sacrament," *Encyclopaedia Britannica* 16, 15th ed. (1975).

17. Edward Brathwaite, *The Development of Creole Society in Jamaica, 1770–1820* (Oxford: Oxford University Press, 1971), pp. 256–7.

18. Rev. Edwin Angel Wallbridge, 1848, *The Demerara Martyr: Memoirs of the Rev. John Smith* (British Guiana: The "Daily Chronicle" Ltd., 1943).

19. M. J. and F. S. Herskovits, *Trinidad Village*, p. 176.

20. Eugene D. Genovese, *Roll Jordan Roll—The World the Slaves Made* (New York: Pantheon Books, 1974), p. 245.

21. Wallbridge, *The Demerara Martyr*, p. 21.

22. Ibid., footnote p. 65.

23. Despatch from Lord Glenelg to Governors of British Guiana, Trinidad, St. Lucia and Mauritius, 15 September 1838, given in *Extracts from Papers Printed by Order of the House of Commons, 1839, relative to the West Indies* (London, 1840).

24. S. P. Smeeton, *Registrar General's Report 1887–8* (Jamaica, 1888).

25. *Report of Commission appointed by Sir. A. Henry to Enquire into the Working of the Marriage & Registration Law. Supplement to the Jamaica Gazette* (28 July 1904).

26. *Report of Committee appointed to Enquire into the Prevalence of Concubinage and the High Rate of Illegitimacy in the Island ...* , (Jamaica, 1941).

27. The Church of England (Anglican) was in fact disestablished over 100 years ago but the term "established" is commonly used to refer to the non-fundamental churches.

28. Oscar Lewis, *La Vida* (New York: Alfred A. Knopf, 1968).

29. E. Bean Underhill, *The West Indies: Their Social and Religious Condition* (London, 1861).

Chapter 2
Quantitative Analysis of Mating Patterns

From discussions of the preceding chapter, it will be evident that demographic and sociological analyses of the family in the West Indies call for much more than the study of marriage. Unlike the situation in European societies, where marriage effectively covers the functioning family, many families of the Caribbean cannot be described as falling within the category married, if this term is taken rigorously as a union enjoying full legal sanction. Indeed two special aspects of the study of the West Indian family have to be catered for. The first is that a classification allowing for types other than formal marriage has to be adopted. The second, following from the first, is that the analysis of dynamic aspects of the family—notably its formation and dissolution—cannot be properly treated in terms of a study restricted to formal marriage.

The small-scale sample on which we are operating cannot be used for a detailed quantitative approach, as the techniques required have to be based on much larger numbers of women. In any event, the material already available from earlier surveys is sufficient to give a satisfactory picture of mating habits in the island, without having to be supplemented by material from the present investigation. In dealing with the position in Jamaica, it is instructive to see whether the situation in this island differs to any degree from that in another society within the region.

In keeping with the above argument, therefore, this chapter, while concentrating on an analysis of the material for Jamaica obtained in an earlier survey, at the same time establishes comparisons with a similar population of the region, the non-Indians of Trinidad.[1] Two surveys have been undertaken to examine quantitative aspects of mating patterns in the region, one in Trinidad in 1958 and another in Jamaica in 1972. And by applying the same method to the analysis of each of these, it is possible to secure an overall picture and at the same time outline any contrasts which appear between the positions of the two populations.

21

The fact that 14 years separate the periods of these two surveys is not thought to affect comparisons made here. Indeed, in view of the evident absence of change in West Indian family forms since the days of slavery commented on in Chapter 1, the 1958 survey probably gives a picture of mating habits which is perfectly valid for 1972.

One limitation of the approach used is, possibly, its restriction to females. While concentration on this sex has obvious advantages, in terms of collection of data as well as in terms of analysis, the experience of males may well prove of critical significance, especially in view of the frequency with which women change partners. But, as will be shown in Chapter 3, there are appreciable difficulties to be faced in incorporating the experience of this sex. Consequently the present treatment of mating completely ignores the experience of males.

The Jamaican material is analysed in precisely the same manner as that used for the earlier Trinidad study. This involves an analysis of the mating experience of women of completed fertility in terms of a gross mating table. This treats the mating pattern of females from age 14 to age 45 in terms of a threefold union classification and assumes that during the childbearing span women participate in no more than three stages or shifts in union types.

This approach assumes that the initial cohort of women, all over age 45 at the time of the field work, are at risk of initiating a family union. This can be done by entry into any one of the three union types recognised: married, common-law or visiting. A small number of women do not enter any family type; they remain genuinely single throughout their childbearing period. Of those women establishing a family in a given union type, say visiting, some will remain in this type up to age 45, while others will move to one of the other two unions or become single before age 45; these constitute women moving to a second union stage. The three groups of women who establish second-stage unions or become single are themselves at risk of establishing a third type before reaching age 45. Thus, in the present illustration, those in second-stage unions of the common-law type are at risk of moving to married, or returning to visiting types; they may also become single. Similarly, second-stage formal marriages are at risk of changing to common-law types or of returning to the visiting type, or of becoming single. Again those single at the second stage are at risk of entering one of the three union types before they attain age 45.

The third union just identified constitutes the terminal stage if it persists up to age 45, and since the vast majority of women conform to the three-stage pattern, this is the model adopted here. However a small proportion of women do experience a shift to another stage, thus involving themselves in four or possibly more stages before they reach age 45. Consequently, in order to maintain the three-stage model in these cases, the stages dealt with are the initial, the second and the terminal, which latter is taken as the type obtaining when the woman reaches age 45 (this may take the form of the single state). It is thus implied that where the woman participates in more than three stages the type or types between the second and the terminal are ignored; her mating history is assumed to be fully covered by treating the three stages indicated. Since in the case of Trinidad only 9% of all the women over 45 have more than three shifts of union type, while in the case of Jamaica the corresponding proportion is 8%, the three-stage model is taken to constitute a fairly accurate description of the basic mating process.

As we are dealing with shifts from one union type to another, the question must be raised whether some form of Markov process can be applied to the analysis of the data. For instance a formulation along such lines is possible if we take the process as involving only movement from the initial to the terminal stages. This approach, however, is greatly complicated by the introduction of the second stage, which is required by the model being followed. Moreover, a particular problem centers around the treatment of the single state. In so far as women remain single throughout their childbearing life, this seems to constitute an absorbing state. But the single state arises in another manner, which also is a consequence of the model adopted. For any woman who establishes a family union is at risk of becoming single, either through widowhood or some form of dissolution of the union. And she may continue in this single state until she attains age 45, or this state may itself give rise to another family type; the latter may even be the same as the initial type. Thus the term single cannot be used in the present context to cover only an absorbing state.

Apart from the foregoing, a basic consideration which seems to rule out the application of Markov chain analysis is that the entire process of shifting from one type of union to another is age-dependent. In other words the probability of movement in this process varies greatly with the age of the woman, an aspect of the situation which has to be taken into account. To do so in terms of Markov chain analysis is too complex. It was these considerations which led to the use of a multiple decrement table approach in the first (1958) study; this is the technique used in the analysis of the Jamaican material.

The probabilities of moving from initial- to second-stage unions, and of moving from second-stage to terminal unions, according to the Jamaican survey, are presented in Tables A and B, Appendix I, which also gives the gross mating table for the Jamaican sample population.

Probabilities of Entering Initial-Stage Unions

The probabilities of women entering initial-stage unions and of moving to second- and third-stage unions form the basis of the gross mating table. The most important of these are those signifying entry into initial-stage unions, as they point to salient features of the population's mating experience. A comparison between the two populations in terms of these probabilities consequently must be made. They are presented in Table 2.1. These bring out clearly that participation in visiting relationships is much greater among Jamaican women than among their Trinidad counterparts in terms of the initial stage. At every age interval this advantage appears, and it is pronounced at ages over 20. Probabilities of entering initial-stage common-law unions do not disclose so firm a contrast. Indeed irregularities in the material make a definitive statement on differentials difficult. It is still evident that for the majority of the age intervals there is a higher chance of contracting these unions among Jamaican females. The other important contrast between the two populations is to be found in the formulation of initial married unions. Here the advantage lies clearly with females from Trinidad. This is most pronounced in the age interval 15 to 25, where the probabilities for Trinidad females are about twice the level of those for Jamaica. While, overall, Trinidad females show somewhat higher probabilities of contracting initial unions, the difference between the two populations is not great. At ages below 20, Jamaica has a slight advantage, but at advanced ages values for Trinidad are at a higher level. The two major contrasts between these populations relate to visiting and married unions. Whereas the former constitute the principal means of entering initial unions among Jamaican females, in the case of Trinidad females marriage is the most frequent means of instituting a family.

In view of the significance of religion in issues of mating in these populations, stressed in Chapter 1, the question may be raised whether differences in terms of religious affiliation between the two populations may account for the somewhat higher frequency of marriage in Trinidad. It is for instance conceivable that the much higher proportion of Catholics in Trinidad than in Jamaica may have a bearing on this.

Ages of Entry into Initial- and Second-Stage Unions

One of the statistics of mating habits derived from the mating tables is the average age at which women enter the initial- or second-stage unions. (Comparable values for terminal-stage unions are not considered here, because of the very small numbers involved.) Average ages at entry into the three types at the initial stage and at the second stage are shown in Table 2.2. Included in the latter is the average age at which initial-stage unions are broken and women become single. This results from widowhood or from some form of separation.

The general similarity of pattern characterising the two populations is evident. Indeed in many cases the values for the two are virtually identical. Considering initial-stage unions, we note that the highest average age is for women whose first union is marriage; this is between 23 and 24 years. The

Table 2.1 Probabilities of entering visiting, common-law and married types at initial stage, Trinidad and Jamaica

Age interval	Probabilities of entering							
	Visiting type		Common-law type		Married type		All types	
	Trinidad	Jamaica	Trinidad	Jamaica	Trinidad	Jamaica	Trinidad	Jamaica
14–15	0.041	0.062	0.008	0.029	0.010	0.007	0.059	0.098
15–20	0.250	0.283	0.087	0.104	0.094	0.053	0.432	0.440
20–25	0.249	0.297	0.127	0.110	0.229	0.111	0.605	0.518
25–30	0.193	0.230	0.078	0.137	0.289	0.145	0.560	0.512
30–35	0.134	0.198	0.134	0.114	0.244	0.158	0.512	0.469
35–40	0.052	0.103	0.034	0.041	0.293	0.138	0.379	0.283
40–45	0.028	0.077	0.083	0.010	0.056	0.077	0.167	0.163

Table 2.2 Average ages at entry into initial- and second-stage unions

Initial type	Trinidad					Jamaica				
	Initial stage	Entering 2nd stage as				Initial stage	Entering 2nd stage as			
		V	CL	M	S		V	CL	M	S
Visiting	20.1	–	25.9	28.2	26.5	20.6	–	25.9	28.3	28.5
Common-law	21.5	28.4	–	32.7	32.6	21.0	29.6	–	30.9	32.6
Married	23.2	29.6	31.4	–	34.3	23.9	31.8	35.5	–	36.9
All types	21.4	29.1	26.4	30.1	29.7	21.3	30.8	26.1	29.2	30.3

lowest average age is for initial-stage visiting unions, between 20 and 21 years. About midway between these two falls the value for initial common-law unions. The average age at entry for all three initial-stage types is very close for the two populations: 21.3 years for Jamaica and 21.4 for Trinidad.

As is to be expected, movement into second-stage unions takes place at ages appreciably above those at entry into initial-stage unions. Despite some differences in levels between the two populations, there is still a common pattern discernible in both. In every case the initial visiting type yields the lowest ages of moving to the second-stage, while the highest are those for initial married unions. Thus Trinidad women moving into second-stage visiting unions do so at average ages of 28.4 years where initially they are in common-law unions, and at an average age of 29.6 years where the initial type is married. Corresponding ages for Jamaican women are 29.6 and 31.8 respectively. Also, women contracting marriage as a second-stage union show a similar pattern, which also characterises movement into second-stage common-law unions. Ages at which Jamaican females dissolve their initial relationships, that is at which they become single, indicate that the lowest age at which this occurs is 28.5 years among the visiting types. For initial common-law and married women, average ages are somewhat higher—32.6

years and 36.9 years respectively. The same relative positions emerge in the case of Trinidad females, but the values are at a lower level. It is possible that differential mortality between the two populations, a product of the time interval separating the samples, may partly account for the age differentials.

A useful extension of the foregoing is the span of years between entry into initial type and movement from that type to another, as revealed in Table 2.2. Thus women in initial visiting types who move into common-law unions do so between 5 and 6 years later, whereas their counterparts moving on to marriage do so after about 8 years. Again, women in initial common-law unions who shift to visiting do so between 7 and 8 years after, whereas their movement to formal marriage takes place after a lapse of between 11 and 12 years. In the case of women initially married, shifts to visiting unions take place between 6 and 8 years after marriage. In the case of initially married women moving to common-law unions, the period elapsing before the contraction of this second stage shows a marked difference for the two populations, the only instance when such departures become apparent. The period is 8 years for Trinidad and 12 years for Jamaica. But in interpreting figures for movement of initially married women to second-stage unions, their very small numbers must be recalled. In summary, the comparison shows a very marked concordance between the two populations as to age at which initial and second stages are contracted.

Aspects of Union Involvement

One of the basic summaries of mating experience obtained from the gross mating table shows the number of women of the original cohort in each of the three types of union or single at successive ages as the cohort is traced from age 14 to age 45. The comparisons of the two populations given in Table 2.3 emphasise again their underlying similarity in mating patterns. A consideration of women never in any union shows that up to age 20 the proportion remaining single is higher for Trinidad women; at age 20 in fact 54% of these women are still not involved in a union, as compared with 51% for Jamaica. But at higher ages it is Jamaican women who show the higher proportions not in unions. At age 45, the proportion of Jamaican women still out of unions is 3.7%, as compared with 2.4% for those of Trinidad. Such a low order of differences is in keeping with the similarity of mating habits between the two populations. Small differences also separate the two in regard to women previously in unions but single at the stated ages. Thus at age 25, there are 9.2% of Trinidad women in this category, as compared with 6.9% for those of Jamaica. At age 45 however the difference is negligible: 20% for Trinidad and 21% for Jamaica.

Also indicative of the essential similarity of mating patterns for the two populations is the degree to which the cohort is involved in the three types at

Table 2.3 Women not in unions and those in unions at various ages according to gross mating tables

Age	Women not in unions			Women in unions			
	Never in any union	*Previously in union, single at stated age*	*Total*	*Visiting*	*Common-law*	*Married*	*Total*
			Trinidad				
14	10,000	—	10,000	—	—	—	—
15	9,405	2	9,407	410	80	103	593
20	5,352	285	5,637	2,195	1,043	1,125	4,363
25	2,113	916	3,029	2,119	2,108	2,744	6,971
30	931	1,358	2,289	1,467	2,535	3,708	7,710
35	453	1,564	2,017	1,085	2,662	4,234	7,981
40	282	1,778	2,060	837	2,406	4,696	7,939
45	235	1,982	2,217	611	2,094	5,077	7,782
			Jamaica				
14	10,000	—	10,000	—	—	—	—
15	9,020	5	9,025	618	278	78	974
20	5,052	229	5,281	2,598	1,371	749	4,718
25	2,416	691	3,107	2,640	2,232	2,019	6,891
30	1,191	1,159	2,350	2,035	2,428	3,186	7,649
35	624	1,512	2,136	1,433	2,210	4,221	7,864
40	451	1,748	2,199	1,037	1,967	4,796	7,800
45	374	2,109	2,483	840	1,609	5,067	7,516

successive ages as we move through the childbearing span. In the case of visiting type unions, proportions increase very steeply between ages 15 and 20: from 4% to 22% for Trinidad, as compared with 6% to 26% for Jamaica. Between ages 20 and 30 the proportions in this type decline slightly, so that at the latter age the proportion remaining in such unions is 15% for Trinidad and 20% for Jamaica. As we move up the age scale, proportions similarly placed decline sharply, to 6% for Trinidad and 8% for Jamaican women. The general pattern of participation in visiting unions therefore is a rapid build-up, followed by a slow and then steadily accelerating shift to other types.

The curve of participation in common-law differs somewhat from that shown by visiting unions, although here as well the pattern is one of increase followed by a decrease. Proportions in this union type increase rather slowly and the maximum proportion is attained at a much higher age than in the case of visiting unions. Thus among Trinidad females the proportion moves up slowly to a maximum of 27% at age 35. The maximum appears somewhat earlier for Jamaican women, at age 30, and the proportion here is slightly lower—24%. As a consequence of movement out of common-law relationships, the proportions remaining in it at age 45 are lower—21% in the case of Trinidad and 16% in the case of Jamaica. The important point is that both populations show that involvement in common-law unions is more pronounced at higher ages than is the case of visiting unions. It is also evident that common-law unions are more prevalent in Trinidad.

Proportions in married unions at various ages emphasise that entry here differs fundamentally from entry into visiting and common-law types. Whereas the significant feature for the last two types is the movement away from them at higher ages, the major feature of marriage is that proportions increase continuously from age 14 to age 45. At ages up to 25 the proportions married are higher among Trinidad females; thus at that age the figure is 27% for Trinidad and 20% for Jamaica. But proportions for the latter move up appreciably at higher ages and by age 45 the proportion is about equal for both populations (51%).

Involvement in all three types, summarised in the last column of Table 2.3, shows basically the same pattern for the two populations. There is a considerable increase between ages 14 and 20 in proportions in unions of all types. By the latter age the proportion in all unions is 44% for Trinidad and 47% for Jamaica. Marked increases occur over the next five years, bringing the proportion to 70% for Trinidad and 69% for Jamaica. For both, the maximum proportion is noted at age 35: this amounts to 80% for Trinidad and 79% for Jamaica. There is a small reduction after this age, but proportions in unions at age 45 still remain substantial—78% and 75% respectively.

Another useful comparison between the two groups can be made in terms of the average number of years a woman passing through the childbearing period (14 to 45) spends in the three types of union or in the single state. Since the gross mating table assumes no mortality, the total number of years lived over this age span is 31. The relative contributions of the three types and of the single state to this total are shown in Table 2.4 and in Figure 2.1. The somewhat greater involvement in visiting unions in Jamaica is evident: this type contributes 5.3 years for this population, as compared with 4.1 for Trinidad. The contribution of common-law type in the case of Jamaica is 5.6 years, as compared with 5.9 for Trinidad, thus bringing out the slightly greater participation in this type by the latter population. The appreciably lower significance of marriage in Jamaica is manifest; here the average number of years contributed is 8.8 for this population, as compared with 9.6 for Trinidad females. The number of years spent outside of any union (that is in the single state) is also slightly higher in the case of Jamaica (8.2) than in the case of Trinidad (7.9). Contributions to the single state come also from women whose unions have been disrupted, and when this is added to the years with respect to women who have never been in any union, the total is the same for both populations (11.4 years). And since this latter figure is 37% of the total span of 31 years, it brings out graphically that a significant factor

Table 2.4 Contribution by various groups of women to average number of years spent by cohort moving through childbearing span

Groups of women contributing to the total	Contribution in number of years by	
	Trinidad females	*Jamaica females*
In visiting union	4.13	5.27
In common-law union	5.93	5.59
In married union	9.55	8.78
Never in any union	7.94	8.16
Previously in union and then single	3.45	3.20
Total	31.00	31.00

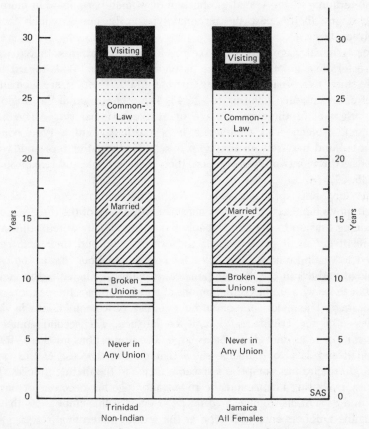

Figure 2.1 Contribution by women in Jamaica and non-Indian women in Trinidad to average number of years spent by cohort moving through the childbearing span

controlling fertility in West Indian populations is the extent to which so much of their life during the childbearing span is passed in the single state.

We next consider at what stage women in a given union type at age 45 enter it, that is whether entry is at the initial, the second or the terminal stage. Periods spent in each of the three types may be considered as originating at the initial stage, at the second stage or at the terminal stage. In other words we may identify positions of the cohort whose initial union is of a particular type and who continue in that type up to age 45; these constitute the contribution of the initial stage. Of women initially in a given type of union some move on to another and then continue up to age 45 in that new type; these constitute the contributions arising from the second stage. Again, some of the women who move into a second union type change to another before attaining age 45; this forms the terminal type and represents the contribution of the terminal stage. A small proportion of women participate in more than three stages; in this case the terminal type is the one in which they are involved at age 45.

The terminal stage may also take the form of re-entrants, that is women whose terminal union is the same as their initial type. With regard to the single state, two broad groups must be identified. The first are women who never enter into any union up to age 45. The other group of the single state may originate at the second stage or at the terminal stage. The former represent women who commence in a particular union type which is disrupted and they remain single up to age 45; the latter represent women who pass through two types of union, then become single and remain so up to age 45.

The foregoing approach makes possible the construction of Table 2.5, which shows numbers of the two cohorts entering each of the three stages and remaining thus up to age 45. Probably the outstanding feature of this table is the relatively small proportion of the cohorts who end their childbearing period in visiting unions. This holds for both populations: 6% in the case of Trinidad and 8% in the case of Jamaica. Equally significant is the fact that most of those who are in visiting unions at age 45 contract these unions at the initial stage. The major component here consists of women initially in visiting unions—53% for Trinidad and 62% for Jamaica. The second component, consisting of re-entrants, also looms large. The proportions for these—29% for Trinidad and 21% for Jamaica—show that only in the case of this type of union do re-entrants comprise a sizeable factor in the mating process. Those initially in visiting unions and the re-entrants together account for between 82% and 84% of all women in this type at age 45; this emphasises that only negligible numbers enter this type at the second or terminal stage.

When we examine the stages of origin of women in common-law unions at age 45, we see that the contributions of the three stages do not vary to the same extent as in the case of visiting unions. But notable contrasts between

Table 2.5 Members of cohort entering a union type at given stage and remaining in that stage up to age 45

Stage of entering	Visiting		Common-law		Married		Single		Total
	No.	% Total	No.	% Total	No.	% Total	No.	% Total	
				Trinidad					
Initial	322	52.7	474	22.6	2,167	42.7	235	10.6	3,198
Second	42	6.9	821	39.2	1,560	30.7	1,446	65.2	3,869
Terminal	71	11.6	614	29.4	1,103	21.7	536	24.2	2,324
Re-entrants	176	28.8	185	8.8	247	4.9	—	—	608
Total	611	100.0	2,094	100.0	5,077	100.0	2,217	100.0	9,999
				Jamaica					
Initial	523	62.3	660	41.0	1,467	28.9	374	15.1	3,024
Second	96	11.4	680	42.3	2,563	50.6	1,667	67.1	5,006
Terminal	42	5.0	209	13.0	993	19.6	442	17.8	1,686
Re-entrants	179	21.3	60	3.7	44	0.9	—	—	283
Total	840	100.0	1,609	100.0	5,067	100.0	2,483	100.0	9,999

the experience of the two populations do emerge. Thus the proportion entering common-law unions at the initial stage among Jamaican women (41%) is nearly twice as great as the corresponding value for women in Trinidad (23%). With regard to the proportion contributed by the second stage, the difference between the two populations is much less: 39% are contributed in the case of Trinidad and 42% in the case of Jamaica. In contrast with the situation for the initial stage, contributions from the terminal stage are much greater for Trinidad (29%) than for Jamaica (13%). In neither case do re-entrants constitute an important proportion of common-law women at age 45.

Again contrasts between the two populations are in evidence when we consider the stage at which women married at age 45 actually contract this type of union. Of the Trinidad women married at age 45, 43% enter these unions at the initial stage, a much higher figure than that for Jamaica (29%). On the other hand a very large proportion (51%) of Jamaican women married at age 45 enter this type at the second stage; this is much higher than the corresponding figure of Trinidad (31%). The proportion contributed by the terminal stage is about the same in both cases: 22% and 20% respectively. Second and higher order marriages contribute very little to the total of married women at age 45—5% for Trinidad and 1% for Jamaica. These suggest very low levels of second and higher order marriage in these populations.

Women who are single at age 45 may be divided into two groups. The first consists of those who fail to enter a family union by age 45; this amounts to 11% for Trinidad and 15% for Jamaica. The second arises from the disruption of an existing union either by the death of the partner or by separation of some sort. These two are responsible for the establishment of the single state at the second or at the third stage. With regard to the second stage, the difference is negligible. Of Trinidad women who are single at age 45, the proportion becoming so at the second stage is 65%: this is very close to the corresponding figure for Jamaica (67%). In the case of women becoming single at the terminal stage, a much larger proportion become so among Trinidad females, 24% as compared with 18% for Jamaica. Since 14 years separate the dates of the two surveys, taken in 1958 and 1972 respectively, the lower proportion single derived from the terminal state in the case of Jamaica may be traceable to its much lower male mortality in 1972 than the corresponding level obtaining in Trinidad in 1958.

Another approach giving a picture similar to the one just outlined is in terms of contributions from each stage of entry to the total number of years spent in each union type and in the single state. This is summarised in Table 2.6. Contributions of the initial stage to the average number of years passed in visiting unions are dramatically depicted in these values. For Trinidad contributions from the initial stage amount to 3.69 of a total of 4.13 years; corresponding values for Jamaica are 4.87 and 5.25 respectively. Also in the case of common-law unions, comparatively large contributions come from initial and second stages, with the former being somewhat more important in both populations. A major contrast between the two groups of women emerges in the case of married unions. For Trinidad, the average number of years arising from entry into initial-stage unions is relatively high (5.8) whereas that for the second stage is less than half of this (2.6). By contrast the amount from the initial-stage union in Jamaica is only 3.5, while the second

Table 2.6 Average number of years spent by women entering a stage as a particular type and remaining in that type up to age 45

Stage of entering	Visiting	Common-law	Married	Single	Total
			Trinidad		
Initial	3.69	2.69	5.76	7.95	20.09
Second	0.17	2.50	2.64	3.10	8.41
Terminal	0.06	0.57	0.97	0.34	1.94
Re-entrants	0.21	0.16	0.19	—	0.56
Total	4.13	5.92	9.56	11.39	31.00
			Jamaica		
Initial	4.87	3.27	3.47	8.17	19.78
Second	0.20	2.04	4.23	2.87	9.34
Terminal	0.02	0.23	1.05	0.33	1.63
Re-entrants	0.16	0.06	0.03	—	0.25
Total	5.25	5.60	8.78	11.37	31.00

stage provides a much greater portion (4.2). Of interest is the similarity in contributions of the several stages to the overall mating position. Thus for both populations the average number of years arising out of involvement in initial-stage unions is 20. The corresponding figure for second-stage shows a range of 8 to 9. In both cases the average arising out of involvement in terminal-stage unions is just under 2.

Union Stability

An index of stability advanced in earlier papers based on the Trinidad study can be used in comparing the relative stability of unions shown by the two populations. This is a purely statistical measure—the proportion of women who enter a type of union at a particular age and remain in it up to age 45.[2] As will be seen from Table 2.7, a common pattern characterises both populations, with the lowest stability being exhibited by the visiting type and the highest stability by the married. The differential is most marked for the initial stages, but appears also in unions established at the second stage, with one exception. In the case of initial-stage unions, the index is slightly higher in Jamaica for visiting and common-law types. When we examine the initial-stage unions, the difference between the indices of the two populations is appreciable only for the married; here the index of stability for the Jamaican females is 83 as compared with 68 for females of Trinidad. The position of second-stage visiting unions following initial common-law unions shows a slight advantage in stability for Trinidad females—47 as compared with 44 for Jamaica.

But second-stage visiting unions following initial married unions show much greater stability for Jamaican women (93) than for their Trinidad

Table 2.7 Indices of stability

| Union type | Initial-stage union | Second-stage unions with initial stage as | | |
		Visiting	Common-law	Married
		Trinidad		
Visiting	6.9	—	22.2	22.6
Common-law	24.8	46.9	—	51.8
Married	67.7	76.4	79.6	—
Single	—	45.9	54.8	56.4
		Jamaica		
Visiting	9.4	—	59.8	58.6
Common-law	29.0	43.5	—	60.7
Married	82.8	93.0	93.5	—
Single	—	63.8	69.5	77.3

counterparts (76). Second-stage common-law unions following on initial visiting unions exhibit a stability index of 22 for Trinidad, which is less than half the corresponding value for Jamaica (60). Again, second-stage common-law unions which follow initial marriages have much greater stability for Jamaican women (94) than for Trinidad (80). Substantial differences appear also with regard to second-stage marriages. Those proceeding from initial visiting unions show a stability index of 23 for Trinidad, as compared with 59 for Jamaica. Where these married unions succeed initial common-law ones, the corresponding indices are 52 for Trinidad and 61 for Jamaica. The general conclusion is therefore that for all types stability tends to be greater among Jamaican females.

Complementary to measures of stability just considered are measures indicative of the extent to which women not initially in a given type terminate their childbearing period in that type. For instance, women in initial visiting and common-law unions are at risk of passing to formal marriage before they attain the age 45. The proportion of women making this shift to marriage constitutes the attractive force of the married type. In this approach, single states, intervening between first and second, between first and terminal union types, as well as single states in which women end their childbearing period, are ignored. Only states representing the three union types are considered in the derivation of the summary indices appearing in Table 2.8. The tendency for women who begin their family life outside of formal marriage eventually to marry is an important factor characterising both populations. Proportions of women initially in visiting and common-law relationships who are married at age 45 amount to 53% for Trinidad and 60% for Jamaica, thus emphasising that by the end of the childbearing period more than half of the females have been married. Much smaller is the tendency for women in initial visiting or married unions to move over to common-law types. Proportions doing so are 23% for Trinidad and much smaller (16%) for Jamaica. Manifestly there is very little chance of women entering initially a common-law or married union terminating their childbearing experience in visiting unions; in fact only between 3% and 4% of these women make a shift of this kind. Thus these measures confirm what has already been established, namely that the general mating process tends to be a movement from visiting to common-law or married; from common-law to married and from visiting to married.

Table 2.8 Attractive force of union types

Union type	Trinidad	Jamaica
Visiting	2.7	4.1
Common-law	23.1	15.6
Married	52.6	59.8

In calculations of measures of attraction just discussed, the single state has not been treated as a condition in which the women participated, that is, not as strictly analogous to a type of union. This modification of the original approach can be pushed further by considering the numbers of women who are involved in a single type of union, in two types of union or in all three. Here, for instance, a movement from visiting to single to married is taken as involvement in two types only. Similarly a movement from visiting to single and then to visiting again is interpreted as involvement in one type. In Table 2.9 the experience of the two populations based on this approach is outlined. These values complement the indicators of stability just discussed.

This table brings out a notable and probably unexpected aspect of mating among West Indian populations. Since so much of the life of the female is spent outside of formal marriage it might be thought that women engage in a large number of changes in their union history. Clearly there is no basis for such an assumption. Taking all women together, we see that in the case of Trinidad 7% of the cohort report being involved in more than two types of unions; a slightly lower figure of 6% obtains for Jamaica. And most of these are women initiating their family life in visiting unions. The proportion of women in initial common-law and married unions involved in more than two unions is negligible for both populations. As is to be expected, the largest proportion of women involved in a given union is noted among women initially married; this is extremely high in the case of Jamaica (96%) and somewhat less in the case of Trinidad (87%). Involvement in one union is much less among those whose initial type is common-law, but it is still appreciable: for Jamaica 48% of initial common-law unions and 45% of such

Table 2.9 Participation in 1, 2 and more than 2 types of union, when single state is ignored

Participa-tion in 1, 2 or more unions	Initial type of union							
	Visiting		Common-law		Marrried		Total	
	Trinidad	Jamaica	Trinidad	Jamaica	Trinidad	Jamaica	Trinidad	Jamaica
	Number in unions							
One union	1,127	1,706	853	1,083	2,784	1,693	4,764	4,482
Two unions	2,877	3,331	1,025	1,172	379	76	4,281	4,579
More than two unions	651	539	31	23	37	2	719	564
	% in unions							
One union	24.2	30.6	44.7	47.5	87.0	95.6	48.8	46.6
Two unions	61.8	59.7	53.7	51.4	11.8	4.3	43.8	47.6
More than two unions	14.0	9.7	1.6	1.0	1.2	0.1	7.4	5.9

unions for Trinidad. The proportion of women initially visiting who participate in one union, that is who do not shift to another type, is much smaller than in the case of initial married and common-law unions. Of all Trinidad females whose initial family experience is visiting, 24% are found in one type only; the corresponding proportion for Jamaican women is 31%.

When we turn to women who have passed through two types of unions, a contrast can be drawn between those initially married and those whose first relationship has been visiting or common-law. Of initially married women, only small proportions are involved in a second type. The proportion is very low in the case of Jamaica (4%), and somewhat higher (12%) for Trinidad. By contrast, considerable proportions of women initially in visiting unions go on to a second type: 62% for Trinidad and 60% for Jamaica. Slightly less, but still considerable, are the corresponding proportions for women whose first unions have been of the common-law type. These are 54% for Trinidad and 51% for Jamaica.

In summary, it can be said that women who are initially married tend to stay married throughout their childbearing life: this is so for both Jamaica and Trinidad. This is in contrast to the position among women whose initial relationship is either visiting or common-law. For these two groups of women the modal number of types of union is 2. But even here proportions who move on to a third stage are not so large: 14% in the case of Trinidad and 10% in the case of Jamaica.

In order to analyse more closely how the initial type influences the woman's overall union history, it is necessary to treat separately the three broad sections of the gross mating table, each of which, it will be recalled, is defined in accordance with a particular initial union type. In other words, the experience of all women whose initial type is visiting is traced up to age 45; the experience of all women whose initial type is common-law is likewise traced up to age 45; and similarly the experience of all women establishing a family in formal marriage is followed through the childbearing span. Such an analysis is best carried out by deriving the average number of years spent by those who pass their entire childbearing span in the initial type, the average number of years spent in second-stage unions to which they may move and the average number of years spent in terminal-stage unions, should they shift from a second to a higher-order stage. The periods spent in each of the second and terminal stages can themselves be decomposed into their component parts (including the single state). Such details of each of the three broad categories appear in Table 2.10.

Because of the lower age at entry the total number of years lived by women in initial visiting unions is the longest for both populations—24.9 years for Trinidad and 24.4 years for Jamaica.[3] Lowest values are for women in initial married unions; these amount to 21.8 years for Trinidad and 21.1 for Jamaica.

What distinguishes the mating pattern of women initially visiting from the

Table 2.10 Years spent in various union types by women in initial, second and terminal stages

Stage and type of union		Initial as visiting		Initial as common-law		Initial as married	
		Trinidad	Jamaica	Trinidad	Jamaica	Trinidad	Jamaica
In initial type union		7.92	8.74	14.07	14.34	18.01	19.58
In second stages	Visiting	—	—	0.40	0.74	0.28	0.17
	Common-law	5.08	3.62	—	—	0.46	0.11
	Married	3.74	5.27	4.72	5.66	—	—
	Single	4.40	3.92	2.41	2.29	1.84	0.91
In terminal stages	Visiting	0.45	0.29	0.17	0.12	0.10	0.02
	Common-law	0.95	0.39	0.81	0.25	0.40	0.07
	Married	1.82	1.71	0.62	0.42	0.57	0.18
	Single	0.55	0.50	0.33	0.18	0.10	0.04
Total from age 15–45		24.92	24.44	23.52	24.01	21.76	21.07

other two broad categories is the relatively short period of time the former spend in that type. The comparatively low value—7.9 years for Trinidad and 8.7 for Jamaican females—stems from the fact that large numbers of these women move on to second-stage unions of common-law and married types. Indeed it is the second stage that contributes most to the experience of women initially in visiting unions. The two types and the single state, in terms of which the second-stage period is broken down, contribute 13.2 years in the case of Trinidad; for Jamaica, the figure is only slightly less, 12.8. Of interest is the fact that among Trinidad women common-law unions contribute the largest component, 5.1 years; the largest in the case of Jamaica is, by contrast, from the married type (5.3 years). For both populations the contribution from the single state is impressive—4.4 years for Trinidad and 3.9 years for Jamaica. Much more modest are the contributions coming from terminal stages, which overall amount to 3.8 years for Trinidad and 2.9 for Jamaica. Because of the appearance of re-entrants at the terminal stage, three components, as well as the single stage, are involved at the terminal stage. But the only prominent amount to be noted here is the married component, which is just under 2 years for each population.

Much greater contributions come from the initial type in the case of women whose initial union is common-law. For females of Trinidad the contribution amounts to 14.1 years as compared with 14.3 for Jamaica. The total number of years lived in the second stage—7.5 for Trinidad and 8.7 for

Jamaica—is much smaller than the relative contributions noted for those initially visiting. And here, much more than in the previous group of women, the dominant union is married, which contributes most to the second stage; the values are 4.7 years for Trinidad and 5.7 for Jamaica. It is of note that the single state contributes much less than it does for the group of women considered above. Here it amounts to 2.4 years for Trinidad and 2.3 for Jamaica. Again in contrast with the other group, the terminal stage does not figure prominently; its contribution is just under 2 years for Trinidad females and just under one year for those in Jamaica.

When we analyse the situation of women initially married, we see the extent to which this type dominates the entire family cycle. Of a total of 21.8 years spent by each woman in this third component of the cohort in the mating table, 18.0 or 83% are passed in marriage in the case of Trinidad; the corresponding figures for Jamaica are 19.6 and 93% respectively. It follows that only token contributions come from second and higher stages. All second-stage unions taken together contribute 2.6 years in the case of Trinidad females, as compared with 1.2 for Jamaican females. In both cases the major component here comes from the single state, but this amounts to only 1.8 years for Trinidad and 0.9 years for Jamaica. Even less significant are the years spent in terminal-stage unions; these total only 1.2 for Trinidad and 0.3 for Jamaica. Most of this, it should be noted, represents re-entrants, that is women initially married, moving into another type (or the single state) at the second stage and then closing their childbearing life in the type in which they began it. But these are of negligible dimensions.

Conclusion

The foregoing comparisons bring out clearly that a common mating pattern is discernible in the samples of non-Indian women in Trinidad and of all women in Jamaica. Since the three-stage mating model describes accurately the situation in both populations, it may be safely concluded that for the populations of the West Indies in general this pattern is valid. Up to about age 25 the dominant union type is visiting, more so in Jamaica than in Trinidad. As we move up the age scale participation in this type diminishes rapidly so that at age 45 less than 10% remain visiting. Although involvement in common-law unions shows essentially the same pattern, the rates of their formation at younger ages are lower than those for the visiting, while at higher ages the shift from them is less pronounced. In contrast to the pattern characterising these two unions, formal marriage exhibits a steady build-up of women to a maximum at age 45. The general mating pattern is therefore one of early entry into unions of relatively unstable nature, accompanied by a progressive shift to formal marriage. We may conclude that most women end their childbearing period in families of the married or common-law type. The proportion of the cohorts in these two types at age 45 amounts to 72% in the case of Trinidad and only slightly less (67%) for Jamaica. By contrast only negligible proportions of the cohorts remain in visiting unions at age 45; it is thus only within the first 10 years of the family cycle that this type attains significance. In terms of single women, that is those who have never established a family as well as those who have become single after having been in one of these unions, the two populations again show a marked degree of similarity.

Uniformity of pattern extends to the ages at which women enter the three union types (or become single) at the formation of initial- or second-stage unions. With regard to the total number of years passed in each of the three union types and in the single state by the average woman from age 14 to age 45, a similarity of pattern again can be noted. In contrast to the situation among East Indians of Trinidad, where marriage is overwhelmingly the dominant union, accounting for two-thirds of the 31 years of the childbearing span, there is much more equal spread among the three unions for the two populations under study.[4] Thus marriage accounts for 9.6 years for Trinidad and 8.8 for Jamaica, that is nearly one-third of the total span of 31 years. Together the other two union types account for just over one-third of the total span. More than one-third of this span, it should be noted, is taken up by the single state, and much of this stems from the dissolution of initial-stage unions.

Despite the importance of visiting types at the initial-stage, both populations emphasise that there is a steady passage from this type to common-law and to formal marriage, so that the latter tend to constitute the major types during the family cycle of the average woman. This is best shown when we compare experience of the three constituents of the gross mating table, that is the experiences of women commencing their family life in visiting, common-law and married unions respectively. Thus the contribution from initial-stage unions amounts to between 8 and 9 years for initially visiting components whereas, in the case of those initially married, this type contributes between 18 and 20 years.

The experience of both populations brings out a factor which may play a part in determining fertility differentials by union type; this is the difference in the period passed in the single state by women according to their initial type of union. Those initially in visiting-type unions spend a substantial proportion (about one-fifth, of the total period up to age 45) single, and most of this is accounted for during the period after the termination of their initial visiting type union. This proportion passed in the single state is much less among women initially in common-law and married unions, ranging from 5% to 12%. The fact that comparatively heavy involvement in the single state by women initially in visiting unions occurs after the termination of the initial-type union, when fertility tends to be highest, seems to be important in any analysis of fertility differentials by type of union.

While the similarities noted are outstanding features of the mating process of the two populations under study, there are differences between the two groups of women calling for some comment. Probably the most notable is that the visiting type, especially at the initial stage, plays a more important role in the family life of women in Jamaica than it does among their Trinidad counterparts. Although in the second stage also the common-law type figures more prominently in the Jamaican family than in the case of Trinidad, this difference does not hold for higher-stage unions, so that in summary the total involvement in unions of this type is greater in Trinidad than in Jamaica. The fact that at the initial stage marriage proves very important in Trinidad may lead to the assumption that unions of this population exhibit greater measures of stability than do those of Jamaica. But the evidence is that there tends to be less shift to second- and third-stage unions by Jamaican women. One inference that may be drawn here is that heavy involvement in visiting unions does not necessarily carry with it greater union instability.

Notes

1. For a discussion of the first study, conducted in Trinidad in 1958, see G. W. Roberts and Lloyd Braithwaite, "Fertility Differentials by Family Type in Trinidad," *Annals of the New York Academy of Sciences* 84, article 17 (December 1960); and "A Gross Mating Table for a West Indian Population," *Population Studies* 14, no. 3 (January 1961). The Jamaican survey was done in 1972 and will be reported on elsewhere.
2. The measurement of stability in the present context is discussed in G. W. Roberts and Lloyd Braithwaite, op. cit.
3. The gross mating table assumes no mortality, but it is possible that differentials in mortality may contribute somewhat to the total years spent in childbearing.
4. See G. W. Roberts and Lloyd Braithwaite, "Mating among East Indian and Non-Indian Women in Trinidad," *Social and Economic Studies* 11, no. 3 (September 1962).

Chapter 3
Organisation of the Study

As the stated aim of this study is an in-depth investigation of mating patterns and reproductive performance in Jamaica, as well as of the social and biological elements surrounding these two variables, the decision has to be taken as to the precise unit in terms of which the material needed for the analysis is to be gathered. In fact a further decision has to be taken: namely whether the unit chosen for the collection of the data should also serve as the basis for analysis. For it is by no means essential for the unit of collection of information to be coterminous with the unit of analysis, although there are manifest advantages in making such an assumption. The procedure followed here is to accept, for both the collection of material and its analysis, the adult female aged 15 to 64 and her children as the unit in terms of which to proceed. And whether or not she and her partner share a common household, the position taken is that the woman and her children constitute a valid family unit for the purpose of this study.

From the standpoint of mating, there is a clear advantage in including the experience of the male partner in investigations of the kind represented in this survey. This means shifting the unit of investigation from the female alone to the couple. The position of the male is of especial relevance in establishing the socio-economic status of the family unit. As will be seen in this study, one of the few seemingly satisfactory measures of social status available from the standpoint of the female is provided by her educational attainment. However the use of occupation and income of the male partner may prove the basis for much sharper delineation of status levels.

Attractive as an approach incorporating the position of the male appears at first sight, there are two problems to be faced in implementing it. In the first place the common changes of partner by females, often accompanied by shifts from one type of union to another, will create interpretational issues, in so far as the basis for determining the socio-economic status of the couple in terms of the male position is not a stable one. Secondly the fact that one of

41

the types of unions being dealt with here, the visiting, is characterised by the absence of the male from the female household means that he is not easily available for inclusion in a survey in which the experiences of both partners of the union are required.

The foregoing considerations have led to the decision to accept the traditional approach of adopting the female as the unit in terms of which material is to be collected as well as the unit of analysis. However a broad classification of the female is used, because two distinct types of experience seem to be called for. In the first place, since the experience of females of childbearing age is needed, it was decided that a major focus of interest should be women aged 15 to 44. And since the complementary study of women of completed fertility seems equally essential, another group aged 45 to 64 is included.

In the course of this study, the value of approaching such problems as mortality among infants, child care and fertility from the standpoint of the experience of family units rather than individual females emerges clearly. It is not merely a case of requiring a satisfactory measure of socio-economic status derived from the position of the male partner, though this remains cardinal. What seems to be required is a means of assessing the position of the family or household as the micro unit within which the experiences are to be studied.

Recording the Information

The questionnaire used in this survey is reproduced in Appendix II. It is 19 pages in length and the information it seeks from respondents has been organised under 43 heads. While emphasis is placed on information relating to the respondent, there is in addition material on her children, her partner, as well as on her parents and the parents of her partner. The major types of data on the respondent covered include: her mating and pregnancy history, the children under 15 years actually living in her household, the several changes in types of union that she undergoes, the number and characteristics of her partners, special treatment of visiting unions, sexual relationships, menstrual patterns, knowledge of reproduction and menstruation, the bond between mother and child and respondent's children living away from her household.

While many of the questions included are precoded, the nature of the questionnaire is such that the majority of questions call for written answers. It was agreed that the best way of administering such a questionnaire was to supplement the written document by a tape recording of the entire interview.

The use of taped interviews presented many problems, mostly of a technical nature. An early consideration was whether respondents would have any objection to their voices being recorded. This happened in only a few cases. In the words of one respondent, "recording my voice would result in someone having power over me"; it was therefore thought best not to conduct the interview with her. Others made various comments on the issue, but did not object. On the whole there was no strong opposition to the use of this technique. Indeed when interviewers resorted to the practice of letting respondents hear a portion of the interview played back, the sound of their own voices proved intriguing to them.

Probably more weighty were the technical problems faced in effecting the recording. Throughout most of the urban areas, households have adequate electricity supplies, which greatly facilitate the use of tape recorders. However some respondents were not happy to have to supply electricity for the conduct of the interview, and this did occasion some inconvenience. In more remote rural areas, not yet electrified, a different procedure had to be followed. Here interviewers had to make use of rechargeable battery packs, or ordinary batteries. Lack of electricity in rural homes posed probably the major problem in the administration of the recorded interview in these areas.

Selection and Training of Interviewers

Because of the nature of the survey being conducted, great care was exercised in selecting interviewers. The professional qualifications required for selection were: nursing, social work or considerable experience in the conduct of social surveys. Of the several applications made in response to a newspaper advertisement for such persons, 18 were selected for training. Some of these had university degrees in addition to other qualifications. Those selected included 11 trained nurses, most of whom had dual qualifications, 5 holding degrees in social work, 2 with other relevant experience.

A two-week training session for those selected was carried out at the University during February 1975. These were full-time training sessions conducted by the authors in association with Dr. Vera Rubin of the Research Institute for the Study of Man. The first week was devoted to the study of the content of the questionnaire, the implications and significance of the material to be collected, and how these fitted into the body of knowledge of these subjects. The second week was devoted to practising how to conduct the interview, to complete the questionnaire and to make the recording. Each interviewer had to complete 7 interviews. Initially the approach was to choose as respondents members of the training session; then respondents unknown to the interviewers were brought in.

Conduct of Field Work

As soon as the training session was complete interviewers began their field work. Most of them were responsible for a single district, but in special cases responsibility for more than one was assumed. These enumeration districts were drawn from those included in the 1972 survey. The selection was made in order to bring into the sample sections of Kingston and St. Andrew, the main metropolitan area, and sections of two towns, Montego Bay and Mandeville, as well as rural areas. In addition 2 enumeration districts from the parish of St. Ann were brought in because of the special fertility features of this parish. The 20 enumeration districts included were drawn from 8 of the 14 parishes in the island. Details of the areas selected are listed in Appendix III. Every household within the confines of the district selected had to be visited in order to ascertain whether they contained persons qualified for inclusion along the lines previously indicated.

By means of three supervisors, careful checks of the first few completed interviews were carried out. Checking these and making comparisons of the treatment of certain questions by all interviewers were necessary in order to ensure as uniform an approach as possible. As has already been indicated, cooperation was good and few refusals encountered. Interviewing was completed in May 1975.

Seminar on Completion of Field Work

On the termination of the field work, a seminar was held at the University of the West Indies to discuss some of the interviewers' experiences in the field and to exchange views on a number of topics covered in the survey. Interviewers' impressions proved interesting, especially with respect to responses on the more intimate portions of the questionnaire. With few exceptions, they were well received by respondents. Some of the latter expressed curiosity as to what was to be gained from a survey of this type, and this might have been behind the abrupt answers interviewers said they received to some of the more intimate questions. As has already been indicated, only two issues seemed to cause any objection from respondents—the use of householders' electricity and the recording of their voices—and these were raised in very few instances. Older women found the interview an occasion for a pleasant talk with someone who could at the same time be counted on to assume the role of a sympathetic listener to many complaints they had to voice about matters that worried them. Typical of some reactions, none of which involved refusal to cooperate, are the remarks of one respondent who claimed, "Jamaica is a small country and there is embarrassment as we are talking face to face and recording." This respondent did not think that "the Jamaican society appreciates a survey of this nature as it is too personal and has left me in doubt."

The only account of people being unwilling to consent to be interviewed came from an interviewer in Portland. But her failure to contact a number of respondents was due to several factors. The scattered nature of the settlement and the difficulties of access were as much involved here as open refusal to cooperate. In any event all of these could have probably been easily overcome by a more enterprising interviewer.

There were one or two unfortunate experiences reported by interviewers. One was actually robbed in the course of conducting an interview in Kingston, although not by the person being interviewed. On another occasion there was an attempt to steal her tape recorder.

An interesting observation concerned the consequences of external migration of members of some families in St. Mary. There were accounts of husbands emigrating and within a year of their leaving their families, their wives or other partners giving birth to children for other men. This did not, however, seem to damage permanently the original relationship, as when the husband returned to Jamaica he again assumed his position vis-à-vis his original partner, and readily accepted and cared for the additions made to the household.

Some interviewers reported embarrassment on the part of a few respondents in answering questions on sexual habits. Some replied, "I am not going to answer that," or "It is too private and no one should know." Generally, however, there was no reserve in dealing with these questions. Most interviewers, it would seem, were able to establish good rapport with respondents.

While accounts of interviewers' experience in the field formed an important focus of discussion at the seminar, much more important from the standpoint of the analysis of the material were the discussions of concepts and topics being studied. Of the several topics taken up, the issue of childlessness called for extensive discussion, and both gynaecological and social aspects of this phenomenon came under scrutiny. Relevant here also were the views of respondents on the question of the value of children and on their general position with regard to large families. Even the cursory examination of the returns at that time made clear the extremely low levels of knowledge of reproduction and of menstruation by respondents. But observations of interviewers could throw little light on these aspects of the island's female population.

Another topic that was extensively examined was the type of union classification adopted. Particular interest centered around the visiting union, which many interviewers tended to hold as standing at the lowest level in the estimation of the society as a whole—a view, incidentally, which is by no means borne out by the findings of this study. Social workers especially held that one aspect of this typology which should be carefully explored was the degree to which any of the prevailing union types proved unfavourable from the standpoint of the development of the child. And again this was an issue which seemed most relevant in the case of children being brought up by mothers in visiting type unions.

The readiness of respondents to discuss intimate matters with interviewers was not unexpected, as this was fully in keeping with their experience with women as a whole. It was nonetheless an important center of discussion. In all portions of the society it seems there were no strong objections to joining in very free discussions with interviewers on intimate topics such as sex and menstruation. This may be as much a tribute to the skill of the interviewers as to the relatively open attitude of the population at large towards sexuality and allied topics.

Processing of Data

The possibility of computer processing of the data was at one time raised, but never seriously entertained, as it was thought that with only 501 respondents, a survey consisting to a large degree of open-ended responses could not satisfactorily be treated by computer analysis. The production of tabulations by simple tallying methods for such a small sample is relatively straightforward, while in many cases the necessity of having to combine quantitative and qualitative material admitted of no other approach.

The first step in processing the material was to check questionnaires for completeness and consistency. This in many cases necessitated interviewers returning to the field to supply missing information or to confirm doubtful entries.

The second step was a lengthy and demanding one, in which tapes were monitored and information they contained merged with the data entered on the questionnaires so that a new document could be produced summarising the material from both media. Listening to the tapes and reducing their contents to a typed form in which are also incorporated data from the written questionnaire called for careful summarising of what respondents actually said. Often the nature of the answer was such that verbatim transfer was impossible. But always the aim was to use as far as possible the exact phraseology adopted by the respondent and to capture the colourful language in which many of their replies were couched.

The total number of women interviewed amounts to 626. While no more than two respondents refused outright to cooperate in the survey, there were 17 who refused to answer some of the questions, on the ground that they were too intimate. It was thought best to exclude these interviews from those to be processed. Also, some of the respondents included, 17 in number, proved, on careful examination of the information they gave, to be over the age of the selected upper limit of the sample (64 years), and these therefore were excluded from the total to be processed.

Although rewarding from every angle, the preparation of documents embodying the information from the questionnaire as well as that secured from the tape recording was a demanding and time-consuming exercise.

Consequently the decision was taken to confine the analysis to 500 interviews; it turned out that the total accepted was 501. This means that about 90 of the completed interviews have not been used. The reason for discarding some interviews was the inability of interviewers to complete the document and the tape recording. The latter may have resulted from a technical difficulty such as the breakdown of the tape recorder, failure of electricity supply or poor quality of the recording. Serious discrepancies and omissions in a few of the questionnaires also resulted in their exclusion from the analysis.

Chapter 4
Properties of the Union Types

This study was not designed to furnish details about union formation, union distribution and characteristics of unions. In fact the small number of women constituting the sample precludes elaborate quantitative treatment of union characteristics. In any event, this has to some extent been covered in Chapter 2, which summarises findings from earlier studies on the subject. The present survey aims at providing information which may make more meaningful some of the accepted features of the three types recognised.

It is convenient to begin this chapter with a discussion of the methods of classification used and some of the problems encountered in applying them. Then follow brief discussions of the major features of the three types of unions. As the challenging issues posed by the visiting union form an important focus of interest, it is essential to consider some of the implications of its principal characteristic—the fact that the partners do not share a common household. Such aspects as the contact between the partners and between the father and his children call for close scrutiny. A further question to be considered is whether there is justification for identifying some unions as casual relationships rather than as visiting unions, in virtue of their very short initial duration and the means of their formation. This of course need not signify a difference in kind between casual and visiting; the former should in the present context be merely a subset of the general visiting type. Of the several factors which may contribute to a woman establishing a particular family type, two which seem important are introduced here. One consists of institutional conditions which may have operated against the formation of marriages in the past, but about which not much is known. The second is an assumption that respondents' assessment of the three types involved may be important deciding factors in guiding their choice of initial and other unions. Another topic discussed is the frequency of sexual intercourse in terms of educational status and union type, as revealed by the present study. As some indication of the relative socio-economic status of the three types is highly

49

relevant to our analysis, this is discussed on the basis of indicators resting on educational status. In a final section a summary of fertility differentials by union type is presented. While the study is too small to yield fertility rates on which extensive enquiries of this nature can be based, there is already available sufficient material on this to form the basis of an adequate summary.

Identification and Classification of Unions

We have already indicated that for a woman to be included in any of the three types of union recognised she must be in a steady sexual relationship with her partner. This however is not to be interpreted to mean that any sexual contact is synonymous with the existence of a union. Presumably many women have been in sexual relationships before these take on a sufficiently stable form and before certain other relationships become sufficiently well defined for the association to be deemed a family. We therefore distinguish between the maintenance of sexual relationships and the existence of a family. This distinction implies that while sexual contact is a necessary condition for the existence of a family union, a variety of relationships other than sexual ones enter into the establishment of any form of family.

Complications such as the change of partners or the interruption of unions and the consequent occurrence of a single state inevitably create difficulties in effecting any kind of classification.[1] Of the different forms of classification which may be applied, the simplest is in terms of the union in which the woman is involved at the time of the interview. And where there is no change in type of union during the woman's reproductive life, this establishes a satisfactory designation for all purposes and is called the pure type. Since we do not carry these classifications beyond the age of completion of fertility (age 45) the safest procedure in respect of women who have already passed the childbearing period is to classify them on the basis of the type in which they are involved when they attain age 45. On this basis age distributions of the female population in terms of the three types of union between ages 15 and 45 can be obtained, and these form the foundation of many analyses of these populations. As will be seen, it is used in many analyses in the present study. Another approach which has been used in a previous study may also be noted.[2] This assigns the type on the basis of the number of years spent in each; here also involvement in one type of union throughout her reproductive life qualifies her for the designation pure. But where the woman has been in two types of union, she will be classified in terms of the union in which she spends more time. Similarly a woman involved in three union types will be classified on the basis of the union in which she passes most of the duration of her union history. This classification is not used in the present survey.

A scheme of classification used in this survey aims at arriving at a "central point" in terms of children of the woman. It is effected on the basis of the type in which the woman finds herself at the time of the termination of a given pregnancy. For women with more than 3 pregnancies, the type in which the median pregnancy occurs forms the basis of the designation. Where the number of pregnancies is even, the parity immediately below the median one is used. For women with 2 or 3 pregnancies, the type designating the woman's experience is the union in which the last pregnancy takes place. In the case of those with a single pregnancy, the type is the one existing when that pregnancy terminates. Where the woman is involved in one type of union throughout her childbearing span, this is the designation adopted. Such unions constitute the "pure" types.

There has recently been passed in Jamaica the Status of Children Act, 1976, (Act 36 of 1976), "An act to remove the legal disabilities of children born out of wedlock and to provide for matters connected therewith or incidental thereto." As its title indicates, it deals with the legal aspects of the status of children, how their paternity is to be determined and their inheritance of property of their parents. It is centered on children rather than on the family unit as a whole; indeed nowhere is there any reference to the family as such. At this early stage it is not possible to judge what will be its effects on current family structure, although its provisions, such as the one stating that "the relationship between every person and his father and mother shall be determined irrespective of whether the father and mother are or have been married to each other ... ," could conceivably influence many familial relationships. Nor can we conclude at this stage whether this law, or any similar law to be passed in the near future, will invalidate, in whole or part, the family typology used in this study.

Summary of Main Features of the Three Types of Union[3]

Visiting

This type predominates at the initial stages, and women entering it are for the most part below age 30. While some of them continue in this type up to age 45—these may be called the pure types—the majority move away from it, usually to establish formal marriage or, less frequently, to enter a common-law union. An appreciable proportion also becomes single. It was shown in Chapter 2 that the average age at entering initial visiting unions in the case of Jamaica is 20.6 years, a figure markedly lower than the corresponding ages for the other two types. As a consequence of this, these women also commence childbearing earlier than the other two. One of the principal features separating the visiting from the other two is the lengthy spacing between births up to about order 5. A differential of this nature constitutes a major contribution to the relatively low fertility level of this type. Equally significant from the standpoint of mating is that this pattern indicates, in the context of the first birth, that many women dissolve the initial relationship after the birth of this child, and that some time elapses before they commit themselves to another association. As will be argued later in this chapter, first births to visiting unions may result from a single sexual contact and may not lead to the establishment of a lasting relationship.

In terms of the dynamic aspect of mating, an important characteristic of the visiting type is the movement from this initial type to married and, less frequently, to common-law unions; this becomes very prominent within the age interval 20 to 25. As a result of this shift away from the visiting type, there is by age 45 a very small proportion of women still in such unions. Another feature of this type which has a bearing on its fertility performance is the comparatively low average age at which these women have their last children. Moreover, it is possible that a measure of selectivity is involved in movements from visiting to married and common-law types, as will be argued in our discussions of the relationship between union status and fertility.

Common-Law

This type of union, having as its principal features the sharing of a common household by the partners and the absence of legal sanction, offers some sharp contrasts with the type just discussed as well as with formal marriage. Unlike the other two, it displays no marked concentration in any age range, so far as entry is concerned; the probabilities of entering this type do not vary much over the ages 15 to 35, although the maximum value occurs in the interval 30 to 35. The average age at entering unions of this type is 21.0 years, which is higher than the corresponding age for initial visiting unions. Again these show a strong probability of being converted into formal marriage. Because of the age at contracting common-law unions, these women have their first child at a higher age than the visiting. Here the birth spacing is much less than it is among women in visiting-type unions, so that the differential with respect to age at first birth is not so decisive in affecting the relative fertility positions. Another feature of the common-law union which tends to enhance its level of fertility is the comparatively high age at the birth of the last child. Again there is movement towards the married category, although it is not so marked as in the case of the visiting-type unions. It also appears that a measure of selectivity is in evidence so far as fertility levels are concerned, as once more women contracting formal marriages tend to be of higher fertility than those who remain in common-law unions.

Marriage

Formal marriage, characterised by the sharing of a common household by the partners and the presence of legal sanction, shows certain distinctive properties. Both in terms of initial and higher stages, ages at contracting marriage tend to be high by comparison with the other two. The average age at which women enter initial married unions is 23.9 years, appreciably higher than the corresponding age for the initial visiting unions and somewhat above that for the common-law type. Consequently the average age at the birth of the first child is inclined to be high. But the interval between the woman's age at successive births is much less than in the case of the visiting unions and close to those for the common-law, which compensates somewhat for the relatively high age at which this type commences childbearing. Also the age at birth of the last child is the highest for the three types; this is another factor contributing to the comparatively high fertility which this union shows. A notable feature of this type is the considerable number of women formerly in visiting or common-law unions who eventually marry.

Some Features of the Visiting Union

In delineating the features of the visiting-type union, one of the main points of interest centers around the degree of contact between the respondent and her partner, what form these meetings take, where they are held and how long they last. A considerable portion of the questionnaire, covering 34 different aspects of the visiting union, is devoted to exploring these issues. These questions have been put to all women who, at any time during their reproductive span, have been involved in a visiting union. The underlying patterns emerging from their answers can be depicted only in broad terms, since, understandably, it is often difficult for the respondent to state with precision how often these meetings take place and to furnish details about them. Whether a respondent who has shifted from visiting to another type is more prone to forget particulars of her initial relationship than one who has not made such changes is debatable. But a study of answers from respondents, especially those who have subsequently married, suggests such a possibility. In Appendix IV the statistical summaries of the replies to these questions are presented, together with relevant comments where these seem to be required.

Limitations to the information collected apply especially to women over 45 whose answers relate to their life during the childbearing span and who consequently may experience difficulty in recalling specific information about contacts with their partners. For these reasons quantification of answers on these topics can give only very broad patterns of an essentially descriptive nature, which cannot be subjected to rigorous statistical analysis. The time interval for recording this information is the average week. Whether dependence on responses from females alone introduces any bias in the answers with respect to these aspects of the functioning family cannot be determined at this stage. But unquestionably supporting material about such unions from the male partners would have helped to improve the precision of answers received on these topics.

While the features by which the visiting union is identified are the existence of a steady sexual relationship between the woman and her partner, the maintenance of separate households and the lack of legal sanction of the union, the functioning family involves a wide variety of contacts between its members. These can be examined from several standpoints. In the first place a general approach seems necessary, one signifying the extent to which the couple meet each other and where these meetings take place. The question put to the respondent here is, "How frequently do you and your partner meet?" Answers to this have been given by more than 90% of respondents. The average number of times these meetings take place in a week is 3.4, but the variation in the number of contacts is considerable. About one-quarter of all respondents see their partners every day of the week and a somewhat smaller proportion do so between 5 and 6 times per week. Frequent meetings between them are the rule when they live near to each other. On the other hand there are unions where very few weekly meetings are possible; sometimes these are down to one a fortnight or even less. Some women attribute such rare contacts to the fact that their partners live far away from them. It is probably extreme separation which accounts for a form of contact in which partners from time to time spend whole weekends together.

Meetings between partners are held at several places, but those at one or other of their homes are numerically the important ones and it is on these that attention will be concentrated. Nearly 90% of the women report receiving visits from their partners during each week. Again the number of these visits shows wide variation, with an average of 3.5 times per week. The length of these meetings also varies widely, and their average amounts to just under 9 hours per week. Somewhat less frequent are the visits which she makes to her partner's home. These occur in 56% of all cases and average 2.3 times per week. Their average duration remains appreciable, being 8.3 hours, that is not much lower than the corresponding average for male visits to respondents.

The functioning family involves contacts between the partners in a variety of fields. Of interest in this respect is the extent to which couples participate in these contacts, in some of which their children are also included. The question on this issue is, "Are there any special occasions, such as Church, Cinema, Sports that you and your partner go to, or to which he takes the children?" While 24 or about 9% of the respondents say that their partners do not take them or their children on such outings, nearly 60% report that these are common practices. The activities in which the family is involved may be grouped into the following six categories:

Cinema	36.5%
Church	22.3%
Clubs, dances, parties	17.2%
Sports of all kinds	16.4%
Beach	3.4%
All others	4.2%

Outstanding in this distribution is the importance of entertainment, both indoor and outdoor. The cinema constitutes by far the most frequently mentioned form of entertainment, and taken in conjunction with the other kinds of an indoor nature accounts for 54% of the joint outings of the family. Outdoor entertainment including sports of all kinds and excursions to the beach account for just under one-fifth of the activities involved. Thus we may conclude that outdoor and indoor entertainment is responsible for 74% of the family's joint outings. Apart from entertainment, attendance at church is the second most important activity in which the family participates, and is responsible for 22% of all joint excursions of the family.

In view of the importance of entertainment as a part of the family's joint commitment a closer examination of this form of participation seems warranted. Those reporting separately on the occasions in which the respondent, and sometimes her children as well, are taken out by her partner indicate that this averages 1.4 times per week and that the average time spent would amount to 4.7 hours per week. A significant aspect of the interaction between the respondent and her partner covers the subjects they usually discuss when they are together. Information on this is collected in respect of what are termed "general visits" in the questionnaire, as distinct from sexual visits or other visits made for specific purposes associated with the maintenance of the family. Answers to these questions have been obtained from 75 respondents, or just over one-quarter of the total in visiting unions. The average weekly number of such meetings is 2.3, while their average duration amounts to 2.3 hours. These take place for the most part (78% of the total) at the respondent's home. Smaller proportions occur at the partner's home, while in some cases meetings at either home are possible; these proportions are 8% and 5% respectively.

The list of topics mentioned as usually forming the basis for discussion at these general visits is interesting. The separate items identified number 22. By far the most frequently occurring topics concern issues relevant to the functioning family. The one most often mentioned is "children" (21%). The fact that "marriage" constitutes the second most frequently mentioned item (16%) emphasises the extent to which women in visiting unions concern themselves with the legalising of their family unions. Another item connected with the home that comes up for regular discussion is described as "planning for the future"; this accounts for 12% of all those mentioned. What are described as discussions of the "home" account for 11% of the total, while only slightly less (10%) deal with "financial items" such as salaries and saving, which are other subjects relevant to the maintenance of the family unit. Also connected directly with the family is the "buying or building of a house" (6%). The business in which the partner is engaged comes up for mention in 6% of total items. In summary it may be said that over 90% of the topics mentioned as forming the basis for discussion between partners in visiting-type unions bear directly on the functioning family: these are support and rearing of the children, the economic maintenance of the union, the provision of a dwelling unit for the family and its future with special reference to the possibility of endowing it with legal sanction. Still there are a few reports of wider fields of discussion between the partners; these touch on subjects of a national and, at times, international character.

It is not always possible for respondents to state specifically what is the purpose of meetings between them and their partners, but many are able to identify visits made mainly for the purpose of having sex. Interviewers report that they encountered no problems in getting information on the sexual experience of respondents. Although a few women thought these questions rather personal—and one expressed the view that they were "impertinent"— the number refusing to give information is negligible. Examination of this form of visit is based on answers to questions on the frequency of sexual visits, on the number of such visits during an average week and their duration, whether any difficulties are faced in organising these meetings and comments concerning their selection of places to meet. These questions are not sufficiently detailed or searching to make possible a distinction between sexual visits and sex acts. Since many sex acts may result from a single sexual visit—especially those described as overnight or weekend visits—the number of sexual visits per week has to be taken as only an approximate indicator of the relative frequency of sex contacts among different groups of respondents.

Answers to questions on the frequency of sex visits vary greatly. Some respondents are not specific, being able to give only answers such as "often," "frequent," "regular," "irregular," "varies," "not often." The proportion of women who gave answers in terms of clearly stated number of times per week amounts to 91%. Only 2 state that these visits are as often as daily, and 1 of these adds the qualification "when possible." Only 3 report frequencies of 5 per week. The modal frequency is once per week while the average amounts to 1.6. Wide variation also characterises the duration of these sexual visits. Here it seems that some answers refer actually to the length of the sexual act rather than the duration of the visit, as these extend to no more than a few minutes. Three report that such visits last overnight, which is interpreted in this survey as of 12 hours' duration. The average duration per visit, with the qualifications already noted, amounts to 2.2 hours. The site of these meetings is for the most part the respondent's home, which is given as the venue in 65% of the cases. But a sizeable proportion (26%) also take place at the home of the male. In 6% of the cases either home is used, while in 3% the site is neither his nor her home. While there may be some difficulties to be overcome in arranging meetings of this nature, 90% of the women reporting on sexual visits state that they encounter no problems in making the necessary arrangements. Of note also are the general comments made concerning these sexual visits. These in general explain the choice of site, usually the home of the respondent, that is the home of her parents if she is young or her own home if she is of more advanced age. The indications are that the site chosen is for one or more reasons convenient, while extension of an answer of this kind is that pointing to the fact that hers is the home selected because she owns or controls it.

The preference for the home of the woman is understandable, as the children live with her and it will be more convenient, from this standpoint, for her not to leave them. In fact in the case of older women, who are heads of their own households, such an arrangement has obvious advantages. In the case of younger women still living in their parents' homes, it is less convenient, but only where the latter are opposed to their daughters' involvement in visiting unions are serious problems of meeting reported. Where their parents approve of the union they may leave the home temporarily so that the daughters and their partners can have privacy for a time.

Complementing the questions on sexual visits are three others relating to the sexual relationships between the partners. One is, "Do (Did) you enjoy having sex with your partner?" The second is, "On the average how many times per month do (did) you have sex with him?" With regard to the first there is virtual unanimity as 97% of the women reply in the affirmative. In terms of the second question, the average number of times per month they had sexual relations is 6.7, and this reduced to a weekly basis is 1.7, that is almost the same as the number of sexual visits per week, already presented. This suggests therefore that in general no distinction is made by respondents between sexual visits and sexual acts.

Information has also been collected on other types of meetings between the respondent and her visiting partner; here interest centers on the form of activity that motivates these contacts. And again the places where these occur and their duration are relevant. Although firm quantitative information has not been obtained in all cases, the answers serve to throw much additional light on the forms of relationship characterising visiting unions. Unlike sexual visits, these less specific contacts are by no means so heavily concentrated at the respondent's home. In fact the proportion which are centered there (55%) emphasise that a sizeable proportion (26%) occur at the partner's residence, while in 15% of the visits either of the homes is involved. In most cases more than one purpose of visit is stated by the respondent, and frequently sexual relationships appear in conjunction with others. The stated purposes fall under 17 heads. Of these by far the most important is sex, which accounts for 26% of the total listed. The second most frequently mentioned involves the father's visit to the respondent in order to see the children; this accounts for 19% of the total. Then follow several categories which taken together constitute the core of the social contacts between members of the family. The most often mentioned of these purposes is "to talk," which accounts for 15%

of the total. Closely associated with this is the purpose described by respondents as "social," which accounts for 13% of the total. Other similar purposes are covered by "companionship" and "being together." When these are combined they may be taken as constituting the contacts made for ensuring the close interrelationship of the members; these are also essential for the proper maintenance of the several functions of the family. They account for 32% of the total meetings of the family group. Another set of purposes of visits which has a bearing on the functioning family covers business and similar topics usually associated with the economic upkeep of the unit; these are mentioned as accounting for 15% of total contacts. The proportional distribution of purpose of visit can be summarised as follows:

Social, talk, companionship, to be together	31.9%
Sex	26.4%
To see children	19.5%
Business	15.3%
Other	6.9%

An important feature of the visiting-type union is the extent to which it ensures adequate contacts between the father and his children. The usual structure of these unions is that the woman and her children live together, but away from the male partner. Cases in which the children live with the father are not unknown, but extremely rare. Contact between children and their father therefore must be made through his visits to the mother's home, through their visits to his home, or through their participation with the father in outings away from the home of either parent. In view of the frequency of his visits to his partner's home, we should expect that much of the contact between father and children occurs in this way. But in addition this survey shows that there is a pattern of visits arranged which makes it possible for the children to spend time at their father's home as well. The question in the survey designed to throw light on this subject is framed thus, "How many hours per week do your child(ren) spend with their father at his home ... at your home ... elsewhere?" Just under one-third of all women in visiting unions give responses which can be readily quantified, and of these, 3 state that the father sees the children daily, while in the case of 10 respondents, the average contact per week between father and children exceeds 20 hours. The average time that the father spends with the children under all forms of contact is 14.5 hours per week. In just over one-half of the cases (55%) the father sees the child at the home of the mother, while in 26% of the cases the child comes to his home. Many respondents report that during weekends children go to see their father and may spend a whole day with him. In 15% of the responses the meetings take place at either home, while in a small proportion of cases (4%) other sites of meeting are mentioned.

These contacts between members of the visiting family emphasise that the union involves much more than the mere sexual relationships between the parents. One important question arising in this context is whether these unions undergo any changes as the partners move through the family cycle. The question put to the respondent on this issue is, "Has the pattern [of your visits] changed as you have grown older?" The proportion of respondents reporting a change in their patterns of meeting amounts to 41%. Those reporting a change indicate several types of change. Some of this takes the form of less frequent meetings, or as some put it the relationship "got worse." But the majority of the change recorded is described as a strengthening of the bond between the partners, and this is accompanied by more frequent meetings and longer duration of such visits.

It is useful to try to summarise the position by giving a rough estimate of the total period which members of a visiting family spend together during an average week. But for reasons that have already been indicated, several qualifications will have to be made to such an estimate. In the first place not all respondents give answers that are readily quantified. Secondly many respondents give no answers at all to these questions. Thirdly the categories of visits discussed here cannot be regarded as mutually exclusive; in most cases they overlap considerably. It is not possible to make allowance for the third factor. But it is still possible to arrive at a rough estimate of the overall period spent together in terms of four categories. This involves simply aggregating the total period spent during these kinds of visits and relating the sum to the 270 respondents who are involved in visiting-type unions. The results are as follows:

General visits	0.9 hours
Sexual visits	1.7 "
Visits to see children	4.0 "
Other visits	16.2 "
Total	22.8 "

This suggests that on the average there is a contact of nearly 3 hours per day between the members of the visiting family, and it is of interest that most of this concerns what may be termed issues centering around the performance of the major functions of the family.

Three concluding questions concerning the visiting unions yield information on whether the respondent feels lonely when not in the company of her partner and on the extent to which she considers herself and her partner should be faithful to each other. Nearly all women reply to the question whether they feel lonely when their partners are not with them. Most of them (62%) state that they do feel lonely, while 29% state that the absence of their partners does not have this effect on them. The remainder claim that they feel lonely in the absence of their partner only on some occasions. With regard to the question on "faithfulness," respondents are almost unanimous about being faithful to each other. Only 2 of the women in visiting unions are of the opinion that they need not be faithful to their partners. Only slightly less strong is their feeling concerning faithfulness on the part of their partners. Here 7 respondents express the view that their partners need not be faithful to them.

The Casual Relationship

The conclusion which can be drawn from the foregoing discussion of the visiting type is that it is by no means as unordered as it is sometimes made out to be. The well defined contacts between the partners, despite the fact that they do not share a common household, their close interrelationships in terms of entertainment and cultural activities, the frequent contact between father and children, the degree to which the various issues facing the functioning family are discussed by the partners—all these seem to depict a type of association which affords adequate care and socialisation of the children. Yet it may be misleading to interpret the situation as entirely to the advantage of the mother and her children. Indeed we must examine more closely one aspect of the visiting relationship, namely its initial stage. For the opinion in many circles is that the initial mating process, especially when accompanied by too early pregnancy, operates to the marked detriment of the woman, that indeed such a brief association may be deemed to be a union only in so far as it results in conception. Often the discovery of the woman's pregnancy spells, so far as she is concerned, the immediate dissolution of the union.

It is therefore necessary to examine more critically the material from the survey in order to see whether a case can be made out for distinguishing a type of initial relationship which, though in gross form (that is in terms of the absence of a common household and lack of legal sanction) conforms to the visiting type, yet does not exhibit much cohesion between the partners. There is some evidence from the present survey justifying the delineation of such a relationship, although, whatever name is used, it seems more appropriate to consider it as a subset of the visiting type rather than as a definite familial category in its own right.

The first condition pointing to the existence of this special type centers around the nature and duration of the initial union which the woman has contracted. It has long been evident that the interval between the births of the first and second children in the Caribbean is greatest in the case of the visiting unions; indeed this relatively long period in visiting unions persists up to the interval following the fifth birth.[4] This has been interpreted as one feature making for fertility differentials by family type. In the present context we concentrate on the interval between the first and second births, which can be illustrated from the material of the survey. And here it is useful to introduce at the same time what respondents think should be the interval between first and second births. A comparison of the actual spacing between first and second births and what respondents report as their desired spacing is as follows:

Union Type	Actual Spacing in Years	Desired Spacing in Years
Visiting	3.09	3.19
Common-Law	2.58	2.91
Married	1.87	2.42

These leave no doubt as to the comparatively long period between first and second births in visiting unions. Moreover, the desired spacing maintains the same ranking as does the actual spacing. In so far as the visiting and common-law types are concerned, the desired does not depart much from the actual, but there is a marked difference between the two in the case of the married, where the actual spacing (1.87) falls 23% below that of the desired.

Comparatively lengthy spacing such as is noted in the visiting union may arise in one of two ways. In the first place it may signify the interruption of the union before or just after the birth of the first child. Secondly it may conceivably arise without the dissolution of the union if the woman makes use of some form of fertility control to postpone the birth of the second child. The latter assumption is however untenable as the phenomenon is evidently of long standing and there are no known methods which in the past could have been used successfully by this section of the population. It seems therefore that the first assumption, the early dissolution of the union, is the operative factor, and this is manifest from the reported union duration.

It would appear appropriate to take as a basic constituent of a casual relationship the birth of a child—in fact the birth of the first child. Presumably such a relationship may exist without being accompanied by a birth, but unless it is a steady and persistent relationship, it would not, within the approaches used in this study, be deemed to be a union. In fact, as has already been argued, a clear distinction must be made between sexual association and the existence of a union. For while the latter of necessity implies steady sexual relationships between the couple, it is possible for a woman to engage in occasional sexual contacts without being involved in a union. A union cannot rest on sexual relationships alone.

In the present context the significance of the extended spacing between the first and second births is the shortened duration of the initial union it implies. In fact it appears that it is the length of the union rather than the spacing *per se* which should be taken as the identifying feature of the casual association. Nevertheless for a better appreciation of the situation it is useful to consider the spacing as well. Likewise mothers who have only one child and for whom spacing between births is not therefore available have also to be taken into account. Another procedure which is relevant to the present treatment is to separate women involved in pure visiting-type unions, that is who have not at any age before reaching 45 been in common-law or married relationships, from the others.

Table 4.1 summarises the material on the basis of which estimates of the number of casual relationships in the sample may be derived. In so far as the pure (visiting) type signifies that the mother has not married nor been engaged in a common-law union, it may be argued that early dissolution of an initial union may not warrant its being separated from the true visiting type, as it is followed by another of the same form. On the other hand, where an initial visiting union of short duration is followed by a different type, the case for its being classified as casual seems stronger. And since the number of pure types with which we are dealing here is small, one line of approach is to prepare maximum and minimum estimates, the former comprising both pure and other types, while the latter is confined to unions not of the pure type. The sum of all mothers whose initial unions have been less than one year amounts to 69, which may be taken as a maximum estimate of the number of casual relationships in the sample. This is equivalent to 20% of the total initial visiting-type unions in the sample. Exclusion of the pure type reduces the estimate to 59, which constitutes our minimum estimate. This is equivalent to 17% of the total initial visiting unions. We conclude therefore that of the total of 340 initial visiting unions in the survey the proportion which may be treated as casual relationships lies somewhere between 20% and 17%. Relating the casual relationships to the entire number of women in the sample who are in unions (464), we see that the range is from 15% to 13%.

These casual relationships arise mainly among young women, for the most part between ages 16 and 19. Respondents' accounts suggest a few basic situations that give rise to relationships of this nature. In the first place a number of them develop when the respondent is still at school and friendship with male schoolmates leads to sexual contact. According to one respondent,

Table 4.1 Mothers in initial visiting unions of less than 1 year's duration, showing spacing between their first and second children, and distinguishing pure from other types

| Duration of initial union | Mothers with spacing between 1st and 2nd children of | | | | Mothers with 1 child only | |
| | Under 30 months | | Over 30 months | | | |
	Pure type	Others	Pure type	Others	Pure type	Others
Under 6 months	—	5	1	8	3	1
6 months to 1 year	4	18	6	17	3	3
Total under 1 year	4	23	7	25	6	4

"It was a school friendship which grew into a love affair." When she got pregnant the relationship ended. It would appear that when such friendships result in pregnancy the girl leaves school and the union breaks up soon after. In many cases the pregnancy is the result of a single sexual contact.

Another group of girls become involved in these relationships through some pressure being exerted on them. A few claim that they become involved in relationships of this nature simply by "rape" or being "forced." While both of these suggest the exertion of pressure on the part of her partner, this aspect of the relationship is seldom elaborated on, but a few seem to have experienced dramatic shock as a consequence of realising that they were pregnant.

In a number of cases these relationships arise seemingly by accident, as is illustrated by the experience of a 19-year-old girl. Sent by her father to collect a pair of trousers from a tailor's shop, she started "fooling around" with an employee and then they "started to play with each other until this thing happen." Relationships between employee and employer are also responsible for some of these associations, as another respondent indicates. According to her, she and her employer "just t'ief a piece" once only, and she became pregnant.

Underlying many of these cases is the respondent's complete ignorance of the reproductive processes, which, as will later be shown, constitutes an important feature of Jamaican women. And inevitably the realisation that she is pregnant results in considerable emotional trauma. The case history at the end of this chapter illustrates the origins and major features of a casual relationship.[5]

Institutional and Other Elements Influencing Mating Patterns

While in the opening chapter of this study the view has been expressed that the three union types identified here have been in existence throughout the post-emancipation period, and we have refrained from being drawn into discussions of their origins, it is still necessary to bring together some observations on factors contributing to the persistence, if not indeed to the origins, of prevailing mating patterns. In the first place there were probably several institutional elements militating against the widespread resort to marriage as a means of initiating family unions. At least one line of evidence pointing to this may be cited. Up to recent years, postmistresses in Jamaica, who also performed the duties of district registrars and many other significant official functions, were not permitted to marry; it was a condition under which they occupied official houses that they should not marry. The reason behind this cruel imposition is not clear, but it is all the more relevant in the present context because these officials were responsible for the registration of births in the island. There were other female-centered occupations—notably nursing, and to a lesser degree teaching—but restrictions against marriage were evidently not in force among them. The reluctance on the part of the colonial civil service to employ married women was well known throughout the Caribbean. The opening of civil service careers to married women has materialised only in recent years.

Perhaps several other institutional factors might have played a part in establishing the existing mating forms, but it is not the aim of this study to pursue these. More relevant in the present context are the views women express about prevailing family types. It is therefore essential to consider briefly their assessments of the three union types. We begin by an examination of what they think of the common-law union. It is curious that there seems to be very little support for this form of relationship. Of the women who gave views on the subject there is only one who comes out firmly in support of it. She is a 64-year-old widow and she states her position as follows, "You are steady and quiet even if things do not work out well, and it is better than running around and having children for different men."

To some women the disadvantages of common-law unions mainly derive from the impact on their children. One claims that if children are involved the partner might not want "to accept responsibilities since it is not legal." Again, another holds that this type of union "don't look proper for children." On financial grounds also the impression is that several disabilities inhere in this type of union. One respondent says that the partner will give an amount of money and "you have to stretch it and cannot ask for any more." Also, in the words of another, the money brought by the partner has to be "shared," whereas in a visiting union "the money they bring is for the woman alone." There is a general feeling among respondents that the common-law union "demands" too much of them and accords them "less freedom" than in the visiting union, while the woman has no certain claim on her partner. As one respondent puts it, "If you live with a man, he will have a girl outside and everywhere you go that girl will laugh at you"; because of this, she prefers just "to talk to them." In the opinion of another, men in these unions usually "stay out late at night." Men in common-law unions also at times ill-treat their partners. In the words of one, "When they come and stay they have too much clue to you. They want to beat you up and tell you not to go outside of the street." And another holds, "When people live together they usually fight and quarrel." Thus there does not seem to be much enthusiasm for the common-law union, which denies the woman much of her freedom, exposes her to ill treatment from a resident partner, does not afford much financial advantage and promises few benefits for her children.

The formal married status is much more acceptable to respondents. Indeed for the most part it appears to be an ideal type to which most women aspire. But it is important to note that many see in it disadvantages which they are anxious to spell out. Thus one argues, "It can be very difficult if one has chosen wrong," and there is "too much responsibility connected." Another is sceptical of marriages because many of them "are not working." And one respondent concludes that the man "leaves you at home and you suffer more."

One of the principal benefits of marriage acknowledged concerns the "respectability" it confers on the family. According to one respondent, it is a "more respectable" form of association and "better for the children." And another expresses her support thus, "People respect you and you are near the person you really like." A married woman, says another, "is more honourable and she is more respected," the union is "binding." In the words of still another, marriage "is more stable and other men do not try to get in so readily." Also, "Marriage is the best thing as you settle down one place." Marriage, several women argue, has definite advantages for children. As one states it, "Marriage is only good for the children's sake, so if their father dies and leaves a little house or land they can get it." Religion has also played a part in inducing some to accept marriage. In the words of one, after "accepting Christ" she "just lay low with everything" and thought marriage was the best way. Also another argues that you cannot be a member of a church unless you are married. "Marriage is the union that God requires," claims a married woman aged 26, who gives her religion as Open Bible. In fact the religious arguments form the basis for extensive support for the married state.

Comments on the visiting type are numerous and far ranging, above all demonstrating the extent to which the women in the society accept such relationships as part of their way of life. In outlining what are advanced as the benefits of this union type it is convenient to consider in the first place the views of respondents who evidently do not contemplate marriage. Their tendency is to stress that the visiting union assures "freedom" and a measure of "independence." This is not to say that they hold that such a position confers licence to any form of conduct on the part of the respondent or her partner.

Underlying many of the views of respondents on the types of union is a lurking fear that living with a man, whether in common-law status or marriage, carries a strong risk of a woman being the victim of her partner's violent behaviour. This theme of violence appears to be another important aspect of the seeming preference for visiting-type unions expressed by many respondents, especially in the early stages of the family. Some even fear that their partners will take their lives, as in the case of one woman aged 51 years, who one night saw her partner with a razor and thought that he was about to kill her. This led to their immediate separation. Another, after remonstrating with her husband because he stayed out late at nights, faced his threat "to break my bones." One respondent in a visiting union and still living in her mother's home was reluctant to set up her own house with a partner, for when "you do this you usually get some lick that you don't suppose to get." Still another in a visiting union comments that she did not want to live with any man; "The men cannot beat you when visiting, but living together they will beat you." It is not surprising therefore to learn that several women see in the visiting union a protection against such violent behaviour. One respondent points out that if conditions do become difficult in the union, the woman "can leave when she wants." This is fully spelled out in another statement, "You can get to know the person and you can break off if it does not suit you." Many women prefer to have short periods of isolation from their partners, and the visiting union assures them this: "It is not every time that you want to see him," declares one respondent. "You can get to know the person without getting tired of him, which might happen if you were living together." This means that the couple remain "sweeter" and the woman has "less work to do; she is free." A poetic assessment is, "It's better being in a visiting union, because 'absence makes the heart grow fonder.'"

Others supporting the visiting type do so from the standpoint of assuming that it is a prelude to marriage. These views dwell less on the aspects of freedom and independence of these relationships. In short, "a visiting union should lead up to something, marriage." "One gets to know a person before marriage," is how another sums up the situation. One, mindful of both marriage and a career, argues that a visiting union "gives one time to get a career before marriage." Another holds that it affords the woman needed experience. She gained so much experience that she "was able to marry a man quite a few years older than herself," which evidently pleased her. Such a marriage could not have taken place if she did not have the necessary experience "about love and so on."

Some disadvantages and drawbacks of involvement in a visiting union are stressed by respondents, but it is by no means the subject of general condemnation. A few express reserve about it on moral grounds. To one, this type of union "does not look decent," while to another it is "not nice." But in none of the views expressing disapproval with this type of union is this position based on or in any way associated with religious principles; the closest to a religious assessment is the view of one respondent that it is "less sinful" than presumably the common-law. Some respondents acknowledge that the freedom of movement which this union type allows to their partners as well as to themselves is not always to their advantage, because "sometimes you think he is gone somewhere and he is somewhere else." Indeed this "coming and going" in visiting unions does not find universal approval.

The implications of this type of union for children are not stressed much by respondents. One claims that she obtained "no good" from her union as she got a child which she had to support herself. More important, very few consider that the existence of this type of union in any way seriously impairs their financial position. One frequent theme is that money received from a partner does not have to be used to support him; it is entirely for her own use.

Another goes so far as to characterise the position of the visiting union in these terms: "It provides ready financial assistance without responsibility of a household."

It seems fair to sum up the general assessment of the prevailing types of union in this way. To many women marriage appears as an ideal with clear advantages of many kinds, but it does not by any means command universal support. Much of the argument in favour of this union rests on religious grounds. There is strong support for visiting unions, the main contention being that it affords the women freedom and independence, as well as protects her from many abuses by her partner. Very important here is that virtually no views against visiting-type unions rest on religious grounds. There is little doubt that the common-law is lowest in the scale of values of the respondents, being disapproved of mostly on religious and moral considerations.

Frequency of Sexual Intercourse

The frequency of sexual intercourse constitutes an important aspect of the relationships between the sexes in the population and have therefore to be examined from several standpoints. The question put to respondents on this topic is, "On the average how many times per month do (did) you have sex with him [her partner]?" Some respondents were unable to give precise, quantitative answers while others seemed reluctant to discuss these intimate matters in detail. Responses such as "often," "frequently," "sometimes," "it varies," prove in the present context just as unsatisfactory as a blunt "don't know," to which also some resorted. Answers of this kind reduce the already small numbers on which averages have to be based, thus imposing further qualifications on discussions of differentials between various groups of women in respect of this statistic.

The first material on frequency of sexual intercourse in the sample to be considered is presented in Table 4.2, which summarises the overall position and compares the situations for two groups, one with primary education and the other with post-primary schooling. For the sample as a whole, the proportion of women giving satisfactory answers to this question ranges from 87% to 60% for women of childbearing age, while the proportion for those of completed fertility stands at 67%. For women under age 40, the average frequency of sexual intercourse for several age groups does not vary much by age, being for the most part just over 7 times per month, that is under twice a week. But the value falls sharply to 4.81 for women aged 40 to 44, then moves up to 6.33 in the case of those of completed fertility.

In the case of women with primary education only, the proportion replying satisfactorily to the question is highest in the age group 25 to 29 (89%) and lowest in the age group 40 to 44 (63%). The frequency of sexual

Table 4.2 Frequency of sexual intercourse per month—women reporting, average and coefficient of variation, by educational attainment and age group

| Age group | Primary education | | | | Post-primary education | | | | All women | | | |
| | Women reporting | | Frequency of intercourse | | Women reporting | | Frequency of intercourse | | Women reporting | | Frequency of intercourse | |
	No.	As % total in age group	Average	Coefficient of variation	No.	As % total in age group	Average	Coefficient of variation	No.	As % total in age group	Average	Coefficient of variation
Under 25	41	85.4	7.82	55.8	43	76.8	6.97	71.6	84	80.8	7.39	64.0
25–29	39	88.6	7.65	56.3	27	84.4	7.83	63.1	66	86.8	7.27	59.3
30–34	31	86.1	7.60	59.7					41	82.0	7.17	59.9
35–39	19	70.4	7.32	66.2	16	66.7	6.00	46.2	22	71.0	7.00	65.6
40–44	15	62.5	4.27	99.5					18	60.0	4.81	86.6
45+	92	66.7	6.18	90.3	24	68.6	6.87	92.7	116	67.1	6.33	90.9

intercourse for the 5-year age groups under 40 ranges from 7.82 to 7.32, but is sharply reduced to 4.27 for the age group 40 to 44. It then moves up to 6.18 for women of completed fertility. Turning to women with post-primary education, we note somewhat smaller proportions of childbearing age reporting usable answers, while the frequency is at times below that for women with primary schooling and at times above it. In fact it is impossible to say from this study definitely whether any differential in respect of frequency of intercourse is observed between the two educational categories of the population.

For the present discussions, the dispersion shown by the various categories of women is as important as the proportion reporting satisfactory answers and their average frequency of intercourse. The coefficients of variation appearing in Table 4.2 emphasise the very high levels of variance encountered. In the case of women with primary schooling, there is a suggestion that the variance moves up with advancing age, being especially high in the age interval 40 to 44 (99) and standing at 90 for those of completed fertility. This pattern however is not repeated among women of higher educational status; here coefficients of variation are very high at ages over 45 (93) and, to a lesser degree, among those under 25 (72), but much lower values obtain within the age range 25 to 44.

We may conclude that two factors impose limitations on inferences which may be drawn from these data. The first is the appreciable proportion of women who do not give satisfactory (quantifiable) answers to the question, while the second is the considerable variation in frequencies given by the women. It is of interest that the lowest frequency of sexual intercourse is found among women aged 40 to 44, and here also the variance is by far the highest.

Another aspect of frequency of sexual intercourse that is relevant to this study concerns its differentials by type of union. Here union signifies the type in which the woman finds herself at the time of the interview, if she is under age 45, or, if she is over 45, the type she was in when she attained age 45. This is the subject of Table 4.3. In view of the very small numbers within the age interval 35 to 44, this is given as a single group, which even in this form affords numbers which are so small that comparisons have to be made with caution. With regard to proportions giving adequate responses, these are lowest for the visiting, with the smallest value (56%) occurring among women of completed fertility. Definitely the highest proportions giving satisfactory answers are women in common-law unions; here the highest value (96%) is shown by those in the age group 25 to 29, while the lowest (71%) is shown by women aged 35 to 44. In the case of married women, the range in the proportion reporting usable answers is from 88% for those aged 25 to 29 to 64% for those of completed fertility.

In terms of frequency of intercourse, the smallest values tend to be those for visiting unions. With the exception of the age interval 35 to 44, where the small numbers indicate a frequency of 7.14 times a month, values are below 7, and in the case of women of completed fertility it is down to 3.87. The average values for women in common-law unions are much greater, being at a maximum of 8.21 within the age interval 25 to 29 and exceeding 7 for all ages under 45. The smallest value is 6.73 for women over age 45. Frequency of intercourse reported for married women is much higher than the level for the visiting, and up to age 35 also in excess of comparable values for women in common-law unions. But at advanced ages married values fall below those for common-law unions. For women under age 25, the average frequency of intercourse is 12.44, the highest value in the sample, while its smallest value (8.59) is for the age group 25 to 29.

With regard to variance also the pattern is complicated. In the case of married unions, there is clear evidence of a rise in dispersion as we move up the age scale. Thus the coefficient of variation for this type rises from 39.2 for women under age 25 to 75.5 with the interval 35 to 44 and to 97 for those over age 45. The level of variation shown by common-law unions tends also to rise with advancing age, but does not reach the levels shown by coefficients of variation for married women. Visiting unions also seem to show a rise in variance with advancing age, but this is only up to age 45. The coefficient of variation for these women over age 45 is actually the lowest of all values for this type of union. The generally high levels of variation throughout all ages and types of unions impose limitations on the inferences that may be accurately drawn from the experience depicted in Table 4.3.

The conclusion is that frequency of intercourse is much lower within

Table 4.3 Frequency of sexual intercourse per month—women reporting, average and coefficient of variation, by type of union and age group

| | | Visiting | | | Common-law | | | Married | | |
| | | Women Reporting | Frequency of intercourse | | Women reporting | Frequency of intercourse | | Women reporting | Frequency of intercourse | |
Age group	No.	As % total in age group	Average	Coefficient of variation	No.	As % total in age group	Average	Coefficient of variation	No.	As % total in age group	Average	Coefficient of variation
Under 25	52	82.5	6.71	66.2	23	79.3	7.04	54.5	9	81.8	12.44	39.2
25–29	17	77.3	5.71	79.7	21	95.5	8.21	49.3	28	87.5	8.59	53.6
30–34	12	92.3	5.21	63.8	13	81.2	7.15	61.8	16	76.2	8.66	49.0
35–44	7	58.3	7.14	72.0	10	71.4	7.25	69.0	23	65.7	5.13	75.5
45+	15	55.6	3.87	53.1	31	81.6	6.73	73.9	69	63.9	6.70	97.0

visiting unions, which is to be expected in view of the separate households maintained by the partners to these unions. The implication here is that this form of relationship, compared with the residential family, permits of a greater degree of control over frequency of intercourse on the part of the woman and therefore, ultimately, greater control over fertility. Likewise the high values shown by married women below age 35 are consistent with the sharing of a common household by the partners. But two factors tend to limit the significance of inferences that can be drawn from data on frequency of intercourse: the high proportion of women who do not give satisfactory answers to the question and the very wide variation of answers given by those who respond in clear quantitative terms.

Socio-Economic Status of Union Types

One of the issues relevant to the study of types of union is their relative socio-economic status. It is essential to explore the possibility of assessing these positions, even though the fact that there is appreciable movement from one to another as women pass through the age span of reproduction creates problems of interpretation. The choice of suitable indicators is limited. The accepted technique of basing socio-economic status of the household on the occupation of the male head cannot be applied here, because of the substantial number of households from which the male partner is absent. The occupation of the female is equally unsatisfactory, largely because of the undifferentiated nature of the occupations in which those who work are engaged. It appears that, in the present context, the most convenient approach is to use the educational attainment of the respondent herself. Information on educational attainment is recorded in this study in two broad categories. The first covers all levels of primary schooling and is subdivided into 7 groups, on the basis of the number of years of primary schooling received. For the purpose of constructing the index, the years of primary schooling are used as weights—a weight of 1 for 1 year of primary schooling, a weight of 2 for 2 years' primary schooling ... a weight of 7 for 7 years' primary schooling. For secondary and higher education a weight of 10 is applied. On this scheme of weighting, indicators of socio-economic status for the three union types and for single women are depicted in terms of three age groups in Table 4.4.

As is to be expected, the highest indicators are those for married women, with those under age 25 having a value of 9.42. This falls to 8.20 for women aged 25 to 44 and to 7.46 for those over age 45. The second highest set of indicators is shown by women in visiting unions. At the youngest age the value for these women stands at 8.91, while the decline is to 7.81 and to 6.38 for the two higher age groups. The fact that the overall indicators covering all ages show the visiting at the highest (8.19) derives wholly from the concentration of young women, whose educational status is relatively high and to their small numbers at ages over 45. The outstanding aspect of these indicators is the position of the common-law union, which for all age groups exhibits lowest levels of socio-economic status. Its highest indicator value (7.64) is for the group under 25 years of age, and this declines as we move up the age scale to 5.68 for those over age 45. Women classified as single, that is, who were in some union previously and at the time of the interview were not in any union, occupy the third position on the socio-economic scale. For these women under age 25, the indicator stands at 8.57 and declines with advancing age to a level of 7.13 for those past the childbearing age. Thus without exception the level of the indicator declines with advancing age.

Table 4.4 Indicators of socio-economic status, based on educational attainment of women, according to union status and age group

Age group	Union type				All women
	Visiting	Common-law	Married	Single	
	Indicators of socio-economic status				
Under 25	8.91	7.64	9.42	8.57	8.59
25–44	7.81	6.68	8.20	7.45	7.65
45 +	6.38	5.68	7.46	7.13	7.03
All ages	8.19	6.78	7.91	7.82	7.70
	Indices, Visiting = 100.0				
Under 25	100.0	85.7	105.7	96.2	96.4
25–44	100.0	85.5	105.0	95.4	98.0
45 +	100.0	89.0	116.9	111.8	110.2
All ages	100.0	82.8	96.6	95.5	94.0

Included in the table are also indices giving the extent to which married, common-law and single women depart from those in visiting unions, in terms of the stated indicators of socio-economic status. It is of interest that although in general the married show the highest levels of indicators, the summary measure falls about 3% below the corresponding value for the visiting union. The finding that the visiting type does not by any means represent the lowest level of economic status has been observed in earlier studies. Similar differentials by union emerged from data on floor space in household and weekly income from 1943 Census data.[6] They are once more observed in the 1960 Census, and here the educational status of the women formed the basis of the indicators.[7]

Fertility Differentials by Type of Union

The interrelationships between union type and fertility present some of the most interesting and challenging aspects of West Indian demography. While detailed investigation of these does not form part of this survey, it is still necessary, for a proper understanding of reproductive processes in the society, to recall some of the principal features involved.[8] To some extent, the complexity of the situation derives from the dynamic nature of the mating process, that is from the shift from one to another type of union by women passing through the age range 15 to 45. It also follows that the form of classification in terms of type of union that we select also determines, to a large degree, the form of these fertility differentials.

It is convenient to begin by considering the form of fertility differential by type of union, when the latter is established on the basis of the status of the woman at the time of the interview. In these terms, the fertility differential takes a distinctive turn. In the first place, we limit the comparison to married and common-law types. At younger ages the level of fertility, in terms of the number of children ever born per woman, shows clearly higher rates of children ever born among the common-law. This position continues through the age scale up to the mid-30s, after which the advantage shifts definitely to the married unions. The age at which this change takes place coincides almost exactly with the average age at which shifts from common-law to married types tend to occur; this at once suggests some links between changes in type of union and the reversal of the fertility differential at about age 35. For the transfer of women from common-law to married at higher ages in the period of reproduction in effect adds to the married type at these ages appreciable numbers who, in virtue of their position in the family cycle, are of relatively high fertility. Correspondingly there should be a reduction of women in the higher ages classified as common-law. For this process to result in the type of differential noted, it must be supplemented by a measure of selectivity, which determines that women who move from common-law to married have comparatively high levels of fertility. Available survey data for the Caribbean fully bear out that a measure of selectivity is involved in the change of union status. In particular, women who begin their reproductive life in common-law unions and then marry have exceptionally high levels of fertility. It is therefore the accumulation of women of comparatively high fertility in the higher ages of the married type that contributes principally to the reversal in the differential at about age 35. This also tends to account for the comparatively high level of completed fertility for those who are formally married.

When we compare the visiting with the married, the picture closely parallels that just outlined in the comparison between common-law and married. Here once more there is a shift from visiting to married as women pass through the family cycle, and this is associated with the form of the differential that we observe. While the majority of family unions contracted at young ages assume the form of visiting, there is a steady transfer to marriage as women move up the age scale; this tends to reduce drastically the proportion of women who complete their reproductive life as visiting and correspondingly to augment the numbers of married women at advanced ages. Again this process is accompanied by selectivity, that is those who begin their family life in visiting unions and ultimately marry have relatively large families. Throughout the reproductive span fertility is higher among the married than among the visiting, but as a consequence of these two elements—shifting from one type to another and the attendant selection in terms of family size—the differential widens appreciably after age 35. And it follows that measures of completed fertility place the visiting-type union much lower than the married.

While the foregoing patterns of fertility cannot be depicted in detail by the present small-scale study, it is still possible to show, in summary form, measures of completed fertility and to discuss how these are related to the processes outlined above. These summary measures appear in Table 4.5. One series of measures represents the completed family size among women who

Table 4.5 Numbers of pregnancies per woman aged 45 and over for visiting, married and common-law unions, distinguishing pure and other types

Pure type or other	Union type		
	Visiting	*Common-law*	*Married*
Pure type	3.50 (18)	3.20 (5)	3.67 (33)
Other	3.00 (4)	4.56 (25)	5.02 (63)
Total	3.41	4.33	4.55

Note: Numbers of women involved are shown in parentheses.

have remained in a given type of union throughout their reproductive life; these may be termed the pure types. Thus for women in visiting unions this amounts to 3.50, which is somewhat lower than that for married women (3.67). The important point here is that there is no marked differential separating the three types. By contrast the corresponding measures for other women, that is for those who, although classified as visiting, married or common-law at age 45 were in their earlier years involved in one or other types of union, show appreciable differentials. Here the low position of the visiting (3.00), as compared with the common-law (4.56) and the married (5.02), is the outstanding feature.

With regard to the differences between the pure types and the others it is relevant to introduce another hypothesis seeking to explain the relationship between fertility and mating patterns in these populations. A comparison of the measures of children ever born for the three pure types shows pronounced differentials, which moreover are in accord with the rates of children ever born per woman, established on the basis of current ages of the women from census data. Indeed for this reason it is possible to argue that the existing pattern may represent a somewhat altered version of the pattern established by these pure types. But this cannot be illustrated from the present study.[9]

Case Study

Respondent 5616

Eloise P. is an unemployed 34-year-old Baptist who is in a visiting union at present. She was born in one of the central parishes of the island but 8 years ago moved to one of those with the lowest fertility. This parish has had a very active family planning campaign but she has never used any method of contraception. Nevertheless she considered family planning "a good thing" which will help to "reduce the population" of the country. Her father, a farmer, was married to her mother who had 17 children. Her 40-year-old partner, the legitimate son of a carpenter and one of a family of 8 children, is a mechanic whose religion is unknown to her.

Eloise was 20 years old when she had her first child. "It was the first time and I wasn't sensible to those things and missing my period, I never know that it was pregnancy." Although the incident could not be considered rape, "it wasn't agree, but him only say to me the night, after him resist me and so, him say that if anything him will say yes." She "used to work with his people" and she was alone at home that night as the family had gone to church to a confirmation service when the baby's father came to the house "for he wasn't living there." That was the only visit that he ever paid to her. When she started to "feel different," a lady told her she was pregnant, so she left the district and "come to town." One of her brothers came to see her and then went home and told her mother about her "condition." Her mother, who had asked the lady with whom she was working not to allow her to go anywhere alone, went to the man but "him say is not true." That same year he migrated to England ... "me hear that him come back last year." He has never given any money for the support of the boy, who is now 14.

Eloise's second child was born 14 months later for another visiting partner. She was then living with her parents and did not consider having any other type of union. The entire relationship lasted only 1 year, ending the month the baby was born. She loved him but she found out that he had another woman whom he was visiting and she asked him about it. In addition, his financial support, which she described as "now and again," petered out to nothing. He also has never maintained his daughter.

Her third union was common-law and lasted for 7 years. Her partner suggested it and she was glad for the change. Another girl, who is now 11, was born of this union, 22 months after her second child. It ended because she discovered that he also had another woman and he used to drink heavily and "come in and want to fight me."

She had no complications associated with the pregnancies or births of her 3 children who were full term and delivered at home by trained nurses. Eloise worked throughout all her pregnancies and breastfed the babies for 5 months, 4 months and 7 months respectively. She does not believe that the fathers of her children love them as they would have supported them. Her present partner looks after her but she has to maintain her 3 children. She has no favourites among them and they call her "Sister" since they heard her older brother call her that. She called her mother "Mamma."

The man who now visits her lives with another woman with whom he has children, so he is able to see her only twice per month. She recently had a spontaneous abortion at a little over 1 month's pregnancy and was treated in hospital by curettage. She says she does not want to have any more children as they both have others already. Eloise has heard of women taking tablets to get rid of a baby and "they have things to drink" but she does not know the nature of these substances.

Her partner takes her out to some form of entertainment once per month for about 3 to 4 hours. Naturally she does not visit his home but he spends 8 or 9 hours with her when he comes to hers and they sometimes discuss owning a shop together. As she lives independently she has no problem in arranging to have sexual intercourse with him and this takes place about 4 times per month and lasts about 20 minutes. When asked if she expected her partner to be faithful to her, she gave the answer "yes," which is surprising as, according to her account, he was then living with another woman. She emphasised that she was faithful to him.

Eloise's attitude towards her various relationships was ambiguous. She claimed that visiting brought her more happiness, but on the other hand she preferred common-law living which was better for the children and for her economically, as well as being approved of by the church.

She thinks "about 2" children constitute a small family and "plenty" is a large one but she could not think of a specific number for the latter. She believes that every man and woman should have a child as the woman who does not have one cannot "enjoy life." She has heard that every woman should have a certain number of children but she does not know how this number can be known. She feels that a woman should have a choice with regard to the number of children she can have, and expressed the view that if a woman is childless it may be because she has not found the "right" partner or perhaps she does not want to have any.

Eloise feels that a second child should follow the first after a period of about 2 years and subsequent intervals should be between 3 and 5 years. When asked if a woman should have a child for each of her partners she replied, "Yes, it depends on conditions," then she continued, "Yes, it would look better." In her opinion, the ideal number of children a woman should have is 4 provided "she can support them."

She was 14 when she had her first period and was frightened when she saw it as no one had explained menstruation to her. She continues to have regular menstrual periods which recently have lengthened from 4 to 8 or 9 days. This however does not seem to bother her. She was against having intercourse immediately before or after the menstrual period and when asked about having it during menstruation she replied, "No sir, that worse." Her partner does "nothing" when she is having her period. She does not "remember" what causes menstruation but prefers having it to being pregnant, and finds it less of a problem than pregnancy. She adds that she feels better when she is not pregnant. Her period does not affect her normal activities in any way but she has heard people say that one must "not use cold water" and "not to lift up heavy things."

Eloise was not told anything about sex either but she gave her opinion about pregnancy as follows: "Either shortly after menstruation or near to menstruation something like so, it easy to get pregnant. After sex when the two sperms meet together and form an egg, something so." She does not know why a woman gets pregnant at some times and not at others.

Notes

1. For a discussion of classification see G. W. Roberts, *Fertility and Mating in Four West Indian Populations* (Kingston: I.S.E.R., University of the West Indies, 1975), pp. 103 et seq.

2. G. W. Roberts, G. T. Cummings, J. Byrne, and C. Alleyne, "Knowledge and Use of Birth Control in Barbados," *Demography* 4, no. 2 (1967).
3. These accounts are based largely on Roberts, *Fertility and Mating*, passim.
4. Ibid., p. 175.
5. Other examples of casual relationships occur in case studies elsewhere in this work.
6. Roberts, *The Population of Jamaica*, p. 305.
7. Roberts, *Fertility and Mating*, pp. 295–299.
8. Ibid., pp. 152 et seq.
9. This hypothesis is discussed in Roberts, *Fertility and Mating*, pp. 152 et seq.

Chapter 5
Aspects of the Menstrual Cycle

An analysis of the several aspects of menstruation is essential in the study of reproduction. Particulars of the main features of the cycle—notably its onset, the characteristics of its flow, its regularity, its termination—have to be taken up, as they have an important bearing on the reproductive performance of the society. These also are essential preliminaries to the analysis of knowledge of the underlying processes shown by respondents, which constitutes the subject of the following chapter. Also to be considered here are respondents' views on the timing of sexual activity with reference to menstruation.

Age at Menarche

The question seeking information on this topic is, "At what age did you have your first menses?" And as this age is collected by means of a retrospective enquiry, it is to be expected that there will be some errors in reporting to be faced. Among older women especially the records suggest some uncertainty as to the age when this commenced. Early tests of the questionnaire made it clear that this event could generally be recalled to the nearest year, so that no attempt was made to collect ages to the nearest month, although this could have been done for the younger women. The effects of recall lapse on the reliability of the material is not considered sufficiently extensive to impair the data on the commencement of this function, the significance of which is fully realised by women of the country, despite their lack of knowledge of its biological basis.

Recent studies of menstruation have shown two important features: there is a tendency for the age at its appearance to decline with modernisation, while there appears as well a differential in terms of socio-economic status of the women.[1] With respect to the first set of findings, we have to examine the present data in terms of the three broad age groups already identified, as these constitute age cohorts, which give the experience of women approximately at 1970, 1955 and 1940. This should suffice to give an indication of changes in age at menarche over a 30-year span. With regard to the second aspect of the topic, we can use the level of educational attainment, previously discussed, in order to get a broad division into upper and lower classes of the society.

Of the 501 women in the sample, satisfactory information on this topic was received from 489. Of the 12 for whom the data have not been obtained, two, both aged 15 years, had not begun to menstruate at the time of the interview. Thus no information was obtained from 10 respondents, that is just under 2% of the total. The distribution of age at menarche is shown in Table 5.1 and Figure 5.1 in terms of present age of women and their educational status. One woman reported an age of 9 years, 3 give ages of 10, and for 24 the age is 11. At the other end of the distribution, there is 1 aged 19, 14 aged 18, and 26 give the age of 17. Clearly however there is a concentration between ages 14 and 15, with the latter being the modal age, and accounting for one-quarter of the total. The average age at menarche for all women amounts to 14.68 years, while the division into those with primary and post-primary schooling yields average ages of 14.94 and 14.17 respectively, thus putting the elementary group at a level which is about 7 months higher than that for women with some secondary schooling.

Ages at menarche in terms of educational attainment as well as age cohorts also given in Table 5.1 make possible an assessment of socio-cultural differentials at different periods, and thus an assessment of movements in the value of this age over time. For the three age cohorts there is a clear advantage in terms of women with secondary education. This is greatest for

Table 5.1 Average age at menarche by present age and educational status

| Age in years | Elementary | | | Post-primary | | | Total | | |
	Under 25	25–44	45+	Under 25	25–44	45+	Elementary	Post-primary	All
9–	—	—	—	1	—	—	—	1	1
10–	—	1	—	2	—	—	1	2	3
11–	3	4	5	7	4	1	12	12	24
12–	8	9	13	16	9	7	30	32	62
13–	16	17	15	20	13	—	48	33	81
14–	11	26	25	14	9	9	62	32	94
15–	17	38	36	9	13	9	91	31	122
16–	2	19	25	3	7	5	46	15	61
17–	1	12	7	2	1	3	20	6	26
18+	—	3	9	1	—	2	12	3	15
Total	58	129	135	75	56	36	322	167	489
Average age	14.21	15.07	15.14	13.69	14.27	15.03	14.94	14.17	14.68
Coefficient of variation	9.51	10.72	11.39	12.29	10.86	12.06	11.05	12.26	11.71

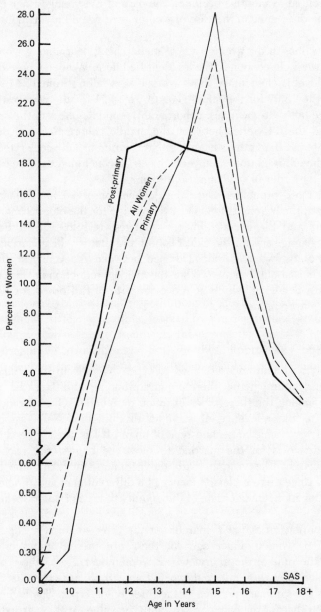

Figure 5.1 Age at menarche—percent distribution by educational attainment

the age cohort 25 to 44, where it amounts to nearly 10 months. The second largest differential (6 months) occurs in the case of the youngest age cohort, under 25. The difference in the case of women over age 45 is small, just over 1 month.

Notable declines in the average age at menarche appear among women in both of the two socio-economic classes identified here. Women whose highest educational level is elementary show average ages falling from 15.14 for the oldest cohort to 15.07 for the middle cohort, to 14.21 for the youngest. Thus the difference between the oldest cohort and the middle one is of the order of 1 month, and the difference between the middle cohort and the youngest amounts to about 10 months, suggesting that the rate of fall accelerated after 1955. Over the entire period of 30 years, it can be concluded that the average decline is of the order of 0.37 month per year.

Somewhat more pronounced are the declines observed for women who have had post-primary education. The average age for the oldest cohort here is 15.03 years and the average for the youngest is 13.69. The difference between the average age for the oldest cohort and that for the cohort aged 25 to 44 is 9 months, whereas the difference between the youngest and the middle cohorts is about 7 months. Thus the average reduction in this context is 0.54 month per year, which is above the rate of fall noted for women with an elementary education.

Age at Menarche by Type of Union

In view of the importance attached to types of union in this study, it is necessary to examine whether there are any pronounced differentials in age at menarche among the three types of union designated. One consideration which adds to the relevance of such an examination is the association between socio-economic status and type of union. It has already been shown that the evidence is for the married to show the highest socio-economic status, followed by the visiting, with the common-law taking the lowest position. And since there is clear evidence of a differential of age at menarche by level of education, an extension of the enquiry to type of union seems fully justified.

The distributions of age at menarche for the three union types appear in Table 5.2. For women under age 45, these are present types or those obtaining at the time of the interview; for women over age 45 the types are those in which they are involved when they attain age 45. First to be considered is the summary position of the three union types. The highest age (14.98 years) is that for the common-law, with the value for the married being very close to this (14.96) and that for the visiting being half a year lower. This pattern does not follow what is to be expected on the basis of socio-economic levels. When the positions of the union types are compared on the basis of the three age cohorts, those over age 45 exhibit the same pattern just indicated,

Table 5.2 Age at menarche by present age and union status

Age in years	Married				Common-law				Visiting			
	Under 25	25–44	45+	Total	Under 25	25–44	45+	Total	Under 25	25–44	45+	Total
9–	1	–	–	1	–	–	–	–	–	–	–	–
10–	–	–	–	–	–	1	–	1	1	–	–	1
11–	1	2	2	5	–	1	–	1	8	5	4	17
12–	2	8	8	18	3	3	3	9	17	7	9	33
13–	1	10	5	16	11	9	4	24	16	9	6	31
14–	1	3	17	21	3	13	7	23	12	18	9	39
15–	2	17	17	36	6	14	13	33	10	20	15	45
16–	1	7	16	24	1	13	7	21	3	6	6	15
17–	2	4	4	10	1	6	–	7	–	3	6	9
18+	–	1	4	5	–	1	2	3	1	1	5	7
Not stated	–	1	1	2	–	2	2	4	–	2	1	3
Total	11	53	74	138	25	63	38	126	68	71	61	200
Average age	14.23	14.79	15.18	14.96	14.26	15.16	15.19	14.98	13.65	14.60	14.98	14.39
Coefficient of variation	18.08	11.70	11.02	11.96	9.12	10.63	9.42	10.23	11.34	10.77	13.38	12.44

that is there is very little between the ages for the common-law and the married—15.19 and 15.18 respectively—but the value is much lower for the visiting, 14.98 years. For the 25 to 44 age cohort, the average age for the common-law (15.16) stands out clearly as above the other two, with the ages for the married and the visiting being 14.79 and 14.60 respectively. In the case of the youngest age cohorts, the rank order of the age at menarche for the three types does not conform to that of their socio-economic status, the highest age (14.26 years) being for the common-law and the lowest (13.65) for the visiting.

From the age cohorts of the three union types can also be obtained a picture of the degree of reduction in age at menarche over a 30-year period. The largest extent of decline is that for the visiting union; here the age at menarche falls by an average of 2.3 weeks per year over the entire period; the other two types of union show declines of somewhat lower magnitude over the 30-year period—1.6 weeks each. It is also evident that for the visiting and common-law types the greatest reduction has taken place in the most recent portion of the period under review. In assessing all of these differentials the movement of women from one union type to another in the course of their family cycle should be borne in mind.

Age at Menarche Among Women Experiencing Irregular Menstruation

Further information collected on menstruation deals with irregularities in the respondents' periods. One question seeks to find out whether any irregularities are experienced, while the following one, relating only to women with such features, asks whether these cause them worry or lead to their seeking medical attention. In another question the respondents are invited to list problems or complications of menstruation that they experience.

Only 10% of the women in the survey report any menstrual irregularities. Of the 50 women involved, 18 state that these have caused them worry, while 28 have been led to seek medical attention. Of interest is the fact that the proportion with irregularities is almost the same for women with elementary education as it is for those whose schooling has been of a higher level, 10% as against 11%.

An issue of consequence is whether there is any association between reports of irregular menstruation and age at menarche. This subject is treated in Table 5.3, which compares the distributions of age at menarche for women who experience irregularities with corresponding ages for those with regular menstrual patterns. In view of the differential between women with elementary schooling and those with some higher education, in regard to age at menarche, it is useful to introduce this distinction once more. There is an appreciable difference (9 months) between the average age of women at menarche for those who experience irregularity and those who do not—15.32 as against 14.60 years. For those with primary schooling, irregularities in menstruation are associated with an average age at menarche of 15.31 years, which is about 5 months higher than the corresponding average for women whose menstrual cycle is normal. A much greater difference separates the

Table 5.3 Age at menarche by regularity of menstruation and educational attainment

Age in years	Irregular			Regular		
	Primary	Post-primary	Total	Primary	Post-primary	Total
9–	—	—	—	—	1	1
10–	—	—	—	1	2	3
11–	1	—	1	10	12	22
12–	3	—	3	25	32	57
13–	2	3	5	44	30	74
14–	7	6	13	55	26	81
15–	7	4	11	80	26	106
16–	8	2	10	36	13	49
17–	2	2	4	17	4	21
18 +	2	1	3	10	2	12
Not stated	—	—	—	8	2	10
Total	32	18	50	286	150	436
Average age	15.31	15.33	15.32	14.91	14.02	14.60
Coefficient of variation	11.18	9.56	10.52	10.96	12.27	11.75

position of women who have had advanced education. These women who report menstrual irregularities have an average age at menarche of 15.33 years, which exceeds the corresponding value for those with post-primary schooling and regular menstrual pattern by 1 year and 4 months. For women whose menstrual cycle is normal there is an appreciable differential between the age at menarche for those with primary schooling (14.91 years) and the corresponding age for women with higher education (14.02). The absence of such a pronounced differential from women experiencing irregularities may be traceable to the very small numbers being dealt with here, but it cannot be ruled out that this may be associated with the menstrual pattern they exhibit.

Duration of Menstrual Flow

Another aspect of menstruation dealt with in the survey is the duration of its flow. The question put to women is, "How many days on the average do you menstruate?" This represents, in the case of those still menstruating, their experience at the time of the interview, whereas for those who have experienced the menopause the reference is to the general menstrual pattern they recall. Whether there is any reason to expect differentials in terms of socio-economic status is not apparent, but it has been considered useful to depict the material on this topic in terms of age cohorts and educational status, which we are using in this context as an indicator of socio-economic status.

From the material on this aspect of menstruation given in Table 5.4, it is seen that satisfactory information has been obtained for 479 women, that is

Table 5.4 Duration of menstrual flow by present age and educational attainment

Days of flow	Primary				Post-primary				All women
	Under 25	25–44	45+	Total	Under 25	25–44	45+	Total	
3	3	10	9	22	6	3	4	13	35
4	21	30	25	76	29	14	5	48	124
5	24	54	53	131	25	31	14	70	201
6	5	18	16	39	8	5	5	18	57
7	3	13	15	31	6	3	4	13	44
8	0	5	8	13	0	1	4	5	18
Not stated	2	3	13	18	3	1	–	4	22
Total	58	133	139	330	77	58	36	171	501
Average period	5.21	5.57	5.71	5.56	5.22	5.39	5.83	5.41	5.51
Coefficient of variation	17.43	21.47	22.31	21.44	19.95	17.75	24.93	20.97	21.31

for 96% of the women in the survey. The range is from 3 to 8 days with a
pronounced concentration on 5 days, which is the period reported by 42% of
all the women. The average duration for the entire sample is 5.51 days. All
women with elementary schooling show a slightly longer duration than those
with post-primary schooling, 5.56 as against 5.41 days. Once more the
evidence is of a small reduction in duration, when the experience of the three
age cohorts is compared. Thus in the case of women with elementary
schooling, the average duration of flow for the oldest cohort is 5.71 days,
which reduces to 5.57 for the middle cohort and to 5.21 for the youngest
cohort. Thus the difference in time between the values for the oldest and the
youngest age cohort is half a day. A similar pattern characterises the three age
cohorts with post-primary schooling. The duration of flow for women of the
oldest age cohort is 5.83 days, which is reduced to 5.39 for the middle cohort
and to 5.22 for the youngest cohort. The reduction of 0.61 day is even greater
than that observed in the case of women with elementary schooling only.

Timing of Sexual Intercourse and Menstruation

A question put to respondents was intended to find out whether they had
any definite opinion on the timing of sexual intercourse with regard to the
menstrual cycle. The question states, "Should a woman have sexual
intercourse: (1) Just before menstruation, (2) During menstruation, (3) Just
after menstruation?" A reply was sought in respect of each of the three of
these. There is no implication here as to a relation between timing of sexual
intercourse and degree of risk of conception. These answers, it appears, can
be related to their knowledge of menstruation. Although respondents'
knowledge of this function will be discussed in the following chapter, it is
convenient to make use of the scores presented there in relation to timing of
sexual intercourse. Small numbers of respondents did not offer opinions on
these questions; these amount to 4%, 2% and 5% respectively.

With regard to those expressing opinions as to whether sexual intercourse
should take place just before or during menstruation, it is convenient to
distinguish two levels of knowledge; this is because of the very low proportion
who evince any satisfactory understanding of the biological processes
involved. The division is between women with scores of 0–1 and 2–5. The
relevant proportions are presented in Table 5.5. There is a general agreement
that sexual intercourse should take place just before menstruation. This is
most strongly marked among women with maximum knowledge of the
process, 90% of whom declare that this is a proper timing of sexual
intercourse. Women with low degrees of knowledge, that is with scores of 0
and 1, are less convinced about this; the proportion agreeing that this is a
time when sexual activity should take place is 57%. As regards the question
whether sexual intercourse should take place during menstruation, the feeling

Table 5.5 Proportion (%) of women answering no and yes to question whether sexual intercourse should take place just before or during menstruation

Average score	Just before menstruation		During menstruation	
	% No	% Yes	% No	% Yes
0–1	42.7	57.3	98.3	1.7
2–5	10.0	90.0	84.7	15.3
Total	37.9	62.1	96.3	3.7

against this is very strong. This is especially so among women with minimal knowledge of the process, 98% of whom state that this is not the time for such activity. Those with a higher degree of knowledge are less strongly averse to this, but even here the proportion against its performance during menstruation is very high (85%).

With regard to the third question, dealing with opinions as to the performance of sex just after menstruation, it is again convenient to discuss the views expressed in terms of the degree of knowledge of the menstrual cycle. Answers can be grouped into three categories: those who say yes without any qualification, those who say no without any qualification, and those who express a qualification, which takes the form of stating how many days should elapse after menstruation before sexual intercourse should take place.

In Table 5.6 the answers are shown in terms of percentages. Among women with very little knowledge of menstruation, the majority (44%) express a qualified answer, while 30% give a clear positive answer, and 27% give a firm negative answer. As will be seen in Chapter 6, some respondents are of the opinion that a woman gets pregnant if she has sexual intercourse "too quick" after menstruation. By contrast, women with some knowledge of the process for the most part agree that intercourse should take place just after menstruation, 75% holding this position. Only 8% of these women are against

Table 5.6 Number and proportion (%) of women giving answers of yes, no, and yes with qualification to question whether sexual intercourse should take place just after menstruation

Average score	Yes, without qualification		No, without qualification		Yes, with qualification	
	Number	%	Number	%	Number	%
0–1	124	29.8	111	26.7	181	43.5
2–5	54	75.0	6	8.3	12	16.7
Total	178	36.5	117	24.0	193	39.5

Table 5.7 Number of women stating number of days that should elapse
after menstruation before sexual intercourse should take place

Average score	Number of days after menstruation when sexual intercourse should take place						Total
	1–2	*3–4*	*5–6*	*7–8*	*9–10*	*11+*	*Total*
0–1	26	75	19	43	7	9	179
2–5	7	3	—	3	1	—	14
Total	33	78	19	46	8	9	193

sexual activity at this time, while a small proportion (17%) gave a qualified
answer. It would appear therefore that a knowledge of the menstrual cycle
induces women to a firm conviction that just after menstruation is a proper
time for these activities.

Opinions expressed by women who consider that some time should elapse
after menstruation before sexual intercourse takes place are worth some
examination. The relevant material is summarised in Table 5.7. Just under
40% of the sample (193) state that after menstruation some time should elapse
before the resumption of sexual intercourse. And, as is to be expected, the
great majority of these women (179) have scores of knowledge of reproduction of 0 or 1. Most of them (78) state that sexual intercourse should not
take place until 3 to 4 days after menstruation. An appreciable number (46)
give a somewhat longer period of about one week, while it is of interest to
note that some put this interval as long as two weeks.

As has been indicated earlier, nothing in the questions posed on this topic
carries any implication as to safe period in terms of days before or after
menstruation. Indeed, because of the very limited knowledge of reproduction
and menstruation, respondents could hardly be expected to have any clear
notion of the safe period. Nor does it necessarily follow that views expressed
by these respondents give clues as to their own preferences in the timing of
sexual activity in relation to menstruation. It so happens that their stated
preferences point, for the most part, to a time in the menstrual cycle which is
outside the period of maximum risk of conception. On the other hand, it
should be noted that a very small proportion give as the preferred period two
weeks after menstruation, which corresponds with the time of maximum risk
of conception. Of course, we must again emphasise that answers to these
questions do not necessarily signify times at which they habitually perform
sexual intercourse.

The Menopause

Gathering information complementary to that on age at menarche—the age
at menopause—forms another aspect of this survey. This material is derived
from answers to a single question, "At what age did you have your last

menses?" It would be expected that recall lapse would be less of a problem here than it is in the case of answering questions about age at menarche. For all menopausal women it will be an event very recent by comparison with the onset of menstruation and therefore more readily recalled. Yet the number failing to give a satisfactory answer amounts to 15 or 12% of the total; this is appreciably in excess of the proportion with unknown age in the case of menarche, which stands at only 2%. Some uncertainty concerning the age at menopause is understandable as periods may taper off gradually and not cease abruptly. It may be this difficulty in identifying the final menses that is at the root of this appreciable proportion of unknown age.

Of the 501 women in the sample, 129 or one-quarter state that they have already had their last menstrual period. The ages at which women attain the menopause show fairly wide variation, as we see from Table 5.8. Of the 129 women involved, 3 report ages of under 33 and 3 ages between 33 and 34. Of interest are the women whose menopause occurs prematurely, that is under age 41; these number 14 or 11% of the total. For the majority this age lies between 45 and 52; those reporting the event within this interval amount to 66, or about one-half of the total. The modal interval is 49 to 50, the number here (30) accounting for about one-quarter of all menopausal women. An

Table 5.8 Age at menopause according to educational attainment and union status of women

Age at menopause	Educational attainment		Union status			All women
	Primary	Post-primary	Married	Common-law	Visiting	
Under 33	3	—	1	2	—	3
33–34	3	—	1	1	1	3
35–36	—	—	—	—	—	—
37–38	1	—	—	—	1	1
39–40	7	—	1	—	6	7
41–42	6	3	3	4	2	9
43–44	6	1	3	2	2	7
45–46	13	1	7	5	2	14
47–48	8	2	5	—	5	10
49–50	24	6	16	2	12	30
51–52	11	1	4	4	4	12
53–54	5	—	1	1	3	5
55–56	4	3	3	—	4	7
57–58	2	—	1	1	—	2
59–60	3	—	1	1	1	3
Not stated	12	4	4	5	7	16
Total	108	21	51	28	50	129
Average age	47.67	48.94	48.38	46.26	48.14	47.86
Coefficient of variation	12.91	9.49	10.96	15.87	12.04	12.43

Note: Included in the visiting category are 2 respondents returned as single.

appreciable number (17) give an age in excess of 52. The average age for all women in the sample stands at 47.86, with a fairly high variance, as is evident from the coefficient of variation of 12.43.

From Table 5.8 it is also possible to compare the average age at menopause for several categories of women, although the very small numbers involved means that these values are subject to wide sampling errors. In the case of the twofold division in terms of educational attainment—primary and post-primary—the former shows a slightly lower age than the latter, 47.7 as against 48.9 years. This may be taken as signifying a lower age at menopause among women of comparatively low socio-economic status. Also of interest is the differential in terms of union status. The highest average age is that for married women (48.4 years) and the second highest is that for women in visiting unions (48.1), while the common-law type shows the lowest average (46.3). Again we may relate this pattern to the ranking in terms of socio-economic status of the three union types. The ranking in average age at menopause—married, visiting, common-law—in fact corresponds to the ranking according to socio-economic status, discussed previously. There are therefore two lines of evidence that the age at menopause is related to the level of socio-economic status, or that the higher the status level, the higher tends to be the menopausal age.

Complementing an examination of ages at which women attain the menopause is a consideration of the age distribution of menopausal women, according to educational attainment and union status. This is the subject of Table 5.9. Only negligible numbers are under age 45, while the proportion within the age interval 45 to 49 amounts to 15%. Nearly one-fifth fall within the age interval 50 to 54 and 64% are over 55. The very small number of women in the post-primary category affects their age distribution, but it is to be noted that the age interval 55 to 59 accounts for 21% of women with primary education, which is one-half of the corresponding proportion for those with higher education.

Considerable difference in the age structure of menopausal women in the three union types appears. Here as well small numbers (especially in the common-law type) may be a factor to be reckoned with in interpreting the differentials. But equally important may be the movement from visiting and to a lesser extent from common-law to married, as women pass through the childbearing span. Since this movement tends to take place towards the end of that period, we should expect a relatively large proportion of menopausal married women in the age interval over 60. In fact 71% of these women are over age 55 and 51% over 60. For the smaller numbers of women in common-law unions, the concentration in higher ages is limited to those over 60, who account for 46% of the total. The age distribution of menopausal women in visiting unions is consistent with a substantial proportion shifting to married unions at higher ages. The age group with the highest concentration

Table 5.9 Age distribution of menopausal women, according to educational attainment and union status

| Age group | Educational attainment | | Union status | | | All women |
	Primary	Post-primary	Visiting	Common-law	Married	
	Distribution of women					
35–39	1	—	1	—	—	1
40–44	2	—	1	1	—	2
45–49	17	2	7	4	8	19
50–54	21	3	11	6	7	24
55–59	23	8	17	4	10	31
60+	45	7	13	13	26	52
Total	109	20	50	28	51	129
	Percentage distribution					
35–39	0.9	—	2.0	—	—	0.8
40–44	1.8	—	2.0	3.6	—	1.6
45–49	15.6	10.0	14.0	14.3	15.7	14.7
50–54	19.3	15.0	22.0	21.4	13.7	18.6
55–59	21.1	40.0	34.0	14.3	19.6	24.0
60+	41.3	35.0	26.0	46.4	51.0	40.3
Total	100.0	100.0	100.0	100.0	100.0	100.0

Note: Included in the visiting category are 2 respondents returned as single.

is 55 to 59, which accounts for one-third of the total, while the proportion over 60 is about one-quarter, that is just one-half of the corresponding proportion for married women.

Further aspects of menstruation emerge from the average ages at which women in the two educational categories and in the three union types attain the menopause. It is also instructive to examine these ages in relation to corresponding ages at menarche. This means that we are limiting the study of menarche to the experience of women who have completed their menstrual cycle. These averages, together with the differences between them, appear in Table 5.10. In the case of educational attainment, there is a marked difference between the two categories in respect of average age at menopause. The value for women with post-primary education exceeds that for women of lower educational status by 2.1 years. By contrast the average age at menarche is somewhat lower among women with post-primary education. The differences between these two sets of ages—34.8 years for post-primary and 32.2 for primary—thus show that the period of potential fertility is greater among women of higher socio-economic status. All of these differentials are consistent with values based on all women in the survey.

When we consider the situation from the standpoint of the three union types, by far the highest average age at menopause is that for married women (48.0) and the lowest that for common-law women (45.3). With regard to the

Table 5.10 Average ages at menopause and at menarche, and differences between their ages for menopausal women, by educational attainment and union status

Category of women	Numbers of women	Average age at menopause (a)	Average age at menarche (b)	Differences (a)—(b)
With primary education	96	46.99	14.75	32.24
With post-primary education	18	49.11	14.33	34.78
Visiting	42	47.67	14.33	33.34
Common-law	24	45.29	14.83	30.46
Married	48	48.04	14.92	33.12
All women	114	47.32	14.68	32.64

Note: Excluded from this table are values for 15 respondents for whom ages at menopause, or ages at menarche, or both, are not available.

average age at menarche, the value for the married is once more highest (14.9), but in this case the lowest is the value for the visiting unions (14.3). The potential fertile period is longest for visiting and married women (33.3 and 33.1 years respectively), with the value for common-law type being appreciably below these (30.5). The relative values of average ages at menopause follow the pattern of differentials shown for all women in the study. In the case of age at menarche however the comparatively low value for visiting menopausal women is a departure from the position shown by all women in the sample.

In dealing with the cessation of menstruation, one factor to be looked into is the number of women who report an artificial menopause. Information on why and how their menstrual processes have been terminated is available for only a few respondents and even where it is available the details are scant. It appears that hysterectomies are mainly responsible for producing the artificial menopause in these women. The total number who have had such a menopause stands at 27, which is 21% of all menopausal women, and the ages at which the menopause occurs are as follows:

Under 35	3
35–39	1
40–44	7
45–49	7
50–54	6
55–59	2
Unknown	1
Total	27

Most of these terminations of the menstrual cycle occur at ages over 45, that is after the completion of their childbearing period. While this suggests that the particular medical technique involved takes place too late in the woman's life to affect her fertility potential, it is probable that the condition which the treatment seeks to correct has been affecting the woman for most of her childbearing span, but became sufficiently serious to warrant medical intervention long after its initial appearance. Of the three women whose artificial menopause is experienced before age 35, one reports a hysterectomy at age 20. This terminated a short pregnancy history consisting of one stillbirth, one miscarriage and one livebirth which, however, died at less than one year of age.

In so far as the distribution of menopausal women is largely determined by the age structure of the sample, a useful summary of the position is in terms of proportions of these women in each group. Table 5.11 relates the natural and artificial menopausal women to the totals in the several age groups. The proportion of these women in the age group 35 to 39 is 3%; this doubles within the next quinquennial age group and by 45 to 49 it stands at 37%. While there is a substantial proportion (65%) in the interval 50 to 54, it is not until after age 55 that virtually all females (97%) conclude their menstrual cycle. The contribution of the artificial menopause, although much smaller than the natural process, is still appreciable at all ages over 40. The proportion it forms of the total is greatest (18%) at the interval 50 to 54 and lowest (13%) at the interval 55 to 59.

Since medical intervention has been sought by 27 women, it is of interest to examine whether there is evidence that they differ from those whose menopause occurs spontaneously. One way of making this comparison is in terms of the average ages at menarche and at menopause for the two groups. These averages are presented in Table 5.12. Probably the very small numbers with which we are dealing have a bearing on the differentials, mainly by affecting the values for the smaller components of artificially induced menopause; these invite caution in assessing this discussion. With respect to

Table 5.11 Women with natural and artificial menopause, showing ages and proportions

Age group	Total women in age group	Menopausal women			% of women at the menopause		
		Natural	Artificial	Total	Natural	Artificial	Total
35–39	33	1	—	1	3.0	—	3.0
40–44	32	2	—	2	6.2	—	6.2
45–49	51	11	8	19	21.6	15.7	37.3
50–54	40	19	7	26	47.5	17.5	65.0
55–59	32	27	4	31	84.4	12.5	96.9
60+	52	42	8	50	80.8	15.4	96.2

Table 5.12 Average ages at menarche and at menopause for menopausal women only, showing natural and artificial, by age groups

Age group	Average age at menarche Years (a)			Average age at menopause, Years (b)			Potential childbearing span (b) — (a)		
	Natural	Artificial	Total	Natural	Artificial	Total	Natural	Artificial	Total
45–49	15.67	12.43	14.25	46.77	41.57	44.50	31.10	29.14	30.25
50–54	14.61	13.57	14.32	47.33	46.57	47.12	32.22	33.00	32.80
55–59	14.96	—	14.96	49.43	—	49.04	34.47	—	34.08
60–64	15.45	14.25	15.22	48.38	45.00	47.78	32.93	30.75	32.56

Note: As there are only 4 women in the age group 55 to 59 reporting artificial menopause, their average ages at menarche and at menopause may be subject to appreciable error and are consequently not included in the table. This means that the corresponding value for the potential childbearing span has also to be excluded.

the average age at menarche, the pattern is for those whose menopause is artificially produced to show lower values. This difference is as great as 3.2 years in the age group 45 to 49. Its failure to appear in the group 55 to 59 probably stems from the very small number of women reporting an artificial menopause. The much lower average ages of menopause where it is artificially produced are to be expected. The difference between the two types of women for the age group 45 to 49 exceeds 5 years, but at ages above this it is not marked. The net effect of differentials with respect to commencement and termination of menstruation is that females who have experienced an artificial menopause have a shorter period of potential fertility than other women.

The foregoing differentials thus suggest that women whose menstrual period has been artificially terminated have also their fertility potential affected. This of course may not be simply a function of premature termination of the menstrual cycle, but of a fundamental aspect of their reproductive capacity. One means of checking on this assumption is to compare the fertility experience for the groups of women. In terms of children ever born, the following is the comparison:

		Pregnancies per Woman	
Age Group	Natural Menopause	Artificial Menopause
Under 50	4.9	3.6
50–54	4.9	4.7
55–59	4.5	3.0
60+	4.4	3.4

Although again small numbers of women may limit the validity of the comparison, the evidence is definitely that the artificial menopause is associated with smaller family sizes. The conclusion therefore is that the artificially induced menopause identifies women whose reproductive capacity is in some way impaired.

Conclusion

The menstrual experience of women in Jamaica, as revealed in this survey, does not depart materially from the general experience emerging from other populations.[2] The decline in average age at menarche shown by successive age cohorts of women, the differentials in this age according to socio-economic status, with the average age being lower for those higher up the economic scale—these are in keeping with findings from other populations. Similarly the differentials in terms of age at menopause seem to be consistent with values for other populations, in so far as higher socio-economic status groups, who presumably enjoy relatively good nutritional and medical care, show a distinct prolongation of menstruation. Although the proportion of artificial menopausal women does not seem to be excessive, it is appreciable. No information on the gynaecological conditions responsible is available, but it is known that a large proportion of women in the society suffer from fibroids, which may be a significant contributing factor.[3] The proportion of artificially induced menopause gives some idea of the extent of impairment of reproductive capacity in general. It may also contribute in some measure to high proportions of sterility, which figured prominently as a factor depressing fertility in Jamaica up to 25 years ago.

Notes

1. For a discussion of these trends see J. M. Tanner, *Growth at Adolescence*, 2nd ed. (Oxford, 1962). For a more recent survey of these trends see Carol J. Diers, "Historical Trends in the age at Menarche and Menopause," *Psychological Reports* 34 (3, pt. 1) (June 1974), pp. 931–937.
2. It should be pointed out however that some recent studies have shown no decreases in average age at menarche. For a recent discussion of such findings, see *Population Reports* Series J, no. 10 (July 1976), p. J–162.
3. J. H. M. Pinkerton and D. B. Stewart, "Uterine Fibroids," in J. B. Lawson and D. B. Stewart, *Obstetrics and Gynaecology in the Tropics and Developing Countries* (London: The English Language Book Society and Edward Arnold, 1974).

Chapter 6
Knowledge of Reproduction and Menstruation

A society's knowledge of human reproductive processes is of itself an important topic of enquiry, as it constitutes one of many indicators of its level of awareness of current issues. Menstruation constitutes a major aspect of a woman's life, literally colouring nearly all areas of social interaction and affecting many patterns of her behaviour. But an even broader value of such an enquiry is that it may assist materially in the development of fertility control programmes making use of modern techniques. For in so far as use of these modern contraceptives entails some disturbances in the menstrual cycle, an understanding of the underlying physiological processes should help to condition users to the changes that will be experienced. For if these are not expected or occur without any clear appreciation that they follow as a normal course of the use of such contraception, their appearance may lead to widespread fear and to termination of the use of the particular technique, thus impairing the entire programme of fertility control.

With full realisation of the value of such an enquiry from both the above standpoints, this study was planned to secure some information on knowledge of this type in three distinct forms. The first seeks to find out the respondents' knowledge of the reproductive processes, and especially how conception occurs. Another question put to respondents asks about the sources of their information on sex, as this may have a bearing on their overall understanding of the topic. A third line of questioning aims at finding out what respondents know about the menstrual cycle, as such knowledge seems highly relevant to the effective practice of modern contraceptive techniques.

Measuring Knowledge of Reproduction

Information on knowledge of the reproductive system is derived from a two-part question. The first part is, "How does a woman get pregnant?" and the second is, "Why at some times and not at others?" The second really amplifies the first and is intended to ascertain whether the woman is aware, even vaguely, of the process of ovulation and how this is linked to menstruation. Initially it was thought that this second question could be dealt with separately, that is, as not dependent on the first. But since so few women evince any clear knowledge of the process of ovulation, this second question is used mainly to throw further light on answers to the first, in order that the respondents' knowledge of the reproductive processes in general can be more properly evaluated.

As respondents were invited to give statements in reply to these questions and not merely yes/no responses, a scheme of coding or evaluation of these statements has had to be adopted. A six-point scale has been used, ranging from 0 (no knowledge) to 5 (adequate knowledge). As is to be expected, scoring these answers presents many difficulties, particularly in deciding whether the curious phraseology used masks some basic knowledge of the processes or really attests to ignorance of the subject. Often answers to these two questions can be effectively evaluated only when they are taken in conjunction with answers to the questions on menstruation. In order to give an idea of how the scoring scheme is applied, the following illustrations are presented.

The lowest score (0) is intended to convey that the respondent has no knowledge whatsoever of the reproductive processes. The most frequent response of this type is simply "don't know." It is possible that a reply of this nature is a consequence of the failure of the interviewer to probe sufficiently. To the extent that this is so, it may result in an overstatement of the number scoring 0. But the general impression is that, in view of the willingness of the great majority of respondents to enter into eager discussion with interviewers on so many intimate aspects of their lives, the relatively large number of "don't know" responses may in fact be consistent with a general lack of knowledge of the subject. And the many statements offered in answer to the question as to how a woman gets pregnant leave no doubt as to respondents' ignorance of the underlying processes. Many answers coded 0 simply equate pregnancy with the cessation of menstruation. Answers of this type are: "When a woman does not see her period she is pregnant"; "By menstruating"; "A woman is pregnant if she does not see her menses and if she has not got a cold then she knows something is 'wrong.'"

A score of 1 is given to any answers which recognise that sexual intercourse is a fundamental aspect of conception, but show no idea of how conception occurs, or of the association between menstruation and ovulation. Examples of this type of answer are: "Sex causes that"; "A woman gets pregnant when she has sex too quick after menstruation"; "A woman gets pregnant by having sex—a woman gets pregnant only if the man fits her"; "By having sex—it depends on whether the eggs are ripe"; "When the man and the woman are having sex and they both discharge at the same time, the two germs meet."[1]

Answers showing something more than a realisation that sexual intercourse is involved in reproduction are given scores of 2. However, the distinction between this score and the one immediately below it (1) and the one immediately above it (3) is not easily made. What is sought here is a recognition, even a vague one, of the process of fertilisation of the ovum. Examples of this type of response are: "When the partner discharges, it goes between the egg and the baby forms"; "When the sperm gets into the womb and the germs mingle a woman gets pregnant"; "They say that a woman gets pregnant within the middle of the month her period comes. Also it must be a special night when sex was 'real good'"; "A germ from the discharge of the man and the woman—they do not get pregnant at certain times because the persons didn't connect at the same time."

The score on the scale representing the midpoint among those with any knowledge of the subject is 3. Answers so coded are taken to indicate that respondents have a tolerable knowledge of the subject. In particular such a score shows the realisation that menstruation is in some way involved in the process of reproduction. Examples of answers coded 3 are: "When the two germs meet they begin to form; a woman gets pregnant by using the safe period—in the first week the eggs have not yet begun to form, the second week anything can happen and by the third week it is safe again"; "When the male sperm finds what he is looking for ... must be one egg"; "Two eggs meet and conceive together."

The two highest scores are 4 and 5, both of which in effect indicate that the respondent has a fairly adequate grasp of the function of the reproductive system, which means that there is, on the part of the respondent, clear awareness of the processes of fertilisation of the ovum by the sperm and that there is a definite relationship between ovulation and menstruation. Examples of answers coded 4 are: "Sexual intercourse. The semen travels up the ovary and fertilises the egg"; "A woman gets pregnant by the male sperr meeting with the female eggs. She gets pregnant at certain times because at certain times of the month the woman's body is preparing to have a baby (every 28 days)"; "The germ from the male goes into the Fallopian tube and remains there and grows"; "When the egg cell from the female gets ripe and the egg is discharged from the male the two eggs meet"; "When the woman's sperm meets the man's. It is not all the time she is shedding an ova." Examples of answers coded 5 are: "Biological process—sperm fertilises the egg. During the month there are some times when one is less likely to become pregnant"; "When the semen of the man gets to the woman's egg and fertilises them a woman gets pregnant"; "The egg and the sperm of the man and the woman have to meet somewhere along the line and if it is fertile pregnancy takes place—after your periods your body gives off this thing [she does not know the name] and if you have sex at that time you are liable to get pregnant easier than before."

From the foregoing examples it will be seen that weighty problems have to be faced in scoring answers to these questions. Not many answers showing deep knowledge of the reproductive processes can be expected, but it is not always easy to determine whether answers given, often in terms of picturesque language, do indeed indicate that respondents have a clear understanding of the processes involved. While scoring does involve a degree of subjectivity, it is believed that a careful study of all answers has made it possible to arrive at a general pattern of prevailing knowledge, in terms of which individual answers can be satisfactorily assessed. For the present analysis of the material, the discussion will center around answers in terms of the six scores recognised, as well as in terms of weighted averages for separate groups of women.

The Overall Position

The summary position of knowledge of reproduction can be studied from Table 6.1. While the overwhelming impression that this conveys is of very low standards among all women, certain special features should be noted. The important fact is that 158 or just under one-third of the women in the sample either do not know, or at least fail to state that they are aware, that sexual relation is involved in reproduction. The number of women in this category (with scores of 0) is very close to the number with scores of 1, who number 162. At the other end of the scale there are 52 women with adequate knowledge of reproduction (that is with scores of 5); these account for 10% of the total. The number of women with a slightly lower level of knowledge (that is with scores of 4) stands at 36 or 7% of the total. In summary therefore it can be said that of this sample of women, 64% evince no knowledge whatsoever or are merely aware of the involvement of sexual contact in the process: these are the women with scores of 0 and 1. By contrast, those showing nearly adequate or adequate levels of knowledge, that is having scores of 4 or 5, amount to 88 or 18% of the total. A summary score for the entire sample in the form of a weighted average is only 1.58, which is just under one-third of the maximum possible in the scheme of scoring adopted.

It is further necessary to consider whether this generally low level is in any way linked to age of respondent. In view of the small numbers being studied here, only three broad age groups are dealt with: under 25, 25 to 44, and 45

Table 6.1 Level of knowledge of reproduction and average scores by age of women

Age group	Scores of level of knowledge							Average score
	0	1	2	3	4	5	Total	
15–24	39	38	17	10	12	19	135	1.81
25–44	47	71	19	19	16	19	191	1.70
45 +	72	53	18	10	8	14	175	1.26
Total	158	162	54	39	36	52	501	1.58

and over. The position of these three age groups can also be examined from Table 6.1. The association between the overall levels of knowledge and age is evident. The three age groups show that the lower the age the higher the overall level of the respondent's knowledge of reproduction. Highest is the level for the youngest age group; the average score for these women (1.81) is 15% above the level for the sample as a whole. The second highest level is shown by the age group 25 to 44 which, with an average score of 1.70, stands 8% above the sample average. Women of completed fertility show the lowest average score (1.26), which is 20% below the level of the sample average score. One outstanding aspect of the level of knowledge among these three age groups is the high proportion (41%) of women of completed fertility with 0 scores. By contrast, the corresponding proportion for women under age 25 is 29%.

Knowledge by Type of Union

For the purpose of this part of the study, the designation of union type follows that outlined in Chapter 4, which aims at arriving at the union midway in the respondents' childbearing period. Levels of knowledge of reproduction for the types of union, as classified in the manner indicated above, appear in Table 6.2. Of the 200 women falling within the visiting type,

Table 6.2 Level of knowledge of reproduction and average scores by type of union and age of women

Type of union	Scores of level of knowledge							Average score
	0	1	2	3	4	5	Total	
Under 45								
Visiting	29	49	18	6	20	17	139	1.93
Common-law	39	31	10	8	–	–	88	0.85
Married	4	21	4	11	6	18	64	2.75
Single	14	8	4	4	2	3	35	1.46
Over 45								
Visiting	24	21	8	5	1	2	61	1.08
Common-law	23	12	3	–	–	–	38	0.47
Married	25	19	7	4	7	12	74	1.80
Single*	–	1	–	1	–	–	2	–
Total								
Visiting	53	70	26	11	21	19	200	1.67
Common-law	62	43	13	8	–	–	126	0.74
Married	29	40	11	15	13	30	138	2.24
Single	14	9	4	5	2	3	37	1.49

*Average score not calculated.

53 report no comprehension whatsoever of the reproductive system, that is have scores of 0, while 70 have only a rudimentary knowledge of the system, that is, have scores of 1. This means that 62% of women in this type of union are without effective knowledge of the biological processes of fertility. At the other end of the scale there are 19 women with adequate knowledge (that is scoring 5), and 21 with somewhat lower levels (scoring 4). Thus about one-fifth of women in visiting unions exhibit a fairly good level of knowledge of the subject. The summary position of knowledge for such women is that the average weighted score is 1.67, which is about 6% in excess of the sample average.

The much smaller number of women in common-law unions shows an even lower degree of understanding of reproductive processes. Of the 126 women so classified, 62 have scores of 0 and 43 have scores of 1; this means that 83% in this form of union have no effective knowledge of reproduction. More important, there are no women in common-law relationships with scores of 4 or 5. The average score of 0.74 for this group is less than half the average score for women in the entire sample.

Appreciably higher levels of knowledge than those for visiting or common-law types are shown by the 138 women who are married. It is true that even here there are 29 women with scores of 0, and 40 with scores of 1, thus indicating that one-half of this type are without effective knowledge of the reproductive processes. But on the other hand, the numbers with scores of 4 and 5 are 13 and 30 respectively, which means that 31% of their number have some adequate idea of the subject. The average score for this union type of 2.24 is by far the highest of the three and stands 42% above the level for the sample as a whole.

There is a fourth category, single, composed of women who are not in any type of union. These number only 37 and their average score stands at 1.49, which is somewhat below the level for the entire sample.

There is a pronounced differential in terms of knowledge of reproduction between women of childbearing age and those over age 45. Among the former, married women display by far the highest level of knowledge. Very few of them (6%) have scores of 0, while 28% reveal adequate knowledge of the reproductive processes. The weighted average score for women in these unions (2.75) exceeds the sample mean by 74%. The second highest level of knowledge is presented by women in visiting unions. Their proportion without any knowledge is 21%, while 35% have scores of 1. The average score for this type amounts to 1.93, which is 22% above the sample average. Women termed single show the third highest level, with an average score of 1.46, that is somewhat below the sample average. By far the poorest characterises the common-law type, 80% of whom have scores of 0 and 1, and none have scores higher than 3. Their average score is only 0.85, that is just above one-half of the value for the entire sample.

When we turn to women over age 45, the same relative positions of the three union types emerge, but their levels of knowledge are lower than those of their younger counterparts. Married women, with 59% of their number scoring 0 or 1, and 16% scoring 5, reveal an average level of knowledge of 1.80, that is 14% in excess of the sample average. The second highest level among women of completed fertility is that of the visiting type. Nearly three-quarters of their number have scores of 0 or 1, while only 3% report adequate knowledge of the subject. Their average score of 1.08 falls appreciably below the sample average. Again the level of knowledge of reproduction associated with common-law unions is extremely low. None of these women have scores higher than 3, and their average score is only 0.47.

The ranking of the scores of knowledge for the three union types is of especial interest when related to the socio-economic status of these three groups of women. The score for the union type with the highest level, the married, is about three times that for the union at the lowest level, the common-law, while midway between these two falls the visiting. This ranking of scores of knowledge is in close accord with the ranking according to their measures of socio-economic status, established, in Chapter 4, on the basis of educational attainment. In other words, the index of socio-economic status puts the married at the highest position, the visiting second and the common-law lowest. And in conformity with the scores of levels of knowledge of reproduction, the same relative positions are maintained by the three types of union.

Knowledge by Educational Attainment

Another important relationship is that between knowledge of reproductive processes and the educational attainment of the women. This emphasises even more forcefully than the discussion in terms of union status the generally low status of understanding of the subject by women in the sample.

Although very few women have had no formal schooling, the general level of educational attainment remains low, largely because of the small numbers who go on to higher schools, so that no detailed breakdowns in terms of years of schooling seem justified. In fact it appears best to adopt a twofold division of primary and post-primary. Most of the former consist of women reporting 4 years or more of primary schooling. Included here as well are 22 women with less than this—some indeed have no formal schooling. Those women with post-primary education report some further exposure to education after leaving primary school. While this may be for the most part attendance at secondary school, there are several forms of training included, because, it is thought, they add in some way to the overall competence of individuals.

Scores for the two broad educational groups adopted are shown in Table 6.3 and Figure 6.1 which also carry breakdowns in terms of three broad age

Table 6.3 Level of knowledge of reproduction and average scores by educational attainment and age of women

Age group	Scores of level of knowledge							Average score
	0	1	2	3	4	5	Total	
				Primary				
15–24	29	18	5	3	3	–	58	0.84
25–44	42	55	12	10	7	7	133	1.29
45 +	68	45	13	7	1	5	139	0.87
Total	139	118	30	20	11	12	330	1.04
				Post-primary				
15–24	10	20	12	7	9	19	77	2.55
25–44	5	16	7	9	9	12	58	2.64
45 +	4	8	5	3	7	9	36	2.78
Total	19	44	24	19	25	40	171	2.63

intervals. With regard to women who have had primary schooling only, two factors stand out: the very low levels of knowledge exhibited, and the relatively favourable position of the age group 25 to 44. Women with primary education falling within the youngest age group have half their number reporting no knowledge of reproduction, and 31% with a rudimentary knowledge of the subject, that is with scores of 1. None of these women indicate knowledge qualifying them for a score of 5, and only 3 have scores of 4. The overall average score for this group is 0.84, which emphasises their low level of knowledge. In the case of women aged 25 to 44, about one-third report no knowledge whatsoever and 41% have scores of 1, so that nearly three-quarters of these women are not effectively informed about the subject. At the upper end of the scale there are 7 with scores of 5, and 7 with scores of 4. The average score for this age group (1.29) is more than 50% in excess of that for women under age 25. Women with primary education who have completed their families show a high proportion (49%) with no knowledge and 32% with rudimentary knowledge. Those with adequate knowledge number 5, while 1 has a score of 4. The average weighted score for this age group is 0.87, that is almost the same as that for women under age 25. The weighted average score for all primary women stands at 1.04, which is 34% below the average score for the entire sample.

Women with post-primary education show very much higher levels of knowledge than those who have not gone beyond elementary schooling. Of women under age 25, only 39% have scores of 0 or 1, while those with scores of 5 and 4 account for 25% and 12% respectively of the total in this age range. The average score is 2.55, which is more than three times that for corresponding women with only primary schooling. In the case of women aged 25 to 44, there is no marked departure from values for those within

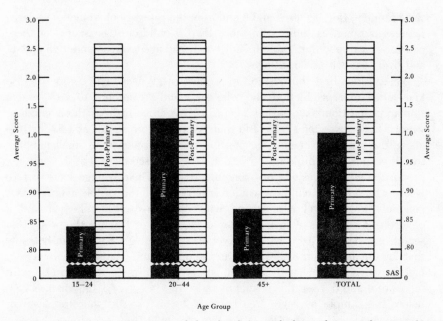

Figure 6.1 Average scores of level of knowledge of reproduction by educational attainment and age group

other age ranges, as is the case when we examine women of primary schooling only. Only 36% of women aged 25 to 44 have scores of 0 or 1, while 21% have scores of 5 and 16% scores of 4. The average score for women aged 25 to 44 is 2.64, which is about twice the level for corresponding women in the lower educational category. Women of completed fertility who are classified as having post-primary education show about one-third their number as having scores of 0 or 1, while one-fifth are scored 4 and one-quarter are scored 5. Their weighted average score of 2.78 is more than three times the corresponding value for women in the lower educational category.

In summary we can say that the weighted average score for all women with primary schooling (1.04) is 34% below the average score for the entire sample, whereas the weighted average score for women with higher education stands at 2.63, which is 66% in excess of the value for the entire sample.

Knowledge by Size of Family

Another relationship to be considered is that between level of knowledge of reproduction and size of family. The latter is treated in terms of four categories. The first represents childless women, the second represents small families with less than 4 children; the third may be described as medium-sized families, that is with 4 and 5 children; the category of women with large families is taken as those with more than 5 children. The scores of these categories are shown in Table 6.4 for two broad age groups—under 45 and 45 and over—as well as for all ages.

We consider first the position of women of all ages. Those reporting no knowledge of reproduction and who are childless amount to 29%, and a similar proportion have scores of 1. Just over one-fifth of these childless women have scores of 4 or 5, and their average score stands at 1.83, or 16% above the sample average. The position among women with small families, that is with 1 to 3 children, shows that 60% have scores of 0 or 1, while the proportion with scores of 4 or 5 amounts to 21%. Their average score of 1.70 is lower than that of childless women and 8% above the sample average. At a generally lower level are women with medium-sized families (4 and 5 children). Two-thirds of their number are scored 0 or 1, while the proportion scored 4 or 5 is only 16%, with the average score being 1.53, or slightly below that for the entire sample. Women in the large family category show a very high proportion (73%) with scores of 0 and 1, and a small proportion with scores of 4 and 5 (8%): this results in an average score of 1.19, which is 25% below the sample average. In summary it can be said that the level of knowledge decreases steadily as the size of family rises.

Table 6.4 Level of knowledge of reproduction and average scores by number of pregnancies and age of women

Size of family	Scores of level of knowledge							Average score
	0	1	2	3	4	5	Total	
Under 45								
No pregnancies	19	25	9	7	7	13	80	1.96
1–3 pregnancies	39	42	14	11	15	20	141	1.87
4–5 pregnancies	16	20	7	7	3	4	57	1.53
6 + pregnancies	12	22	6	4	3	1	48	1.31
Total	86	109	36	29	28	38	326	1.75
Over 45								
No pregnancies	8	1	2	1	–	1	13	1.00
1–3 pregnancies	25	21	7	5	2	6	66	1.33
4–5 pregnancies	14	10	1	1	3	5	34	1.53
6 + pregnancies	25	21	8	3	3	2	62	1.10
Total	72	53	18	10	8	14	175	1.26
All ages								
No pregnancies	27	26	11	8	7	14	93	1.83
1–3 pregnancies	64	63	21	16	17	26	207	1.70
4–5 pregnancies	30	30	8	8	6	9	91	1.53
6 + pregnancies	37	43	14	7	6	3	110	1.19
Total	158	162	54	39	36	52	501	1.58

The pattern with respect to women of childbearing age follows closely the overall position of women of all ages just considered, but the general level is higher. One-quarter of these younger women are childless and these show the highest level of knowledge. An appreciable proportion (55%) of these women are scored 0 or 1, while the proportion with scores of 4 or 5 is relatively high (25%). The average score of knowledge for childless women under age 45 of 1.96 is 12% above the average for all women of childbearing age. More than half of the women with 1 to 3 children (57%) have knowledge scores of 0 and 1 while women with adequate knowledge, that is showing scores of 4 and 5, comprise one-quarter of these women. The average score for women with 1 to 3 children (1.87) is 7% above the average for all women of childbearing age. Of women with medium-sized families, those scoring 0 or 1 with regard to knowledge of reproduction constitute 63% of the total, while the proportion with scores of 4 or 5 amounts to 12% of the total. The overall average score for these women (1.53) is below that for all women of childbearing age. When we turn to women with 6 children and more, the proportion without adequate knowledge amounts to 71%, while only 8% show scores of 4 or 5. The weighted average score for this group is down to 1.31, which is 25% below the average for all women under age 45.

The pattern of level of knowledge for women of completed fertility differs from that characterising women of childbearing age and for all family sizes stands at lower levels than do those for women under age 45. Much larger proportions of women in this age range have no knowledge of the subject, while correspondingly the proportions evincing any adequate knowledge are very small. The average score for all women of completed fertility is 1.26, which is 20% below the level for the entire sample. The pattern of knowledge by size of family takes the form of a rise from those without children up to a high point of 1.53 for women with medium-sized families. Then the average falls to 1.10 for women with large families. This rise to a maximum followed by a fall in level of knowledge as family size increases, in marked contrast to the pattern shown by women of childbearing age, poses several issues. It is possible that it is, to some degree, an artifact of the small numbers in some categories, notably those without children and those with families of medium size. On the other hand, the very low level for women with large families (1.10) conforms to a situation in which older women will be expected to have less knowledge of the basic details of reproduction.

Knowledge by Religion

Although there exists a wealth of religions in the island, these can be conveniently classified into 6 groups. Apart from the miscellaneous groups in which a host of sects are included and which account for 35% of the total, the largest religious groups are the Baptist, which accounts for 17% of all women, and the Anglican (15%). As will be seen from Table 6.5, when we con-

Table 6.5 Level of knowledge of reproduction and average scores by religion and education

Religion	Scores of level of knowledge							Average score
	0	1	2	3	4	5	Total	
				Primary				
Baptist	20	25	3	3	–	1	52	0.87
Anglican	18	11	4	5	1	4	43	1.35
Roman Catholic	5	7	3	2	2	2	21	1.76
Moravian	14	18	4	2	3	2	43	1.26
Church of God	10	14	5	–	2	–	31	1.03
Other	64	36	10	8	3	3	124	0.86
None	8	7	1	–	–	–	16	0.56
				Post-primary				
Baptist	8	8	5	3	4	5	33	2.06
Anglican	2	9	4	5	5	9	34	2.85
Roman Catholic	1	6	2	3	6	8	26	3.19
Moravian	–	5	4	–	1	2	12	2.25
Church of God*	2	2	2	1	–	2	9	–
Other	6	12	5	7	9	12	51	2.73
None*	–	2	2	–	–	2	6	–
				Total				
Baptist	28	33	8	6	4	6	85	1.33
Anglican	20	20	8	10	6	13	77	2.01
Roman Catholic	6	13	5	5	8	10	47	2.55
Moravian	14	23	8	2	4	4	55	1.47
Church of God	12	16	7	1	2	2	40	1.27
Other	70	48	15	15	12	15	175	1.41
None	8	9	3	–	–	2	22	1.14

*Average scores for these categories are not calculated.

sider the level of knowledge for the total women within each of the six religious groups, the Roman Catholics stand out as the group with by far the highest level of knowledge. Although 40% of these women have scores of 0 and 1, the appreciable numbers with scores of 4 and 5 (18) account for 38% of the total, and is sufficient to force up the average score to 2.55. The second highest level of knowledge is shown by the Anglicans, 52% of whom have scores of 0 and 1, and one-quarter of whom have scores of 4 and 5; the average score for this group is 2.01. Lowest levels of knowledge are shown by Baptists and Church of God followers, with average scores of 1.33 and 1.27 respectively, that is at about one-half the level shown by women of the Roman Catholic faith.

When religious knowledge is treated in conjunction with the two broad educational categories already established, the primary group appears as definitely lower than those with some exposure to higher education. Roman Catholics show the highest level of knowledge: with 57% scoring 0 and 1 and 19% scoring 4 or 5, the average score stands at 1.76. The second highest level is that for Anglicans (average score of 1.35). Lowest score of the religious groups being considered is that of Baptists, 87% of whom have scores of 0 and 1, and only 1 with a score of 5. The average score (0.87) is only about one-half of that of the Roman Catholics.

At a much higher level is the knowledge of reproduction assessed for women with post-primary education. The outstanding group is the Roman Catholic, which, with an average score of 3.19, has one of the highest scores of any group in this survey. Only 27% have scores of 0 and 1, while the proportion with scores of 4 or 5 is as high as 54%. The second highest average score is that of the Anglicans (2.85), which is 11% below that of the Roman Catholics. The outstanding feature of scores of knowledge for women with post-primary education is that there is a very small range in the average scores, compared with women with only primary schooling. Apart from the two groups—Others and Church of God—the ranking of the religious groups is the same for both levels of educational status. It can be said that knowledge of reproduction is much higher among the "established" religious groups, especially so among Roman Catholics, whereas the fundamentalists exhibit much lower levels of knowledge.

Knowledge by Information Received About Sex

Relevant to the discussion of knowledge about reproduction is the degree of information which women receive about sex. Limited clues on this issue can be gleaned from the present survey. The question on the schedule being relied on in the present context is, "Did anyone ever explain sex to you?" Affirmative answers to this question may conceivably signify that information gained about sex covers, to some extent, the reproductive system in general, although this assumption may be reading much more into these answers than the form of the question really warrants. In any case it is instructive to consider the relationship between the level of understanding of reproduction and whether or not the respondent was ever told about sex, and, if so, by whom.

From the summary situation of this relationship presented in Table 6.6, the outstanding feature is the large proportion of women who receive no formal information about sex from any source at all. When we consider the sample as a whole, we see that nearly one-half of the respondents report having had no information on the subject, while the largest source of information on the topic, mothers of the respondents, accounts for only about one-quarter of the total sample. Teachers and other relatives contributed 7% each to this information. The fact that respondents are unable to state a specific source of

Table 6.6 Level of knowledge of reproduction and average scores by source of information on sex

Source of knowledge of sex	Scores of level of knowledge							Average score
	0	1	2	3	4	5	Total	
Under 45								
No source reported	48	55	16	13	5	12	149	1.38
Books	1	1	–	1	3	–	6	2.67
Mother	16	23	11	8	8	11	77	2.03
Other relatives	6	7	1	1	4	6	25	2.32
Teacher	5	11	7	2	5	4	34	2.09
All other	10	12	1	4	3	5	35	1.80
Over 45								
No source reported	47	24	10	3	4	7	95	1.09
Books	2	–	2	–	–	2	6	2.33
Mother	15	19	1	4	2	3	44	1.27
Other relatives	5	1	1	3	1	1	12	1.75
Teacher*	–	1	1	–	–	1	3	–
All other	3	8	3	–	1	–	15	1.20
All ages								
No source reported	95	79	26	16	9	19	244	1.27
Books	3	1	2	1	3	2	12	2.50
Mother	31	42	12	12	10	14	121	1.75
Other relatives	11	8	2	4	5	7	37	2.14
Teacher	5	12	8	2	5	5	37	2.14
All other	13	20	4	4	4	5	50	1.62

*The average score for this category is not calculated.

information on sex does not necessarily mean that they are without such knowledge. From a variety of sources which they could not identify at the time of the interview they may have received bits of information which when put together constitute some body of knowledge of the subject. So that although they cannot identify any definite source for their information about sex, it is not surprising that they evince some knowledge, even though this is at a much lower level than that shown by respondents who have identified definite sources of knowledge. Of these women 39% have 0 scores of knowledge of reproduction, and 32% have scores of 1. But there is still a sizeable group reporting some knowledge of the subject; in fact the proportion scoring 4 and 5 amounts to 11% of the total. The average score for this group of women (1.27) is below the average for women reporting any source of knowledge.

When we turn to women acknowledging some source of knowledge, those with the highest average score report books as the source of their information

(2.50), although the small number of women involved here (12) reduces the significance to be attached to this score. As sources of such information, teachers and other relatives are associated with reasonably high scores of knowledge; both show averages of 2.14. Although a substantial proportion of women receive information about sex from their mothers, the understanding they display of reproduction is not high, their weighted average score being only 1.75. The average score shown by women reporting all other sources of information is 1.62. It is important to note that of the six categories of source of knowledge under consideration here, only one, that relating to women identifying no source, shows an average score falling below the sample average. Here the average score falls 20% below that of the sample. In the case of the other categories of source, the average scores range from 58% in excess of the sample average to 3% above it.

In view of the very small numbers falling within some of the categories, comparisons between women of childbearing age and those who have completed fertility have to be made with caution. In the case of women of childbearing age, the lowest average score (1.38) is that for women identifying no source of information on sex, while the highest is the source termed books; women in the latter category show an average score of 2.67, which however has to be used with reserve, since it is based on replies from only 6 women. The second highest score (2.32) is that relating to other relatives, with teachers (2.09), mothers (2.03) and all others (1.80), following in that order.

With the very small numbers in the six categories for women of completed fertility, scores of knowledge are subject to appreciable margins of error. In fact only women reporting no source of knowledge (95) and those reporting mother as the source (44) are large enough to be compared with levels for women of childbearing age. Both of these show average scores considerably below the values for younger women—1.09 and 1.27 respectively.

This analysis yields an interesting conclusion that women who receive information on sex, from any source whatever, have more understanding of the reproductive processes than those who report that no such information on sex has been imparted to them. This suggests that prevailing forms of popular instruction in the subject do contain some outlines of reproduction and of the menstrual cycle.

One unexpected aspect of these scores is the low level shown by women who receive information on sex from their mothers. Their scores of knowledge are much lower than levels for those who receive such information from other relatives or from teachers. Whether it is justified to ascribe this to the mother's inability to pass on satisfactory knowledge to their daughters is not clear. On the other hand, the fact that generally levels of knowledge for younger women are much higher than corresponding values for women of completed fertility is not unexpected; it strongly suggests an overall improvement in knowledge of the subject within recent years.

Measuring Knowledge of Menstruation

Even more arresting than the low level of knowledge of the general reproductive processes is the widespread ignorance of the menstrual cycle among most groups of women. In view of this level of ignorance of the subject, scoring of the answers obtained presents some problems. Again a six-point scale is used, with 0 representing no knowledge and 5 representing adequate knowledge. It is relatively easy to identify answers qualifying for scores at either end of the scale. Identification of respondents without any knowledge of menstruation is easy. Most of them are content to give a simple "don't know" response. But there are large numbers of replies in the form of statements, which leave no doubt as to respondents' total lack of understanding of the processes involved. Likewise it is comparatively easy to identify answers which qualify for a score of 5. But evaluation of answers falling within intervening points on the scale is much more difficult than is the scoring of answers to the general question of reproduction. Evaluating answers to questions on the menstrual cycle has to be done by considering, in addition, answers to the broader question of reproduction. Although the six-point scale is adopted here, the high concentration at its lower end and the difficulties of assigning scores to answers qualifying for intermediate positions make it more reasonable to discuss knowledge of menstruation in terms of three levels, those with no knowledge (coded 0), those with some knowledge (codes 1 to 4) and those with adequate knowledge (coded 5).

It is instructive to illustrate the kinds of answers collected, in terms of the above-mentioned three-level assessment. Responses coded 0 emphasise the wide range of ignorance of the topic, as can be seen from the following answers: "Caused by the food you eat and the waste matter has to pass out"; "A sign that you are healthy. It is also caused by how you work and how you eat"; "Waste matter coming"; "You are made of flesh and blood and born a woman so you are supposed to see your menses"; "Some bad blood you had to pass out ... from the blood vessel"; "Waste matter"; "Part of your health"; "Waste blood coming away"; "It is a sign that you have enough blood to make a baby"; "Oh, God, I don't know, just a way, a way of life"; "Don't know, but it is a sign from the Lord"; "It was ordained"; "A flow of excess blood you must have"; "Egg fertilises and bursts and menstruation comes on"; "The Lord work out that"; "Normal course for women." While it does not seem necessary to analyse in detail these notions about menstruation, some recurrent themes may be noted. A large number of women accept it as a part of their normal bodily functions—as something ordained by nature—and do not seek to explain it. Also recurrent is the theme that the process is a discharge of waste matter from the body. Often this is taken to mean that the woman is healthy; in fact to a large number of women, menstruation is a sign of their "health."[2]

A few examples from the small numbers showing some vague knowledge of the menstrual cycle may now be noted: "It is like a wheel going round (cycle) and you have two weeks and when it reaches red your period comes"; "The walls of the uterus sheds"; "This happens to show you are now of age to have children"; "The egg ripens and bursts if not fertilised and the woman menstruates"; "The egg comes down monthly."

We now give three answers showing adequate knowledge of menstruation. Incidentally two of the respondents supplying these answers are teachers and the other is a midwife. The answers are: "The body each month is getting ready for a new child and if the egg is not fertilised, the lining of the womb comes out in the form of menstruation"; "Shedding of decidua of the uterus"; "Biological reason: failure of the egg to fertilise."

Summarised in Table 6.7 is the knowledge of menstruation among women with primary and post-primary education. The great majority of these women are without any clear understanding of menstruation. For the sample as a whole, 413 or 82% have no knowledge of the subject, while those with only vague comprehension (that is with answers coded 1 to 4) amount to 62 or 12% of the total. Thus only 26 or 5% of the entire sample give answers indicating a satisfactory understanding of the menstrual cycle. The resulting overall score of knowledge in terms of a weighted average is only 0.60; this is equivalent to 38% of the average score of knowledge of reproduction.

This unsatisfactory state of knowledge of menstruation extends to both educational categories of women, but is especially depressing among women with only primary education. As many as 94% of these women have no knowledge whatsoever of the underlying processes of menstruation, and only 4 or 1% evince any adequate knowledge of the subject. The situation is much better among women with post-primary education. Of these, 104 or 61% have 0 scores, while those with adequate knowledge number 22 or 13% of women within this educational level. The average score for this group (1.40) is nearly eight times that for women with primary education only, signifying the vast difference between the two in terms of knowledge of the subject.

Table 6.7 Level of knowledge of menstruation and average scores by education

Educational level	Scores of level of knowledge							Average score
	0	*1*	*2*	*3*	*4*	*5*	*Total*	
Primary	309	4	6	3	4	4	330	0.18
Post-primary	104	9	5	13	18	22	171	1.40
Total	413	13	11	16	22	26	501	0.60

Knowledge of Menstruation by Type of Union

Differentials of knowledge by family union, appearing in Table 6.8, stress the deplorable position of the women in common-law unions, none of whom have any adequate knowledge of the subject, and who show a weighted average score of only 0.03. Women in visiting unions have a much higher score than their common-law counterparts, although here also overall levels are extremely low. Of the 200 women classified as visiting, 172 or 86% have 0 scores, while the proportion scoring 5 is only 4%. The weighted average for this union type (0.50) is very low, although it is many times the corresponding value for women in common-law unions. At a much higher level of knowledge are women in married unions. A substantial proportion (65%) report no knowledge of menstruation, but the proportion with adequate knowledge (12%) is much higher than corresponding values for other union types, thus resulting in an average score of 1.25, by far the highest for all the categories of union.

Table 6.8 Level of knowledge of menstruation and average scores by type of union

Type of union	Scores of level of knowledge							Average score
	0	1	2	3	4	5	Total	
Visiting	172	4	3	4	8	9	200	0.50
Common-law	124	1	–	1	–	–	126	0.03
Married	90	6	4	10	12	16	138	1.25
Single	27	2	4	1	2	1	37	0.70
Total	413	13	11	16	22	26	501	0.60

Levels of Knowledge of Menstruation by Size of Family

The low state of knowledge of menstruation is again evident when we consider the differentials by size of family, as in Table 6.9. There is a definite pattern here—a fall in the general level of knowledge as we move up the scale of family size. Women without children show 71% of their number without any knowledge of the subject, but the proportion with adequate knowledge (9%) is the highest for the 4 categories of family size; the summary position of childless women is an average score of 0.92, which is 53% above the sample total. Women with 1 to 3 children also show a large proportion scoring 0 (80%), while only 5% have scores of 5, and the resulting weighted average score is 0.72, which is 20% in excess of the corresponding sample total. The position in the medium-sized families shows a sharp fall below the two preceding family categories. Here the proportion of women with no knowledge of the subject moves up to 88%, while the proportion scoring 5 is

Table 6.9 Level of knowledge of menstruation and average scores by number of pregnancies per woman

Number of pregnancies	Scores of level of knowledge							Average score
	0	*1*	*2*	*3*	*4*	*5*	*Total*	
No pregnancies	66	6	4	4	5	8	93	0.92
1–3 pregnancies	166	2	5	9	14	11	207	0.72
4–5 pregnancies	80	3	1	2	1	4	91	0.38
6+ pregnancies	101	2	1	1	2	3	110	0.27
Total	413	13	11	16	22	26	501	0.60

only 4%. The average score of knowledge for women of medium-sized families is down to 0.38, just over one-half the value for women with small families. Even lower levels of knowledge of menstruation characterise women with more than 5 children. The proportion of these women with knowledge scores of 0 amounts to 92%, while less than 3% show adequate knowledge of the subject. The average score for women of this family size (0.27) is only 45% of the corresponding sample total and is less than one-third of the level shown by childless women.

Women's Opinions About Menstruation

Low levels of knowledge of the menstrual processes do not preclude women having particular beliefs concerning them, some of which in fact may have a strong bearing on aspects of their behaviour. Beliefs about this subject, as distinct from knowledge expressed about it, have come to constitute an important topic for study.[3] This seems fully justified as beliefs may have just as significant an impact on the acceptance and successful practice of contraception as actual knowledge of the bodily functions involved. In this survey the question put to the respondent on this point is, "What beliefs do you know about menstruation?" This does not therefore limit the answer to the views of the respondents themselves; any current opinion, whether or not she shares it, is in fact being sought. And some opposing standpoints on issues concerning menstruation are advanced. Answers to this question cannot be quantified in the same way that answers in respect of knowledge can, but they do constitute an important qualitative complement to the quantitative analysis of knowledge.

With the exception of a few respondents who express the view that menstruation is a normal bodily function, that consequently no extraordinary activities are called for and that no usual activities need be curtailed, the general impression is that this condition sets the woman apart and calls for her taking special precautions. Menstruation, in the expressive language of one respondent, is "God-sick." In many instances, these views are reported as prevalent within the community, although not necessarily shared by the respondent. To what extent either set of admonitions is heeded is not clear, but presumably many women observe them. They all serve to show the degree to which menstruation is regarded as setting the woman apart from others in the community.

It is convenient in discussing the answers to the question to group them into catogories, each of which deals with a particular aspect of the subject. These aspects are: uncleanness of menstruation, its effects on sexual relations, its implications with regard to food, the mobility of women in this condition, and miscellaneous phases of the menstrual state.

Many respondents hold that the menstruating woman is unclean.[4] Evidently there is no way of making such a woman clean; cleanness will return only after the period is over. Since menstruation is so strongly associated with uncleanness, it is curious that so many women maintain that during their period bathing should be avoided, especially bathing in cold water. It is to some extent permissible if done in warm water. Even if it does prove necessary for the woman to bathe, she is not supposed to sit in the water. One proviso advanced by a respondent is that the use of lime is recommended by women who bathe during menstruation. On the other hand, another respondent cautions against drinking lime during the period. One form of washing which is not advocated by many respondents is washing the hair. Indeed should the menstruating woman wash (or indeed comb) the hair of another woman, the latter may well face the disaster of losing her hair.

With few exceptions, the state of menstruation is regarded as one in which the woman is to abstain from sexual intercourse.[5] Some see this presumably as an extension of the unclean state previously noted. One goes so far as to claim that during her period the woman should not share the same bed with her partner. Some dire consequences of sexual intercourse during menstruation are possible; it may, one contends, result in disease. A few urge that this may make the woman "become pregnant quicker." More serious are the results if a woman does become pregnant as a result of sexual intercourse while she is menstruating. Two respondents maintain that a child of such a pregnancy would be an albino, and in the opinion of one a freak of some sort. It would appear best therefore to avoid sex during the period and even for a few days following the cessation of the flow. But an opposing position should be noted, according to which, painful menstruation is a sign that "the woman requires sex." This advice was in fact advanced by some members of the medical profession in Jamaica up to recent times.

The general belief that the menstruating woman is unclean has important implications with regard to the preparation of food and eating habits.[6] The women are supposed to keep out of kitchens, presumably because they may contaminate the food. In the words of one respondent, "Whatever you use, only you alone should use it. Keep away from other people, according to the Bible." One respondent holds that the menstruating woman should not cook, though the more widespread belief is that it is baking that should be avoided. Even the mixing of a cake is not advisable, as it may "flop." Another claims that liver should not be eaten by menstruating women. Also, if boiling guava jelly the menstruating woman should not look into it, while meat must not be handled by her. More curious are the admonitions against eating jackfruit and soursop; the possible consequences of eating such fruit are not spelled out. The warning against eating cabbage has a more direct bearing on menstruation, as in the words of one answer this "will cause the menses to smell unpleasant." Several women contend that menstruating women should not drink alcohol, as this may cause the blood to clot. Drinking ice water, it is argued, has a similar effect.

There are widespread beliefs concerning the mobility of women who are menstruating.[7] In many cases it is held that they should be immobilised, or at least that their activities should be greatly reduced. They are not supposed to walk without shoes, or to go out in the rain, according to one answer. Opinions are expressed against such women going to the cinema, to the beach or to dances. Nor should the menstruating women go to church, "especially communion, as she is unclean." She is not to make an appointment. All contact with the dead must be avoided. Walking over graves is extremely dangerous; equally so is the attendance at funerals. Even to look on the dead is fraught with serious consequence. "You should not look at the dead because while the dead is rotting your body will go away the same way and can't stop," in the words of one respondent. Another puts the consequences of looking at the dead in similarly disastrous terms: "Your stomach will rot." One seemingly inexplicable warning is against "walking over a pumpkin," as it is difficult to associate this with any untoward implication.

A number of general beliefs about menstruation, mostly expressed in the form of precautions to be taken, should be noted. The menstruating woman should not look into a mirror or "her face will get spotted."[8] She should not use a foot-driven sewing machine. The cleaning of the house is to be put off, as scrubbing especially is not good for her. Nor should she "handle anything young and blooming," such as plants. Allied to this is the advice against holding someone else's young baby, as the infant may be adversely affected. A further warning is against the extraction of teeth, as this may lead to a haemorrhage.

While these opinions for the most part spell out restrictions placed on the menstruating female, there are other courses of action advocated, generally with the aim of ensuring an easing of discomfort during the period. Perhaps the strangest of these is the advice to drink "blue water" as this is supposed to stop excessive menstrual flows. Another urges women to drink "red water grass," which is supposed to produce similar effects.

Knowledge of Reproduction by Use of Contraception

Further aspects of knowledge of reproduction and menstruation center around their relationship to the use of contraception. In the first place such knowledge may play a part in inducing women to make use of family-planning techniques. In the second place, an understanding of the processes of reproduction and of menstruation may help users to appreciate the disturbances in the menstrual cycle which may be associated with the use of certain modern contraceptives.

Table 6.10 shows the relationship between knowledge of reproduction and use of contraception for women of childbearing age as well as for those of completed fertility. Taking first the experience of women of all ages, we note the appreciable number who have not stated whether they have used contraception or not. Nearly one-fifth of the sample fall within this not-stated category, while there is a large proportion (59%) who have never used contraception, thus showing that the proportion who definitely make use of these devices is 22%. Users show by far the highest level of knowledge. Nearly half of their number have scores of 0 and 1, while those with scores of 4 and 5 amount to one-third of the group. The average score for this group of 2.29 is 45% higher than the sample average. By contrast non-users show a very high proportion (71%) with scores of 0 and 1 and a low proportion (11%) with scores of 4 and 5, so that their weighted average score is only 1.28, which is about one-fifth less than the sample total. Of interest is the position of the group who do not indicate whether they have ever made use of contra-

Table 6.10 Level of knowledge of reproduction and average scores among users and non-users of contraception by age of women

Use of contraception	Scores of level of knowledge							Average score
	0	1	2	3	4	5	Total	
Under 45								
Users	19	26	7	8	9	16	85	2.12
Non-users	48	58	19	14	14	11	164	1.52
Not stated	20	25	9	7	6	11	78	1.83
Over 45								
Users	1	8	2	2	6	6	25	2.88
Non-users	61	43	13	7	1	7	132	0.98
Not stated	10	2	3	1	–	1	17	0.94
Total								
Users	20	34	9	10	15	22	110	2.29
Non-users	109	101	32	21	15	18	296	1.28
Not stated	30	27	12	8	6	12	95	1.67

ception. With a proportion of 60% having scores of 0 and 1 and 19% having scores of 4 and 5, their average score is 1.67, which is midway between the levels of users and non-users, and which is only slightly above the average score for the entire sample.

The position of women of childbearing age shows the same general order as that revealed for the entire sample. Of the 26% of these women who report having made use of some contraception, just over one-half are scored 0 and 1, while those scored 4 and 5 amount to 29% of the total, thus resulting in an average score of 2.12. This is equivalent to 34% above the sample average. Much lower is the level of knowledge of reproduction shown by non-users, who, with 65% scoring 0 and 1, and 15% at 4 and 5, have an average score of 1.52, which is slightly lower than that for the sample as a whole. Again we see that the not-stated category has an average midway between the users and the non-users (1.83).

The pattern of knowledge for women of completed fertility differs considerably from that shown by younger women. There is a small proportion (14%) of this age group who report having used contraception. But of this group only 36% have scores of 0 and 1, while the proportion registering 4 and 5 is very high (48%). This results in an average for this group of 2.88, which is 82% above the sample value and in fact constitutes one of the highest levels of knowledge in this study. At a much lower level of knowledge are women who report not having used any contraceptives in their lives. Most of them (79%) have very low scores of 0 and 1, while the proportion at the 2 highest levels is only 6%, thus resulting in an average score of only 0.98, equivalent to 38% lower than the sample average. Moreover, unlike the position with younger women, the not-stated category is comparatively small, and is slightly below the level of non-users in terms of knowledge, with an average score of 0.94.

It may be concluded that, according to the sample, users of contraception have appreciably higher scores of knowledge of reproduction than non-users, throughout the population. But at this stage no attempt can be made to state the precise causal connexion between the two.

Knowledge of Menstruation by Use of Contraception

As is to be expected from earlier discussions, there is, with one exception to be studied presently, very little understanding of this subject among any of the groups that can be identified in the sample. While there is some similarity with the pattern of knowledge of reproduction in so far as users exhibit much higher levels than non-users, there are differences, some of which however may follow from the very small numbers of women in some of the categories. As is seen from Table 6.11, the position of women as a whole indicates that among those reporting the use of contraception, 64% have absolutely no knowledge of the subject, that is are scored 0, whereas scores of 5 are given to

Table 6.11 Level of knowledge of menstruation and average scores among users and non-users of contraception by age of women

Use of contraception	Scores of level of knowledge							Average score
	0	1	2	3	4	5	Total	
Under 45								
Users	57	3	3	6	9	7	85	1.15
Non-users	150	–	–	1	5	7	163	0.36
Not stated	55	6	4	2	4	7	78	0.91
Over 45								
Users	13	2	–	4	2	4	25	1.68
Non-users	122	2	4	2	2	1	133	0.22
Not stated	16	–	–	1	–	–	17	0.18
Total								
Users	70	5	3	10	11	11	110	1.27
Non-users	272	2	4	3	7	8	296	0.29
Not stated	71	6	4	3	4	7	95	0.78

only 10%. The resulting average score of 1.27, although very low, is about twice the level for the average of the entire sample. In the case of non-users, 92% are scored 0 and only 3% are scored 5, so that the average score stands at 0.29, or less than half that of the sample average. As in the case of knowledge of reproduction, those who have not stated whether or not they used contraception have an average score midway between users and non-users.

For users among women of childbearing age, 67% of whom show no knowledge of the subject and only 8% of whom score 5, the average score is only 1.15. This, however, is still nearly twice the level for the sample as a whole. In the case of non-users, the vast majority (92%) are without any understanding of menstruation, while only 4% have any adequate knowledge; consequently the average score is only 0.36. It is strange that those women who do not indicate whether or not they have used contraception show a much higher level of knowledge than non-users, having 71% at the lowest level (0), and 9% at the highest (5). The average score of 0.91 is also appreciably above that of the sample level.

Levels of knowledge for users who are over age 45 are somewhat higher than corresponding ones for users at younger ages. Here the proportion in the 0 category accounts for 52% of the total, while 16% evince adequate knowledge. On the other hand, hardly any of the non-users show adequate knowledge of the subject, while the great majority (92%) have no understanding whatsoever, thus resulting in an average score of 0.22, which is less than half of the sample average. In the case of women for whom there is no indication of use of contraception also, virtually all are without any understanding of the menstrual cycle, with the result that the average score is no more than 0.18. In assessing the position of users and the not-stated category among women over age 45, their very small numbers, 25 and 17 respectively, imply that they are subject to appreciable sampling errors.

Once more a measure of some understanding of the biological processes of reproduction—in this case the menstrual cycle—is associated with a somewhat higher degree of resort to contraception. It is tempting to conclude that such higher knowledge is, in some way, responsible for the greater use of contraception. On the other hand it seems equally acceptable that their relatively high level of knowledge of the menstrual cycle has been acquired after the resort to contraception and may indeed have been gained in the course of their attempts to understand the effects of the methods used on their menstrual cycle.

Knowledge and Use of Various Methods of Contraception

Another aspect of the use of contraception in its relation to knowledge of reproduction and menstruation is the level of knowledge shown by users of the methods reported by respondents. Just over one-fifth (110) of the whole sample report the use of one or more contraceptives in their reproductive life. Since several report using more than one method, either together or in sequence, the approach here is to treat each method reported as an event to be related to the knowledge shown by each respondent. Thus a woman who has used 3 methods in her life and who has a knowledge score of 4 contributes this value to each of the 3 types concerned. On this basis there are 133 reports of the use of contraception by the 110 contraceptors in the sample. The methods used have been divided into four categories and a residual group covering all other methods which are reported.

The relation between levels of knowledge and the methods used is summarised in Table 6.12. In considering this position it must be recalled that contraceptors have much higher levels of knowledge of both reproduction

Table 6.12 Average scores of knowledge of reproduction and menstruation and standard deviation of scores, by type of contraception used and number of users

Contraception used	Number of users	Average scores of knowledge of		Standard deviation of scores of knowledge of	
		Reproduction	Menstruation	Reproduction	Menstruation
Pill	61	1.95	1.20	1.85	1.78
Condom	19	3.16	2.58	1.86	2.06
Cream, foam tablets, jelly	18	2.50	0.89	1.86	1.75
Injectibles	8	1.88	0.50	1.81	1.41
All others	27	2.44	1.41	1.80	1.99

and menstruation than non-contraceptors. Dealing first with knowledge of reproduction, we see that the method associated with the highest score is the condom, which is the technique reported in 14% of the cases recorded. The average score for these women amounts to 3.16, which is the highest level obtaining in any of the groups of women recognised in this study. It is 63% of the possible maximum obtainable under the present scheme of scoring, and 38% in excess of the average score for all contraceptors. The group of methods showing the second highest score consists of creams, foam tablets and jelly, which account for 14% of all users; the average score here of 2.50 is again in excess of the value for all users. The third highest occurs in the case of users of the pill. The mean score for these women (1.95) is, however, 15% below that for the whole level of users. A fairly high level of knowledge is observed for women using miscellaneous methods (2.44), which itself is in excess of the average for all users. One important feature of these levels is their extremely large dispersion. As will be seen from Table 6.12, the standard deviation for these average scores are all of the order of 1.8, thus attesting to the very high concentration within the 0 categories.

It is to be expected from the previous discussion that knowledge of menstruation will be at a much lower level than that of reproduction and this is also well brought out in Table 6.12. The average score of knowledge of menstruation is highest again for women who depend on the condom; these show a mean of 2.58, which is more than twice the corresponding level for all contraceptors. Unlike the pattern of differential observed in the case of knowledge of reproduction, knowledge of menstruation is second highest among users of the pill, who show an average score of 1.20, which is only slightly below that for the level for all users of contraception, and about one-half of the value for women who rely on the condom. Third highest is the level shown by users of cream, jelly and foam tablets; here the average score of knowledge of menstruation (0.89) is equal to 70% of the corresponding value for the entire sample. Again the evidence is of considerable variance in all cases, and this is clearly visible from the standard deviation for the means of knowledge of menstruation. These are in fact much greater than those for scores estimated on the basis of data for knowledge of reproduction. Here standard deviations range from 1.4 to 2.1, and again the concentration in the 0 categories contributes heavily to this.

Another context in which knowledge of reproduction and menstruation seems to be relevant is in regard to the time when the women make use of contraception. This is best assessed in terms of interpregnancy intervals, rather than actual date of commencement. For although women may be uncertain about this date, they are in general able to state the interval during which they commenced use of a particular contraceptive. The first interval is that between the commencement of the initial union and the termination of the first pregnancy; the second is the period intervening between the first and second pregnancies; the third interval is the period intervening between the termination of the second and third pregnancies; and so on.

Entered in Table 6.13 are the average scores for reproduction and menstruation shown by women in the sample, according to the intervals during which contraceptives have been used. In terms of knowledge of reproduction, by far the highest average score (3.19) is that shown by women who use the methods before the birth of their first child. This is the most favourable score of all the groups of women treated in this survey. It is in fact slightly higher than the score recorded by women who rely on the condom (3.16), and is 1.4 times the level of knowledge of reproduction shown by contraceptors in general. The second highest is that for women who have used contraception between the first and second pregnancies. This score, although 17% below that shown by those who commence use of contraceptives before their first pregnancy, is still appreciably in excess of the average for all users. The relationship between time of use of contraception and score of knowledge is not wholly linear. Although the level of knowledge for the next interpregnancy interval (1.90) continues to decline, it is followed by one exhibiting an appreciably greater level of knowledge (2.50). But higher interpregnancy intervals, up to the sixth, conform to the pattern of a decline.

Table 6.13 Average scores of knowledge of reproduction and menstruation, and standard deviation of scores, by interval of commencement of use of contraception

Interval	Number of users	Average scores of knowledge of		Standard deviation of scores of knowledge of	
		Reproduction	Menstruation	Reproduction	Menstruation
Between form-ation of union and 1st preg-nancy	26	3.19	2.62	1.84	2.00
Between 1st and 2nd preg-nancies	39	2.64	1.46	2.03	1.92
Between 2nd and 3rd preg-nancies	20	1.90	0.75	1.51	1.37
Between 3rd and 4th preg-nancies	14	2.50	0.71	1.80	1.44
Higher inter-pregnancy intervals	34	1.53	0.65	1.29	1.57

When we turn to levels of knowledge of menstruation, there is a marked linear relationship between knowledge and time of use of contraception. In other words the highest level of knowledge (2.62) appears among women employing contraceptives before the initial pregnancy, and women who make use of the several methods at higher intervals show a progressive fall in level of knowledge of menstruation. A very low level of knowledge is shown by women who commence the use of contraception between their third and fourth pregnancies (0.71) while an even lower value appears among those who begin contraception at later intervals (0.65). The wide variation in the scores again appears from the high standard deviations shown. These range from 2.03 to 1.29 in the case of knowledge of reproduction and from 2.00 to 1.37 in the case of knowledge of menstruation.

Conclusion

In these discussions of the degree to which the society understands the fundamental aspects of the biology of reproduction, we have taken the position that its level is very low, especially in the case of the menstrual cycle. But manifestly part of an assessment of this nature will involve comparisons with other studies, of developing societies as well as of highly industrialised ones which have already experienced the transition to a low fertility regime. It may be that such comparisons will lead to a modification of some of the norms implicit in our discussion of these topics.

Comparisons with the position in societies which have experienced marked reductions in fertility will be especially relevant. An examination of the position in European societies suggests that the widespread resort to contraceptive practice during the nineteenth and early twentieth centuries was not accompanied by any significant spread of accurate knowledge about reproduction. What was involved was the widespread use of a limited range of traditional methods, for the satisfactory use of which no profound knowledge of the reproductive processes was called for. Indeed it seems that up to the late nineteenth century both the medical profession and the church remained opposed to the spread of contraception and presumably to the dissemination of current knowledge of the reproductive processes.[9] In fact the satisfactory use of methods current at the time—coitus interruptus, the condom, douche and various occlusive devices—did not call for any understanding other than the realisation that sexual intercourse led to conception. And their use long antedated the elucidation of the phases of the reproductive system, particularly the relationship between ovulation and menstruation, which was not achieved until the late 1920s.[10] It cannot be said that the spread of family-planning methods in European populations was to any extent impeded by lack of knowledge of the reproductive processes.

While the successful application of the rhythm method was impossible without a full comprehension of the relationship between ovulation and menstruation, we have to raise the question whether this holds for the successful use of the pill, the injectibles and the IUDs. In any event it is not clear whether the philosophy underlying programmes for the spreading of modern techniques of fertility control assumes the position that some understanding of the reproductive system is essential for the efficient practice of contraception. There is in fact ample discussion of the promotion of sex education in schools, but whether the curricula involved are intended to cover an adequate treatment of the reproductive system or are to be merely limited to the propriety of resorting to family-planning methods is not always manifest. Of course the evidence from the survey is that information about sex from any source conduces to enhanced knowledge of reproduction and menstruation.

Our emphasis here is not so much on knowledge as mere information, or as an indicator of the cultural level of the society, although these remain significant in their own right. Rather we are interested in knowledge in the sense of individual awareness, or, more properly, awareness that will ensure appropriate action. This is not to assume that such knowledge necessarily induces persons to make use of contraception, but it seems reasonable to urge that it should constitute a part of the intellectual equipment of any adult, in a society which is aiming at reducing its level of fertility.

The steady rise in resort to contraception with the rise in the degree of knowledge of both reproduction and menstruation strongly suggests that such knowledge is one measure essential to ensure the spread and, possibly as well, the continued and efficient use of modern contraceptive methods. This argument of course rests on the premise that an understanding of reproductive processes will prepare users for any changes in their menstrual cycle that may appear; these will probably be less alarming, as they are expected. But the possibility cannot be ruled out that knowledge of this nature may not always induce women to resign themselves to any form of bodily change that a contraceptive may induce. Indeed the possibility has to be faced that an increase in knowledge may make some women less likely to accept drastic changes in their menstrual patterns, or other bodily functions, which use of a given method may entail. Whatever the ultimate effects of such knowledge, there seems to be on balance a strong case for ensuring the spread of adequate knowledge of reproductive processes in general and of menstruation in particular.

Notes

1. Views of this nature are widespread, as is shown for instance in James Leslie McCary, *Sexual Myths and Fallacies* (New York: Van Nostrand Reinhold Co., 1971), pp. 62–63.

2. This concept of "health" in relation to menstruation goes back to the days of Aristotle, as is shown in Raymond Crawford, "Of Superstitions concerning Menstruation," *Proceedings Royal Society of Medicine (Section Historical Medicine) 1915*, 9, pp. 49–66. Modern writers also deal with this association between "health" and menstruation, see for instance Janice Delaney, Mary Jane Lupton, and Emily Toth, *The Curse: A Cultural History of Menstruation* (New York: Dutton, 1976), passim.

3. The literature on taboos associated with menstruation is vast; especially important are the writings of anthropologists. Convenient recent discussions can be found in Delaney, Lupton and Toth, *The Curse*. Part One; and Paula Weideger, *Menstruation and Menopause: The Physiology and Psychology, the Myth and the Reality* (New York: Alfred Knopf, 1976), especially Chapter 4; McCary, *Sexual Myths*, pp. 16–17.

4. Delaney, Lupton and Toth, *The Curse*, Chapter 4; and Weideger, *Menstruation and Menopause*, Chapter 4.

5. Delaney, Lupton and Toth, *The Curse*, Chapter 2; Weideger, *Menstruation and Menopause*, Chapter 4; and McCary, *Sexual Myths*, pp. 12–13.

6. Many of the taboos mentioned here have their parallels in other cultures, as is shown in Delaney, Lupton and Toth, *The Curse*, pp. 9–13.

7. Customs isolating menstruating and immobilising menstruating women are widespread. See especially Delaney, Lupton and Toth, *The Curse*, pp. 5–13.

8. This is an old belief, as is shown in R. Crawford, "Of Superstitions", pp. 49–66.

9. J. A. and Olive Banks, *Feminism and Family Planning in Victorian England* (Liverpool University Press, 1964), pp. 97–100.

10. K. Ogino, "Ovulationstermin und Konzeptionstermin," *Zentralbl. f. Gynak.* 54 (1930), p. 464; and H. Knaus, "Eine neue Methode zur Bestimmung des Ovulationstermines," *Zentralbl. f. Gynak.* 53 (1929), p. 2193.

Chapter 7
Pregnancy Outcome, Child Mortality and Replacement, and Twins

An important part of the survey centered around the securing of information on pregnancy histories of respondents. These include not only the outcome of each pregnancy, but also its duration, the month and year of termination, type of attendant at delivery, place of delivery and complications of pregnancy. Further data relevant to this topic deal with mortality experienced by the children born to respondents. With a sample of 501 women no detailed studies of losses among their children can be carried out. But it is believed that the broad categories dealt with present an adequate pattern of some aspects of child mortality in the society. Two other subjects dealt with in this chapter are the frequency of twins and the replacement hypothesis.

Pregnancy Outcome

The total number of pregnancies to the 501 women in the sample is set out in Table 7.1, which shows their outcome, their place of delivery and the type of person in attendance at delivery. Of the total of 1,699 pregnancies, 1,537 result in livebirths, 35 in stillbirths and 127 in miscarriages. The latter are assumed to include some induced abortions, although information on this is not easily obtained, and in fact was not specifically sought in this survey.

The majority of confinements take place in homes (63%), and it is of interest to note the type of persons attending at these deliveries. One-half of these are delivered by trained nurses or midwives, some of whom may be attached to hospitals and making domiciliary deliveries under the auspices of these institutions. Other types of nurses in attendance at home deliveries are public health nurses or trained nurses in private practice. The second largest category of attendants at delivery consist of so-called nanas.[1] These are untrained birth attendants, who operate almost exclusively in rural areas. This group account for 26% of all deliveries in the survey and for 41% of all home

Table 7.1 Pregnancy outcome, place of delivery and attendants at delivery, numbers and proportional (%) distribution

Pregnancy outcome	Home delivery by:				All attendants	Hospital delivery by:		All attendants	Total deliveries
	Nurse	Nana	Doctor	Self		Nurse	Doctor		
					Numbers				
Livebirths	525	420	23	–	968	437	130	569**	1,537
Miscarriages	4	13	7	58	83*	14	30	44	127
Stillbirths	9	9	–	–	19*	7	9	16	35
Total	538	442	30	58	1,070	458	169	629	1,699
					Proportional distribution %				
Livebirths	97.6	95.0	76.7	–	90.4	95.4	76.9	90.5	90.5
Miscarriages	0.7	3.0	23.3	100.0	7.8	3.1	17.8	7.0	7.5
Stillbirths	1.7	2.0	–	–	1.8	1.5	5.3	2.5	2.0
Total	100.0	100.0	100.0	100.0	100.0	100.0	100.0	100.0	100.0

*Includes 1 delivery for whom the attendant is unknown.
**Includes 2 deliveries for whom the attendants are not stated.

deliveries. Very few home deliveries are made by doctors, who evidently are called upon to deal only with deliveries of this nature which present special obstetrical problems.

Of the two types of attendants responsible for hospital deliveries, it may be assumed that nurses are engaged in routine cases, while doctors take charge of the more difficult ones. The former account for 73% of hospital deliveries and the latter for 27%.

When we consider the outcome of pregnancies, we note that the percentage distribution in terms of livebirths, stillbirths and miscarriages is the same in home deliveries as those in hospitals, with 90% being livebirths, 8% miscarriages and 2% stillbirths. In the case of nurses performing home deliveries, as much as 98% are livebirths; the corresponding proportion in the case of nanas is also very high (95%). It is interesting to note that deliveries made by nanas are not associated with unduly high rates of stillbirths. But for doctors making home deliveries, where there are presumably many difficult cases, the proportion of livebirths is much lower (77%). In terms of the survey definition, home deliveries with the term "self" in attendance constitute miscarriages of one form or another.

Of the two forms of hospital delivery, that by nurses puts 95% as consisting of livebirths, which is slightly lower than the corresponding proportion for home deliveries made by nurses. Hospital deliveries by doctors, who again will be responsible for complicated cases, show 77% livebirths, the same as in the case of doctors making home deliveries. And 18% of these deliveries are miscarriages, while the proportion recorded as stillbirths is the highest for all forms of delivery (5%).

In summary, it can be said that trained personnel—doctors and nurses—are in attendance at 1,195 deliveries, that is 70% of the total. Livebirths account for 93% of all deliveries by trained personnel, which is much higher than the corresponding proportion for untrained personnel (84%). And it follows that proportions of miscarriage among the former class of delivery is much lower than it is for delivery made by untrained personnel, 5% as against 14%.

Foetal Mortality and Perinatal Mortality[2]

Foetal losses in the form of miscarriages and stillbirths can be expressed in terms of rates of loss, when related to the relevant number of pregnancies. Two such types of loss are discussed here. The first, termed late foetal loss, consists of stillbirths, while the second, termed total foetal loss, is made up of stillbirths as well as miscarriages. These rates are presented in Table 7.2. The position with regard to two forms of home deliveries is that the lower rate of late foetal loss is that of deliveries made by nurses (17), while the corresponding loss among deliveries for which nanas are responsible amounts to 21. Turning to hospital deliveries, we note that those done by nurses again show the most favourable level (16), while doctors, who doubtless encounter the more serious deliveries, show a level of loss of 65 per 1,000.

Slightly different relative levels emerge when we examine the rates of total foetal loss. Thus whereas rates of late foetal loss in the case of both categories of nurses—those making home deliveries and those engaged in hospitals—are

Table 7.2 Stillbirth rate, foetal death rate and perinatal death rate per 1,000 by place of delivery and person in attendance

Persons responsible for delivery	Stillbirth rate	Foetal death rate	Perinatal mortality rate
Home delivery by:			
Nurse	16.9	24.2	33.7
Nana	21.0	49.8	37.3
Doctor and self	—	738.6	173.9
All attendants	19.3	95.4	37.5
Hospital delivery by:			
Nurse	15.8	45.9	31.5
Doctor	64.7	230.8	107.9
All attendants	27.3	95.4	49.4
Total	22.3	95.3	42.0

Note: The stillbirth rate is obtained by relating stillbirths to live and stillbirths. Foetal death rate relates miscarriages and stillbirths to total pregnancies. Perinatal mortality relates stillbirths and infant deaths of less than 1 week to live and stillbirths.

about the same, in the case of total foetal loss, the level among deliveries performed by nurses in hospital is nearly twice that for nurses responsible for home deliveries—46 as against 24 per 1,000. Losses resulting from deliveries attended by doctors (as well as those termed "self" in the case of home deliveries) emphasise the higher level of miscarriages, some of which probably consist of induced abortions. These are extremely high for home deliveries because of the category termed "self," but the losses among hospital deliveries are also considerable. At the same time, it is of interest that on the overall basis, the total foetal loss is about the same for home as for hospital deliveries.

A measure complementing rates of foetal loss is the rate of perinatal mortality which relates stillbirths and deaths in the first week of life to live and stillbirths. The rationale of this rate is that pregnancy losses in the form of stillbirths and deaths occurring among infants within the first week of life may be traceable to the same causes. These rates again show that pregnancies attended by doctors are subject to exceptionally high levels of wastage and here also this may be attributed to the fact that they are inherently difficult obstetrical cases which by their very nature have to be handled by doctors. Unlike the overall foetal rate, however, rates of perinatal mortality among deliveries made by nurses are higher when they occur in homes (34) than when done at hospitals (31). The perinatal rate for all home deliveries (37) is appreciably lower than the rate for all hospital deliveries (49).

Probabilities of Dying Among Infants

In order to present a more detailed picture of loss of life among the different categories of deliveries, probabilities of dying within successive intervals of infancy are calculated from the data. This is done by taking all livebirths in the particular category as a cohort and subjecting it to losses over three intervals of age under 1, and also during the interval 1 to 2 years. Because of the very small numbers involved, this can be done only for three of the categories recognised—home deliveries by nurse, home deliveries by nana and hospital deliveries by nurse. By grouping women of different ages we are presenting a composite picture of infant mortality, extending over a period exceeding 30 years. These probabilities of dying are given in Table 7.3.

The probability of dying under one week, that is within the early neonatal period, is lowest in the case of deliveries made by hospital nurses (11) and highest in the case of home deliveries made by nurses (19), with deliveries by nanas showing an intermediate level of 17. For the probability of dying within the late neonatal period as well, the lowest level is that among hospital deliveries made by nurses (7), while corresponding values for home deliveries are much higher: 17 for infants delivered by nanas and 12 for those delivered by nurses. The same form of differential obtains for probabilities of dying at 1

Table 7.3 Mortality (probabilities of dying per 1,000 at commencement of age interval) by place of delivery and person in attendance

Age interval	Home deliveries by:			Hospital deliveries by:		All deliveries
	Nana	Nurse	Total	Nurse	Total	
Under 1 week	17	19	18	11	19	18
1–4 weeks	17	12	15	7	9	15
1–12 months	35	27	31	19	18	23
Total under 1 year	67	55	64	37	46	55
1–2 years	13	6	9	8	18	14

to 12 months, when the rates are 19, 35 and 27 respectively. The summary picture in terms of probabilities of dying within the first year of life shows the appreciable difference among the three groups. For infants delivered by nurses in hospital, the level of mortality is 37 per 1,000, whereas the value for infants delivered in homes by nanas is 67, or 81% higher; the probability of dying within the first year of life among infants delivered by nurses at home amounts to 55, which exceeds the comparable value for hospital cases for which nurses are responsible by 49%.

A summary comparision—hospital deliveries versus home deliveries—shows that with the exception of the early neonatal period, where the probabilities of dying are the same, the hospital values are more favourable than those revealed by home deliveries. The summary position under 1 year shows a value of 64 for all deliveries in the home, which is 39% above that for hospital deliveries (46). Also included in Table 7.3 are probabilities of dying within the second year of life, although the very small numbers of deaths reported in this interval make comparisons somewhat uncertain. The probability for all home deliveries (9) is one-half the comparable value for hospital deliveries. No causal factors can at this stage be advanced for this differential. In the case of home deliveries, probabilities of dying are high among those delivered by nanas (13), while the value for pregnancies for which nurses are responsible is just under half this level (6).

Two features of infant mortality revealed in these data call for further comment. One is the mortality status of infants delivered by nanas. In the case of mortality within the first week of life, their experience compares favourably with that of the other category of infants. In fact it is lower than all except the losses among infants delivered by nurses in hospitals. Thus, before environmental factors begin to impinge seriously on the health of the infants, those delivered by nanas are not at a disadvantage compared with those delivered by trained medical personnel. However at all higher ages mortality among infants delivered by nanas moves up appreciably compared with the position of other infants. One possible reason for this is lack of appropriate post-natal care among infants for whose delivery nanas are responsible. The latter may be remiss in advising mothers on the necessity of having their children immunised and of carrying them to clinics; it may indeed be beyond their competence to do so. Thus these infants remain largely unprotected against diseases which begin to take their toll after the first week of life.

Secondly, while the adverse experience of children delivered by nanas within the later months of infancy stands out, there is also a differential with regard to deliveries made by nurses. Such deliveries when effected at home are associated with much higher mortalities at ages where environmental elements begin to influence the child's health. Once more it is possible that mothers delivered at hospitals receive better advice concerning the care of their babies than do those who are delivered at their homes. Another possible factor is that mothers seeking hospital deliveries are in fact more motivated to follow the advice they receive concerning post-natal care.

It must however be stressed that neither of the two foregoing arguments can be substantiated from survey material, as questions on children's attendance at post-natal clinics and on their immunisation status were not included in the questionnaire.

Summary of Pregnancy Wastage and Child Mortality

The picture of pregnancy loss and mortality under age 2 outlined in detail above can be conveniently summarised by means of a life table application. Here the total of livebirths, stillbirths and miscarriages are taken as the sum of all pregnancies experienced by the 501 women in the survey. These amount to 1,537, 35 and 127 respectively, thus yielding a total of 1,699, that is 3.39 per woman in the sample. As must again be emphasised, the principal limitation of this estimate of total pregnancies is clearly the component termed miscarriages. These represent exclusively events reported by respondents. Since estimates of induced abortions in the population at large are very high, the number of miscarriages reported in the survey is used here with the qualification that it is by no means to be construed as a satisfactory estimate of this component.

From the available material, pregnancy losses suffered, as well as neonatal mortality, mortality under age 1 and mortality from age 1 to age 2, can be determined. The total of recorded pregnancies to all women of the sample (1,699) has been used as the starting point, as in fact a cohort of known pregnancies whose outcomes can be traced and whose wastage and mortality can also be studied. This is best done however in terms of a cohort of 1,000 and consequently the experience of the total pregnancies is corrected to this more convenient form, as is shown in Table 7.4. It is seen that, on the basis of a total of 1,000 pregnancies, wastage due to reported miscarriages, which are

Table 7.4 Summary of pregnancy loss and mortality to age 2

Description of pregnancy loss or deaths	Interval of time (months)	Pregnancy loss or deaths	Survivors of the total of 1,699 pregnancies to beginning of stated interval	Survivors of the total of 1,000 pregnancies to beginning of stated interval	Probabilities of loss or deaths per 1,000 survivors in stated interval
Reported miscarriages	0–6	127	1,699	1,000	75
Stillbirths	6–9	34	1,572	925	22
Early neonatal deaths	9–9.25	28	1,538	905	18
Late neonatal deaths	9.25–10	22	1,510	889	15
Post-neonatal deaths	10–21	34	1,488	876	23
Deaths during 2nd year of life	21–33	20	1,454	856	14
Total pregnancy losses	0–9	161	—	—	95
Total deaths under 1 year	9–21	84	—	—	55

Note: Survivors of the total of 1,699 pregnancies to the end of the second year amount to 1,434. The corresponding value on the basis of a cohort of 1,000 is 844.

taken as the types of loss experienced up to the sixth month of pregnancy, reduces the cohort to 925. Stillbirths bring it down further, so that livebirths represent 90% of total pregnancies, as defined in the present context. Early neonatal deaths involve a loss of 16 infants; and late neonatal deaths, a loss of a further 13. Thus of the original cohort of 1,000 pregnancies, the number of infants alive at the end of the first month of age is 876. This indicates a loss up to this stage of 12% of the original cohort. Post-neonatal deaths, amounting to 20, bring down the number of survivors to the end of the first year of life to 856, and this indicates an overall rate of infant mortality of 54 per 1,000. There are 12 deaths in the second year of the cohort's life, that is up to the 33rd month after conception; this indicates a probability of dying of 14 per 1,000.

Thus of the total cohort, pregnancy wastage accounts for a loss of 95, infant mortality a loss of 49 and deaths in the second year of life a loss of 12. It is therefore within the first 6 months of pregnancy that the greatest decrement is sustained, but of course the period in which it reaches its greatest intensity is the first week of life.

Impact of Child Mortality on the Family[3]

One of the aims of the study of mortality among young children was to try to find out how these tragic events influence the functioning family. Besides the emotional disturbances they produce, they may also affect such aspects of family life as the decision to replace dead children, and some study of these also formed part of the survey.

Since we are investigating the effects of infant deaths on parents, on their other children and generally on the conditions within the family, we are in fact treating mortality not in the general statistical sense as the relationship between events (deaths) and numbers at risk of experiencing such deaths (the appropriate population), but rather as events having a complex impact on the group of individuals making up the family units. Questions put to respondents on this topic are designed to find out their views on how deaths of young children affect the family in various ways. Did such deaths make her or her partner ill or cause either of them any emotional disturbance? Did they engender any feeling of guilt, that is did respondents feel themselves in any way responsible for deaths of their children? Did these deaths have any effect on the sexual relationships between them and their partners? Did respondents consider replacing these children? Then there was a specific question to find out how the father was affected and a further one aimed at ascertaining the mother's interpretation of the impact on her surviving children. Finally the respondent is asked how she thought the entire family was influenced by the loss. As in other aspects of this survey, a few respondents are uncertain as to details concerning deaths of their children, but the general impression gained is that these events make an indelible impact on their memories; this is strongly emphasised by the fact that recall of the precise circumstances surrounding the death prove often very painful to them.

Expressions of grief at the death of young children are recorded by virtually all women who experience such losses. Indeed, of the mothers who lost children only 3 come out with statements which do not contain overtones of sadness or consider the death a tragic occurrence. One mother said she was happy because the maintenance of the child "wasn't pretty" and she felt the child "would punish" and she "would punish" also and she would be getting older "so fast." But even here her reaction was more an expression of resignation than one of happiness. Another mother who did not directly report any feeling of sadness claimed that she did not even cry, and was not affected at all. Although "it was hard" when she lost the first child, she still did not "fret." In the words of a third mother who lost one of twins, the family was not affected much. She did not "feel any way about the death of the child." The father was not concerned, nor did the death affect the family in any way.

But apart from these 3 mothers, the reaction to deaths of young children was sadness, dismay and emotional upset, which all members of the family usually share. One mother "cried day and night up to a year after." In some cases the mother showed great distress when asked about the death of her children. One asked the interviewer, "Please don't remind me [of the death]," as she still reacts badly to discussion of the subject. Another mother "went out of my mind for about 6 months after. Sometimes I would find myself 10 miles from home and did not know how I got there or what I was doing there .... I felt walled in and separated from everybody." It so happened that this mother was pregnant at the time of the death of her child. Illness of several kinds accompanied these emotional upsets.

A pathetic picture is painted by one mother who lost her first child. She and her partner were sad as it was their first child and she was looking forward to having it, but she "did not let it beat us down." She believes that "nothing can happen unless the Lord permits it." Once when she went to the bathroom she squeezed her breast and milk came and then she "felt very, very badly and cried a little but not for long." The father reacted to the death in the same way, and encouraged her "to think of replacing it."

In some cases this feeling of sadness, loss and despair extends to the fathers. Terms such as "very upset," "very sad," and "sorry" are used in describing the reaction of fathers to deaths of their children. One father "was very sorry and talked about it every day that he has no boy." Sometimes he consoles his partner at the loss and in many cases where replacement is mentioned he fully shares in this desire to replace the lost infant.

Although the reactions of the children are by no means so widely reported as those of parents, there are very many families in which the sadness was expressed by surviving children as well. Many cried and missed their lost brothers or sisters, although they are by no means so greatly affected as their parents. Very often they are too young to feel the loss deeply and where expressions of sorrow are reported, these seem to be of short duration.

While mothers express reactions of sorrow and distress at the death of their children, these expressions are in some instances accompanied by resignation at the loss. Usually this resignation has religious overtones. In the words of one mother, "The Lord giveth and giveth away." In another family, consolation is found in the position, "God knows best." Resignation also appears in such terms as, "God's will," "the Lord's will," "God's work," "God's plan," in discussions of deaths of children.

Many mothers went in for soul-searching, wondering whether any measure of guilt attaches to them because of their remissness in not seeking medical attention, or doing so too late to save the child's life. One mother felt guilty over the death of her child whom the doctor said should have been hospitalised but whom she begged to be allowed to take home. Another felt guilty because of the delay in seeking medical aid for her sick child.

One of the aims of this study is to explore the relationships between the woman and her partner under varying conditions within the three types of unions recognised. Deaths of children within the family represent very disturbing occurrences which should shed some light on the cohesion of the family unit. One question seeks explicitly to find out whether the death of a child in any way affects the relationships between partners, the sexual relationships being particularly stressed here, as this may also have some bearing on the question of replacing the child. Very few mothers offer any information on the impact of death on their sexual activity. One mother reports that the sexual relationships between her and her partner remained unchanged as they "did not want another child then." Another states that she "did not enjoy sex for a while" after the child's death. Similarly another had "no sex for a long time as I had lost the desire." A mother of 11 children, 4 of whom died, reports that after the death of one, these sexual relationships increased as they wanted "a baby to hold." None of the comments of respondents show that relationships between the parents are greatly strengthened or significantly weakened as a result of a death of a child. But the fact that respondents almost universally report that grief was shared by their partners suggests that no weakening of the family bonds takes place as a consequence of such losses.

Infant Mortality Among Families

So far the discussion of mortality has followed the usual approach in which rates are derived by relating deaths treated as single events to appropriate births at risk. However a case can be made out for analysing mortality in terms of events occurring within a given environmental unit, such as a household or a family. There are definitional issues to be faced here, but in the case of the family unit these may be resolved simply by taking as a family all children ever born to the respondent.[4] Several characteristics of the individual family units can be taken as the bases for analysis in this context. Here we are especially concerned with the number of deaths occurring in family units of different sizes. And there are a variety of characteristics in terms of which deaths to families of different sizes may be treated. Such aspects as union type, educational status and age are of relevance. But elaborate breakdowns are precluded because of the very small numbers involved. A major limitation of the approach which has to be followed is that combining the experience of women of all ages results in a picture of mortality extending over a period of a generation.

Conceivably rates of mortality calculated on the basis of families may be affected by at least three elements. In the first place the size of family may play a dominant part. Statistically, it seems reasonable to assume that the larger the number of children ever born to a woman, the greater the number of deaths among such children. This will hold whether or not the probabilities of death are functionally linked to size of family. For even the existence of the same probabilities over families of all sizes would entail larger numbers of deaths among larger families, because of the greater numbers at risk. Secondly, variations in conditions within the family units may imply differential impacts of environmental factors affecting mortality. Indeed, on this basis it is probable that unfavourable social and economic conditions within the family units may expose them to severe mortality, especially from diseases which have their origin in environmental conditions. One type of information which should illuminate this aspect of mortality bears on the cause of death, but this cannot be utilised here because of the very small numbers involved and because of the comparatively high proportion of cases which do not supply cause of death information. Thirdly, there is the possibility that the risk of mortality among children within a family unit may be a function of their genetic make-up, which in turn derives from their parents. In other words, more than one child in a family may succumb to diseases transmitted from their parents. This however seems to be of less importance in the present context than the factors of family size and environmental conditions mentioned above. In any event genetic implications are greatly complicated by the prevailing types of mating. It is not at all clear how the genetic make-up of children is affected by the woman's involvement in a succession of relationships with different partners. It is of course conceivable that all three factors may be operative in producing the pattern of mortality by families which can be gleaned from the present survey.

Here, as in the earlier analysis, we consider only deaths under 3 years of age. Deaths experienced by respondents in this survey can be classified into five categories. Four of these are based on the numbers of deaths each family experiences—that is families with 1, 2, 3 or 4 deaths. The fifth designates families in which the single death experienced is one of twins. In Table 7.5 the number of families experiencing different numbers of deaths are shown, together with the numbers of children they have, and appropriate rates derived from the basic information. Figure 7.1 shows the relationship

Table 7.5 Characteristics of families experiencing deaths of children under 2 years in terms of size, numbers of deaths and proportion dying

Number of deaths under 2 years in a family	Number of families experiencing these deaths (a)	Total number of children dying in families (b)	Total number of children ever born in families (c)	Proportion dying (b)/(c)	Average size of family (c)/(a)
1	53	53	282	0.188	5.32
2	19	38	144	0.264	7.58
3	6	18	46	0.391	7.67
4	3	12	34	0.353	11.33
Deaths among twins	5	6	29	0.207	5.80
Total	86	127	535	0.237	6.22

Note: Records of deaths among 5 sets of twins show 4 cases in which 1 of the twins died and 1 case in which both of a set of twins died.

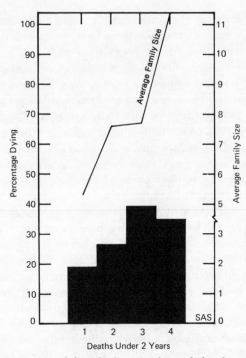

Figure 7.1 Average size of family by number of deaths under 2 years in family and proportion (%) dying·by number of deaths under 2 years in family

between numbers of deaths and the average size of family in which these take place.

According to the distribution of families by the number of deaths each has suffered, it appears that of the total of 86, 53 or 62% experience a single death, while those suffering 2, 3 or 4 deaths amount to 28 or 33% of the total. In a small proportion of families (6%), a single death (or 2 deaths) experienced is one of (or a set of) twins. These 86 families contribute in all 127 deaths under 2 years of age, that is an average of 1.48 per family. Thus had the 86 families involved each contributed a single death there would have been 86 such deaths to women in the sample, that is 41 less than the total actually experienced.

In considering the family-size aspect of the picture, the important point to note is that all families which suffered losses of children are much larger than the average for the whole sample. The latter value is 3.07, which is about half the average size for all families who have reported deaths (6.22). In other words, the families in this sample who contribute to deaths of children under 2 years of age are also those who contribute heavily to the number of children ever born. Thus size of family may be taken as an important component determining the loss through deaths in families. This may not fully warrant the generalisation that the larger the size of family the greater the number of deaths under age 2. But the fact that families experiencing a single death show an average size of family of 5.32 and that this value moves up fairly regularly with the numbers of deaths experienced to a maximum of 11.33 in the case of those losing 4 children seems to support such a proposition.

By relating the numbers of deaths experienced in each family category to the total family size of each such category we obtain a measure of mortality which enables us to compare the rates of loss each experiences. These rates should reflect differentials that may originate as a consequence of any or all of the three factors indicated above, that is size of family, environmental conditions or genetic features. These rates show clearly a rise with the number of deaths contributed. Thus in the case of families contributing a single death, the rate of loss is 0.19, and this moves up to a maximum of 0.39 among families that experience 3 deaths. The slight decline to 0.35 in the case of the small number of families that experience 4 deaths is still consistent with a general tendency for mortality to rise as family size increases.

There is therefore strong indication that family size is in some way associated with the level of mortality within the family. It would have been useful to pursue this analysis further, in order to ascertain for instance whether socio-economic status differentials or aspects of union types are in any way involved. But unfortunately the very small numbers of women with whom we are dealing preclude any more detailed examination of the topic. The complex nature of the relationship between mortality and family size has been stressed by Brass and Barrett in their simulation study of the problem.[5]

Child Replacement[6]

The question whether the death of a child leads its mother consciously to entertain the notion of replacing it and, possibly, taking steps to do so is now of interest from several angles. It appears to be of special relevance in view of marked falls in infant mortality noted in many societies where fertility is high. For the extent to which women in these societies replace dead children has some effect on levels of fertility. Many approaches to this question take the form of macroanalysis, which seeks to infer from studies of mortality and fertility patterns among large groups of people or from entire populations whether parallel movements in these two vital processes can be discerned.

It may be contended that results already made available in this analysis afford some support for the replacement hypothesis. For it has been already shown that when the mothers are classified according to the number of children in their family who have died, there is a clear association between family size and level of mortality. Women in whose families are found lowest levels of infant mortality have also the lowest level of fertility, and as we move up the mortality scale, so the level of fertility also tends to rise. Suggestive as this macro approach is, it seems essential to examine the survey data more critically and to rely on what can be gleaned from the records concerning fertility patterns and mortality levels within each family unit experiencing one or more deaths during the first 5 years of life of the children involved. In this survey an attempt is made to relate answers to a specific question on the topic to some relevant information on family building patterns and child mortality. This moves the examination from the macro to the micro approach.

The relevant question on this topic is, "Did you consider replacing the [dead] child?" Answers to this fall into three categories. The most frequent is in effect a no-response to the question, and is interpreted as a negative answer, that is to indicate that no consideration was given to replacing the dead child. A much smaller group of mothers who experience deaths among their family claim that they considered replacing dead children; these constitute the second category. A still smaller number of respondents explicitly deny having considered replacement of their dead children. In the present context, the first and third categories are taken together to represent all women who do not claim to have considered replacement of such children.

The limitations of the claim of the second category as a measure of replacement are manifest. In the first place, it is by no means certain whether at the time of the death of the child the consideration of replacement took the form of definite behavioural patterns aimed at ensuring the birth of a child. Probably the process involves no more than the maintenance of certain family size norms that had come to be part of the society. Nevertheless the acknowledgement of such a consideration by a respondent seems to suggest a readiness on her part and, possibly, on her partner's as well to try to ensure another birth. By contrast, her failure to consider replacement may be interpreted as signifying that no course of action was taken to ensure further births, although it does not necessarily follow that steps were taken to avoid additional births. These data have to be treated with caution and we have to be careful not to read too much into them. For in view of the very few women with any adequate knowledge of the reproductive processes and the modest numbers who report ever having used contraception, it remains highly unlikely that many of them were in a position consciously to set out to build families in accordance with decisions to replace or not to replace dead children.

As a first step in the examination of the hypothesis of replacement, two categories of women who have experienced deaths of children may be established. The first consists of women claiming to have considered replacing children who have died, and the second covering women who advance no claim of this nature. In order to gain fuller insight into the question of replacement, a further dichotomy of women who have lost children is required. The first of these consists of women who have had children after the death of the infant which is the subject of analysis. Falling within the second are women for whom the dead child is the last. Whereas women in the first category continue childbearing after the death of their children, those in the second have no further children after the death occurs. If it can be shown that women who continue to have children after the death of the child are also those for the most part claiming to have considered replacement, this would constitute some support for the replacement hypothesis. Moreover, if the majority of women making no replacement claim consist of those who have no further children after the death occurs, this would be another line of support for the replacement hypothesis.

A simple approach to this hypothesis is to compile a fourfold table, with relevant subsections; this is the subject of Table 7.6. It gives the position of all women who experience deaths of children, as well as those who suffer a single death and those who lost more than one child. Of the 90 women in the survey who report deaths of young children (including some over 2), 26 or 29% claim

Table 7.6 Women experiencing deaths within their families according to whether or not they claimed to have considered replacement

Categories of families experiencing deaths among their children	Women claiming they considered replacement	Women not claiming they considered replacement	Total
Families experiencing 1 death			
Women bearing further children after child's death	14	36	50
Women bearing no further children after child's death	5	7	12
Total	19	43	62
Families experiencing more than 1 death			
Women bearing further children after child's death	7	17	24
Women bearing no further children after child's death	—	4	4
Total	7	21	28
All families experiencing deaths			
Women bearing further children after child's death	21	53	74
Women bearing no further children after child's death	5	11	16
Total	26	64	90

Note: The total number of families in this table (90) differs slightly from the number in Table 7.5 because the former includes deaths of children over 2 years of age.

to have considered replacement. This proportion is somewhat higher for those reporting a single death in the family (31%) than it is for those reporting several deaths (25%).

It is at once evident that by far the majority of mothers who report deaths in their families continue bearing children after such deaths have occurred. For women in the survey as a whole, 82% fall within this category. The corresponding proportion for women with one death in their family is 81%; for the smaller numbers with more than one death, the proportion is 86%. While these very large proportions of women who continue childbearing after suffering deaths within their families suggest some support for the replacement hypothesis, it is by no means conclusive. Only if the proportions prove to be .much higher among women claiming to have considered replacement could they be taken as definitely supporting the hypothesis in question. As it is, the differentials between the sets of proportions in no way confirm that replacement does take place. Both those who claim to have considered replacement and those who make no such claims show high proportions who continue family building after the death of their children. It should also be emphasised that the relative ages of the respondents have little effect on the situation. Of the women involved, 14 are over 35 and thus may be approaching the end of their childbearing period; of these, 4 claimed to have considered replacement. Thus the exclusion of these does not materially affect the proportions already quoted.

Despite the fact that at the macro level the survey data furnish some evidence supporting the replacement hypothesis, there is no confirmation of this from the micro approach. True, 29% claim to have considered replacing the children who died, but there is no evidence that their pattern of family building differs to any degree from that characterising mothers who advance no such claims.

Twins

Throughout the ages the occurrence of multiple products of conception has proved a constant source of fascination irrespective of the multiple involved. The most frequent is of course that of 2 or twins and it is this group with which we are here concerned.

There are 26 pairs of twin conceptions among the 1,700 pregnancies of the women in the study. The ages of the mothers at the times of these events range from 18 to 38 years. The modal age group is 25 to 29, with 9 pairs being born to women between these ages, and the average age of the entire group is 27.7 years. The ages of 6 fathers are unknown but for the remaining 20 their average age is 37.3 years with the peak of the age group being bimodal with 5 at 25 to 29 and 6 at 40 to 44 years. The 2 youngest fathers are in the group 20 to 24 and the oldest in 50 to 54. Eleven sets are born to married women, 9 to those in visiting unions and 6 to mothers in common-law unions.

These 26 pairs and 52 products are produced by 21 women. The majority (17) have only 1 set, while 3 women have 2 and 1 woman has 3 consecutive sets in 5 years. These 26 sets give a ratio of 1 in 65 pregnancies. The rate of twinning differs among races and is highest for negroes as a whole and the Yorubas of Nigeria in particular, with a rate of 1 in 22 pregnancies.[7] This racial difference is largely in respect of fraternal twinning as the rate of identicals is similar in most populations of whatever racial group.

The terms identical and fraternal refer to the basic units of conception, that is all multiples from 1 egg are identical and with very rare exceptions these are always of the same sex, 2 boys or 2 girls. Fraternals on the other hand are the products of 2 separate eggs being fertilised within a short period of each other. These simultaneous conceptions therefore permit of a threefold combination in respect of sex. Thus we may have a boy/girl pair, the most obvious fraternals, 2 girls or 2 boys. The 2 latter combinations, while appearing similar, are in fact 2 quite distinct individuals, as is the case with singleton births.

It is evident therefore that the designation of true identical twins is not a straightforward one based on sex. However since the rate of identicals is, as has been pointed out earlier, similar for most racial groups, the rate which shows true racial difference is that of the fraternals. According to Weinberg's formula the proportion of identicals can be calculated by doubling the percentage of known fraternals and subtracting this from 100. This gives the total percentage of fraternals and the differences are the identicals.[8] On this basis we can calculate the percentage of identical twins born to the 1946 to 1950 motherhood cohort as follows:

Known fraternals—3 sets	= 33.33%
(Other like sex pairs—6 sets)	
Total fraternals	= 66.66%
∴ Identicals	= 33.34%

The 26 pairs consist of 11 all male, 10 all female and 5 male/female sets. These pregnancies resulted in one male set miscarrying at 4 months while 5 others were stillborn. Of these the 2 female sets were full term and no cause of death is given. One of the all male sets was full term, but the respondent suffered a post-partum haemorrhage and in the other case the mother was 5 months pregnant when she slipped and fell on the floor which resulted later in the delivery of stillbirths. In the case of the only boy/girl set the mother slipped and fell on her abdomen when she was 7 months pregnant and she was subsequently delivered of stillbirths. Of the remaining 20 sets, all liveborn, 18 are full term and two are of 7 months gestation.

Since it is evident that twins require more uterine space it is expected that high parity will enhance the ability to carry twins due to the increase in uterine size achieved from multiple pregnancies. In addition the propensity to twinning increases with age and parity. Thus we see that the majority (16) of these are born to women of parity 4 and above. Again, more than half (16) of these deliveries are in the mother's home while 10 are born in hospital—the high rate of hospital deliveries thereby attests to the special problems inherent in multiple births. This is further borne out when we note that 20 sets are delivered by nurses, either in the woman's home or in hospital and 4 by hospital doctors. In only 1 case is a nana responsible for the delivery and one of the twins died at age 1 month from respiratory problems. The only women who miscarried had no assistance.

With the exception of one set who were "weak" and had to be bottle fed all others were breastfed for periods ranging from 2 months to 18 months with the average period of breastfeeding being 6.7 months. In the majority of cases both twins were breastfed for the same length of time.

Although the number of twins in the sample is much too small to admit of the calculation of any meaningful rates of loss through mortality, it is still of interest to note the actual numbers and other features of deaths reported among the group. Of the 40 livebirths involved, 7 died before attaining the age of 1 year. By far the greatest toll is among early neonates, as 4 succumbed within 24 hours of birth. It is worthwhile to note further details of these 4 deaths. Two girls died within 15 minutes of birth, but no cause of death is available. One female of a male/female set died within 1 hour of birth and the cause is given as "stifled." The fourth case is the younger of an all girl set and she died after 15 hours and the cause is put down to prematurity. The infant reported as being "stifled" was a home delivery, with a nurse in attendance, while the other 3 were hospital deliveries.

Two deaths, both females, occurred in the late neonatal period and in both respiratory factors are listed as the cause. In the case of 1 girl who died at 12 months of age, no cause of death is available.

It is striking that all the deaths of the twins are females, even in the case of male/female sets. Only 1 other death, at a much later age, is recorded: this is of a boy who was "stuck" by a nail and developed tetanus after receiving no medical attention.

Another aspect of these twins calls for comment. This is the degree to which these children are given "twin" names. Thus we see that 10 sets, including the 4 liveborn boy/girl sets, are named in conformity with this tradition. Seven have nonrelated names and 8 sets which are either foetal or infant deaths are unnamed. One liveborn set have yet to be named.

Notes

1. According to F. C. Cassidy, "*Nana*, which in the Twi language means a grandparent of either sex, means in Jamaica a grandmother, an old woman, and therefore also a midwife (compare dialectical 'granny-

woman' in the United States). But the most usual sense in the cities is probably nursemaid ... ." F. C. Cassidy, *Jamaica Talk* (London: Macmillan, 1971), p. 166.

2. For a fuller discussion of mortality at young ages in Jamaica see G. W. Roberts et al., *Recent Population Movements in Jamaica* (Paris: Census Research Programme, University of the West Indies, C.I.C.R.E.D. Series, 1974), pp. 105 et seq.

3. It seems this subject is most generally treated by psychologists, as for instance in E. James Anthony and Cyrille Koupernik, eds., *The Child in His Family: The Impact of Disease and Death*, International Yearbook for Child Psychiatry and Allied Disciplines, vol. 2 (New York: John Wiley & Sons, 1973).

4. Some of the issues in defining size of family are examined in Samuel H. Preston, "Family Sizes of Children and Family Sizes of Women," *Demography* 13, no. 1 (February 1976), pp. 105–114; and L. Herberger, "The Demographic Approach to the Study of Family Health," *Social Science and Medicine* 8 (1974), pp. 535–544.

5. William Brass and J. C. Barrett, "The Measurement of Fertility and Child Mortality to Investigate Their Relationship in Studies of Aggregate and Family Data," in C.I.C.R.E.D., *Seminar on Infant Mortality in Relation to the Level of Fertility* (Paris, 1975).

6. The literature on child replacement is extensive. A recent general examination of this hypothesis appears in Carl E. Taylor, Jeanne S. Newman and Narindar U. Kelly, "The Child Survival Hypothesis," *Population Studies* 30, no. 2 (July 1976), pp. 263–271. Several technical papers on the subject are presented in C.I.C.R.E.D., *Seminar on Infant Mortality*.

7. J. B. Lawson and D. B. Stewart, *Obstetrics and Gynaecology in the Tropics and Developing Countries* (London: The English Language Book Society and Edward Arnold, 1974), p. 255.

8. Amram Scheinfeld, *Twins and Supertwins* (New York: Penguin, 1973), p. 64.

Chapter 8
Changing Patterns of Breastfeeding

Breastfeeding demands close attention in any analysis of reproduction because of the important role it plays in many aspects of child care. It constitutes a vital part in maintaining the proper nutritional status of the infant and several studies of health among children have implicated reduced breastfeeding in the appearance of certain diseases among them. Many studies have also demonstrated the association between duration of lactation and several causes of death among infants.[1] Further, the contention that prolonged lactation tends to be accompanied by an extension of the period of amenorrhoea has led to the hypothesis that it may constitute in effect a type of fertility control.[2] Neither of these two important phases of the subject is being taken up in this chapter. We are here wholly concerned with tracing the length of time that mothers nurse their infants and relating duration of nursing to a few of their salient characteristics.

General Patterns

One of the questions about the respondent's children deals with periods over which each was breastfed. This is recorded in terms of numbers of months for each liveborn child. Here, as in other fields of the survey, there is the possibility of recall lapse resulting in errors of various kinds, notably among older women and in respect of children of large families.

A feature of the replies is that there appears to be a series of patterns adopted by mothers. In some cases a particular pattern is reported for all of the respondent's children. In other cases patterns of breastfeeding may vary from one child to another, so that we have within a given family examples of several of the broad patterns noted. It is convenient to base the present analysis of this topic on children of orders 1 to 6, who number 1,264 or 82% of all livebirths in the survey. This suffices to give a reliable picture of nursing habits of the population.

The distributions of periods of breastfeeding display wide variation and have several modes. At their lower ends are infants who, for one reason or another, have not been breastfed. These amount to 56 or 4.4% of the total being analysed here. At their other ends are infants breastfed for periods in excess of 14 months. These number 17 or about 1.3% of all babies being studied here. More important is the emergence of patterns, showing concentrations on certain durations. By far the most arresting of these is the 9-month pattern. There appears to be a general belief that this is a desirable period to follow, but no satisfactory expression as to the basis for its widespread adoption has been offered by respondents. Two other patterns of shorter length are also prominent: one is of moderate extent, between 6 and 7 months, while the other is of short duration, that is 3 months. Six months, it should be noted, is the minimum period for breastfeeding recommended by some authorities.[3] It is therefore necessary to examine the relative concentration on these patterns or modes; the summary measure which is most appropriate to distributions of this nature is the median, and this is used throughout.

The first aspect of breastfeeding to be treated consists of medians and concentrations on the 3 patterns noted in terms of 2 broad age bands of mothers and order of birth of the children; these form the subject of Table 8.1 and Figure 8.1. With regard to women over age 45, the outstanding feature is the virtual equality of the median values of breastfeeding they reveal. These values, with one exception, lie between 9.7 and 9.8 months. The exception is in respect of infants of order 3, for whom a slightly longer period of 10 months is recorded. Associated with this median of between 9 and 10 months is a very high proportion of mothers who follow a period of exactly 9 months. The proportion reaches its highest value (39%) in the case of third-order

Table 8.1 Median periods of breastfeeding and % of children breastfed for 3, 6-7 and 9 months—infants of first to sixth order, mothers under 45 and over 45

Birth order	No. of children with mothers		Median period of breastfeeding (months) by mothers		% Children breastfed for 3 months		% Children breastfed for 6 to 7 months		% Children breastfed for 9 months	
					Mothers at ages					
	Under 45	Over 45	Under 45	Over 45	Under 45	Over 45	Under 45	Over 45	Under 45	Over 45
1	230	129	7.00	9.74	16.1	11.6	13.0	17.8	16.1	31.0
2	183	110	7.47	9.69	15.3	8.2	14.2	18.2	16.4	28.2
3	129	95	7.57	9.95	14.7	8.4	11.6	11.6	12.4	38.9
4	94	75	9.17	9.75	10.6	5.3	14.9	17.3	18.1	29.3
5	68	56	9.33	9.76	10.3	8.9	8.8	16.1	22.1	33.9
6	41	54	9.00	9.76	9.8	11.1	19.5	13.0	14.6	35.2

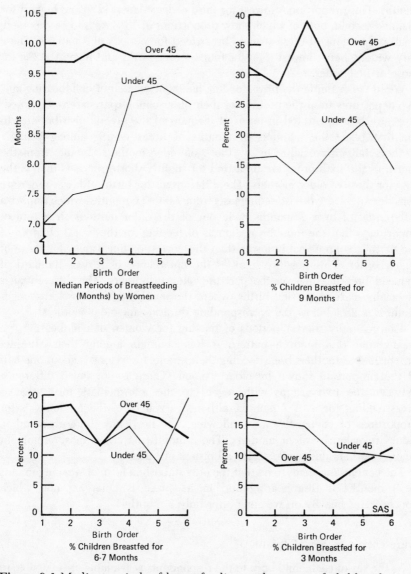

Figure 8.1 Median periods of breastfeeding and percent of children breast-fed for 3, 6–7 and 9 months, infants of first to sixth order, mothers under 45 and over 45

infants, and is lowest for those of the second order (28%). Much smaller proportions of these women of advanced ages report durations of 6 to 7 months. This proportion is lowest for third-order infants (12%) and highest for first and second, both of which show proportions of 18%. As is to be expected, small proportions of these women breastfeed for periods of 3 months. These vary widely, being lowest (5%) for fourth-order births and highest (12%) for those of first order.

When we examine the breastfeeding habits of women of childbearing age, two departures from the position of their older counterparts are to be noted; these are best illustrated in terms of medians of the several distributions. In the first place the numbers of months of breastfeeding among younger mothers falls appreciably below those of older mothers. Infants from the fourth to the sixth order are breastfed for slightly shorter periods than is the case for those of older mothers. The differentials for births of lower order are considerable. Here breastfeeding lasts from 7.0 to 7.6 months, which implies a differential of over 2 months in favour of the older mothers. It is also of importance that the number of months of feeding for the first 3 children of the mother is appreciably lower than the corresponding values for those of higher order. This possibly signifies the emergence of a new standard of reduced breastfeeding on the part of younger mothers. The differential is especially marked for first births, where the number of months for younger mothers is 28% below the corresponding duration for older mothers.

The generally shorter periods of nursing for women of childbearing age means that the 9-month pattern is less common among them. In fact proportions of mothers breastfeeding their infants for so long is about one-half of the proportion shown by older women. There is not much difference between the two groups with regard to the intermediate form, that is breastfeeding for 6 to 7 months, although, even here, the tendency is for proportions of younger women following it to be below the corresponding values revealed by older mothers. The 3-month pattern is most prominent among mothers under age 45 for all orders of birth.

The conclusion seems to be that the old established form of weaning infants at 9 months is disappearing and in its place is emerging one which concentrates heavily on weaning after only 3 months.[4]

Differentials by Sex of Infant

As the sex of each child born to the respondents is available, it is possible to ascertain whether there are any differentials with regard to the treatment accorded the two sexes in this matter. Using the same measures as in the previous discussion, we can compare feeding habits for the two sexes of infants, and again it is necessary to distinguish between women of child-bearing age and those of completed fertility. Both of these age cohorts of

Table 8.2 Median periods of breastfeeding and % of children breastfed for 3, 6-7 and 9 months—male and female children, mothers under 45 and over 45

Sex of child	No. of children with mothers		Median period of breastfeeding (months) by mothers		% Children breastfed for 3 months		% Children breastfed for 6 to 7 months		% Children breastfed for 9 months	
					Mothers at ages					
	Under 45	Over 45	Under 45	Over 45	Under 45	Over 45	Under 45	Over 45	Under 45	Over 45
Male	367	274	8.84	9.78	12.3	9.1	13.6	15.0	19.3	35.8
Female	378	245	7.50	9.80	15.9	9.0	13.0	17.1	13.2	28.6

mothers report a total of 641 male and 623 female births of order 1 to 6, and these form the basis of Table 8.2.

In terms of medians of the distributions, very little separates the patterns of nursing of male infants from those of females, when the analysis is confined to mothers past the childbearing span. The median period amounts to about 9.8 months for each sex. There is a strong concentration on the 9-month duration in the case of males, 36% of whom are nursed for this period. This pattern is somewhat less strongly represented in the experience of female infants, 29% of whom are breastfed for such a period. Appreciable numbers of both sexes enjoy breastfeeding for 6 to 7 months; these account for 15% of all male infants and 17% of all female. An examination of the short duration form (3 months) shows no differentials between the sexes, both indicating about 9% of their number nursing for so short a time.

The younger age cohort exhibits features similar to those outlined above. These mothers depict a much smaller reliance on lengthy breastfeeding, and the emergence of a much shorter period of nursing than that which characterises their older counterparts. The summary position, in terms of median values, shows a higher level for males than females, 8.8 as against 7.5 months. Associated with this is the somewhat higher proportion of male infants (19%) receiving breastfeeding for 9 months than is the case among females (13%). The proportion of infants enjoying breastfeeding for an intermediate period of 6 to 7 months is about the same for both sexes, approximately 13%. The greater proportion of female than male infants who have been breastfed for 3 months—16% as against 12%—is in accord with the appearance of a slightly higher median duration for male infants.

The general conclusion is that although there is evidence of a somewhat extended duration of breastfeeding for infant males, the sex differential is not pronounced. The important aspect is that both sexes show that younger mothers are tending to reduce the time they nurse their infants.

Differentials by Type of Union

Of interest is the question whether any differentials in duration and form of breastfeeding can be found among the three types of union identified. There are several ways of establishing types of union for such an analysis. The one seemingly most suited in the present context is to tabulate on the basis of the type of union in which the mother was involved at the time of the birth of each of her liveborn children. This in effect takes into account her family experience at the time of every birth she reports up to that of order 6, which means that some information on her union history and fertility is excluded. This approach, however, gives adequate representation of the prevailing nursing habits of each union type.

It is useful to link with the family typology other variables: women of childbearing age and those of completed fertility, early births (first and second), later births (third to sixth), as well as the sex of each infant. The medians according to these variables appear in Table 8.3. Perhaps the outstanding feature of this table is the appreciably longer period of breastfeeding shown for high order births as compared with that for births of first and second order. This differential is most marked among infants of married mothers. First- and second-order infants of these women over age 45 receive some 2 months less nursing than those of higher order, the differential being greater for female than male children. Married women of childbearing age show an even more pronounced differential in period of breastfeeding, according to the order of the infant. Thus for infants of both sexes of orders 3

Table 8.3 Median periods of breastfeeding (months) for 2 sets of children, by sex of child and union status of mothers under 45 and over 45

Sex of child	Mothers under 45		Mothers over 45	
	First and second children	Third to sixth children	First and second children	Third to sixth children
		Married		
Male	5.00	8.50	7.67	9.52
Female	4.79	8.50	7.06	9.50
Both sexes	4.86	8.50	7.21	9.51
		Common-law		
Male	8.83	9.76	9.00	10.04
Female	7.75	9.62	9.83	10.32
Both sexes	8.06	9.71	9.62	10.16
		Visiting		
Male	8.06	8.12	9.96	10.06
Female	7.94	7.00	10.12	10.06
Both sexes	8.00	7.68	10.02	10.06

to 6, the period is 1.7 times that of children of lower order. Accompanying this important differential, it should be noted, is a development commented on earlier, namely that an appreciable shortening of the period has been witnessed among the younger age cohort. This is as high as 2.4 months for infants of orders 1 and 2, and smaller (1 year) for those of orders 3 to 6.

Similar, but less marked, are the differentials for infants of mothers designated common-law. For older women first- and second-order infants receive between 1 month and one-half of a month less breastfeeding than do those of third and higher order. Infants of younger common-law mothers also present a well-defined differential, with early male births receiving about 1 month less than those of higher order, the medians being 8.8 and 9.8 months respectively; the corresponding differential for females is just below 2 months, with medians of 7.8 and 9.6 months respectively. Again, as in the case of married women, the general duration of breastfeeding has declined; thus for infants of orders 1 to 3 the reduction in the case of children of both sexes is 1.6 months, on the basis of the medians. By contrast, the corresponding reduction in medians shown for infants of orders 3 to 6 is only 0.4 month.

In contrast to the situation characterising infants born to married and common-law mothers, the position of those born to mothers in visiting relationships reveals minor differences with respect to birth order. The pronounced differences in time of weaning between infants of low and high birth order, so prominent in the case of children of married mothers, is absent from those of visiting mothers. Thus in the case of those born to mothers over age 45, median periods of breastfeeding do not depart much from 10 months, so that there is virtually no difference in terms of birth order or sex of infant. When we turn to infants of younger mothers, we see that, far from those of low order being weaned much earlier than those of higher order, there is in the case of females a definite advantage of nearly 1 month in favour of those of low birth order. The differential with regard to male infants of younger mothers is negligible. Reductions in periods of breastfeeding as shown by median values for the two age cohorts of mothers are appreciable. In the case of infants of orders 1 and 2, the reduction in median values is 2.0 months, while for those of higher order it reaches 2.4 months. The latter value is by far the highest for the 3 types of union.

Feeding habits characterising the three union types can be examined also by means of the extent to which they conform to the 9-month pattern, which is the subject of Table 8.4. Here is emphasised the high proportion of infants of orders 3 to 6 born to married mothers over age 45 who receive breastfeeding for such a period, as compared with the period enjoyed by those of orders 1 and 2. Infants born to women over age 45 who are in the other two types do not experience this form, as in this case very little separates the age at weaning for early and late infants. In fact common-law

Table 8.4 Proportion (%) of children breastfed for 9 months, by sex of child, and union status of mothers under 45 and over 45

Sex of child	Mothers under 45		Mothers over 45	
	First and second children	Third to sixth children	First and second children	Third to sixth children
		Married		
Male	19.44	10.86	24.24	36.23
Female	5.00	7.41	13.89	33.87
Both sexes	11.84	9.00	18.84	35.11
		Common-law		
Male	19.64	27.27	30.43	31.11
Female	11.63	16.00	25.00	27.50
Both sexes	16.16	21.71	27.66	29.41
		Visiting		
Male	16.81	20.51	42.42	42.11
Female	18.40	9.76	29.82	34.62
Both sexes	17.65	15.00	36.59	39.06

mothers report a proportion breastfeeding female infants of orders 1 and 2 which is greater than the corresponding values for infants of higher birth order. Another feature that seems to characterise mothers over age 45 is their tendency to follow the 9-month pattern more in the case of male than female infants; this is marked among those in married and visiting unions.

For mothers under age 45, there is much less of a regular differential between children of low and high birth orders, although a much smaller proportion of them receive breastfeeding for 9 months than is the case with those born to mothers over age 45. Male infants of orders 1 and 2 born to married mothers show a much higher proportion breastfed for 9 months than those of higher order (19.4% as against 10.9%), but the reverse is the case for female infants where the proportions are 5.0% and 7.4% respectively. When we turn to infants of common-law mothers under age 45, we see a greater concentration on the 9-month pattern for those of orders 3 to 6 for both sexes. On the other hand, the position in the visiting unions shows a higher proportion with 9 months breastfeeding among male infants of orders 3 and higher, but this is the reverse of the differential for females, where the proportion for the first and second born is nearly twice that for those of higher order. Overall, the proportions conforming to the 9-month habit are much lower among women under age 45 than is the case among those of completed fertility.

Summary positions for the three family forms are of interest, especially in terms of the ranking they show according to ages of the mothers (See Table 8.5). For those over age 45 very little separates the median values for visiting

Table 8.5 Median periods of breastfeeding (months) and % of children breastfed for 3, 6-7 and 9 months, by union status of mothers under 45 and over 45

Union status	Median period of breastfeeding (months) by mothers		% Children breastfed for 3 months		% Children breastfed for 6 to 7 months		% Children breastfed for 9 months	
	Mothers at ages							
	Under 45	*Over 45*	*Under 45*	*Over 45*	*Under 45*	*Over 45*	*Under 45*	*Over 45*
Married	6.33	8.22	18.75	11.50	10.80	22.50	10.23	29.50
Common-law	9.18	9.96	12.35	10.53	15.14	14.29	19.53	28.57
Visiting	7.88	10.04	12.89	4.81	13.21	13.37	16.98	37.43

and common-law types, which amount to about 10.0 months each. Much lower is the corresponding value for married mothers (8.2 months). Turning to the younger age cohort, we see that their medians fall below the levels of their older counterparts. Most marked is the differential in the case of visiting mothers, which is some 2 months below the value for older women in this union. Also appreciable is the differential with respect to married mothers, which is just under 2 months. By contrast, the median age at weaning for common-law mothers in this age range is only slightly below the corresponding value for mothers over age 45.

Associated with these differentials with regard to median values are concentrations on the 3-month patterns which have already been identified. There is, among older women, a marked concentration on the 9-month pattern by those in visiting unions, 37% reporting this duration, while about 30% of the other two union types report a similar duration. Those who follow the 6–7 month pattern are most strongly represented by the married type (22%), while the proportions for the common-law and visiting are 14% and 13% respectively. Only 5% of the visiting women over age 45 conform to the 3-month breastfeeding pattern, which is about half of the level that characterises the other two.

Shifts from long to short durations of breastfeeding constitute the main aspect of the experience of women under age 45. The prevalence of the 9-month duration is reduced from 30% to 10% among married and from 37% to 17% among the visiting. Appreciable falls also appear among the common-law unions where the proportions decline from 29% to 20%. With regard to the 6–7 month duration, the proportion for married mothers under age 45 is one-half that of the value for older women. The shift over to the short duration of 3 months is marked among women in visiting and married unions, being double for the former and increasing by one-half for the latter.

By contrast, the proportion of common-law mothers under age 45 following this reduced period (12%) is only slightly in excess of that for older women.

Probably the principal features here are the considerable falls in the duration of breastfeeding that younger mothers in visiting unions have made, and the relatively short term of breastfeeding which married mothers have adopted.

Differentials by Educational Attainment

Of special interest is a comparison between breastfeeding patterns adopted by women with primary schooling and by those who have had some higher education. If educational attainment is taken as an indicator of socio-economic status, this comparison serves, to some degree, as a measure of differentials between two broad classes of the society in regard to this important aspect of child care.

Differentials in the form of breastfeeding shown by these two broad categories are summarised in Table 8.6, which also compares the position of those under age 45 with those who have passed the childbearing period. Manifestly the time of feeding is much greater among those with primary schooling, especially in the case of women under age 45. For women of completed fertility, those with primary education show a median period of 9.7 months, which is 33% in excess of the corresponding period for those with some further education (7.3 months). For younger mothers, the median value, 9.1 months, is more than twice that for women with post-primary schooling (4.3 months). The fact that the periods for mothers over age 45 are so much in excess of those for younger ones again points to substantial reductions in the age at weaning in recent years.

Further light on the position summarised by median values comes from proportions of infants breastfed for the three periods in which we are here

Table 8.6 Median periods of breastfeeding (months) and % of children breastfed for 3, 6-7 and 9 months, by educational attainment of mothers under 45 and over 45

Educational attainment	Median period of breastfeeding (months) by mothers		% Children breastfed for 3 months		% Children breastfed for 6 to 7 months		% Children breastfed for 9 months	
	Mothers at ages							
	Under 45	Over 45	Under 45	Over 45	Under 45	Over 45	Under 45	Over 45
Primary	9.07	9.73	11.45	8.97	13.16	15.38	19.32	30.56
Post-primary	4.32	7.31	21.14	6.00	12.00	17.00	5.71	27.00

interested. Considering first the 3-month pattern, we see that, in the case of infants of mothers over age 45, the proportion weaned after this period is 50% higher for those whose mothers have elementary schooling than it is for those whose mothers are of more advanced educational status. By contrast, a comparison for children of younger mothers puts those whose mothers have had some advanced schooling twice as high as those children whose mothers have not attained this status. This demonstrates the marked reduction in duration of breastfeeding that has taken place in recent years, and especially the dominance of the 3-month pattern in the feeding practice of the more highly educated members of the society. With regard to the 6–7 month pattern, there is much less change, but even here the proportion of children of mothers with post-primary education is much lower for younger mothers (12%) than for their older counterparts (17%). Unquestionably the outstanding aspect of shifts in forms of breastfeeding emerges from a consideration of the 9-month pattern. For children of mothers with primary schooling, the proportion weaned after this interval of time in the case of the older age cohort stands at 31%, whereas for children of the younger cohort this proportion is reduced to 19%. Even more striking is the reduction in the proportion of children of mothers with post-primary education who have followed this pattern. The proportion for infants of older mothers stands at 27%, whereas it is down to 6% in the case of infants of mothers who are under age 45.

The conclusion is therefore that the 9-month pattern is rapidly disappearing and giving place to the 3-month practice. There have been some reductions in the proportion of children weaned after 6 or 7 months, but these are by no means as prominent as appears for the 9-month period.

A more detailed analysis of breastfeeding habits among the two educational classes of mothers is afforded by median values given in Table 8.7. These demonstrate that women with primary schooling report a much longer time of breastfeeding than those who had had some further education. Mothers over age 45 whose schooling has been no higher than the primary level report breastfeeding their first and second male children for an average of 9.9 months, and female children for 9.8 months, both of which are appreciably in excess of corresponding values for women with higher education. In the case of female infants, the difference is as high as one-half. Differentials in ages at weaning for children of orders 3 to 6 are of similar dimensions. Women with post-primary schooling spend 15% less time breastfeeding their male infants; the differential in the case of female infants is greater, one-third.

An examination of the situation among women under age 45 discloses two important features. One is that these women spend much shorter times breastfeeding than their older counterparts. We consider in the first place the position with regard to infants of orders 1 and 2. Mothers with primary schooling report an average breastfeeding period which, for male infants, is

Table 8.7 Median periods of breastfeeding (months) for 2 sets of children, by sex of child and educational attainment of mothers under 45 and over 45

Sex of child	Mothers under 45		Mothers over 45	
	First and second children	Third to sixth children	First and second children	Third to sixth children
	Primary			
Male	8.75	9.69	9.86	9.65
Female	8.50	8.88	9.80	10.20
Both sexes	8.62	9.42	9.67	9.76
	Post-primary			
Male	5.21	4.08	8.44	8.17
Female	4.25	3.87	6.64	6.90
Both sexes	4.57	3.96	7.31	7.61
	Post-primary as % of primary			
Male	59.54	42.11	85.60	84.66
Female	50.00	43.58	67.76	67.65
Both sexes	53.01	42.04	75.59	77.97

about 1 month less than that for older women, 8.7 as compared with 9.7 months. The differential in the case of female infants is less, 0.4 month, that is 8.5 as against 8.9 months. Turning to women with post-primary schooling, we see that those under age 45 show much shorter periods. The median for male infants of orders 1 and 2 falls below the corresponding values for women of completed fertility by 3.9 months in the case of males and by 2.4 months in the case of females.

When we consider the age at weaning of infants of orders 3 to 6 by mothers with elementary schooling, no marked differences separate the position of the two age cohorts. Medians are the same for male infants of both age groups (9.7 months), while for females the differential in favour of younger mothers is only 1.3 months. Much more in evidence are differentials between younger and older females with post-primary education. Their male infants of orders 3 to 6 receive an average of 4.1 months where the mothers are under age 45, which is just over one-half the corresponding duration for infants of mothers over 45. The corresponding differential is somewhat smaller for female infants: 3.9 as against 6.9 months.

The second feature, brought out by examining the position of infants of women under age 45, is that the difference between medians for the two educational levels is much more pronounced among them than it is among women of completed fertility. Thus those with primary schooling nurse their first and second male children for 3.5 months more than do mothers with

Table 8.8 Proportion (%) of mothers breastfeeding children for 9 months, by sex of child and educational attainment of mothers under 45 and over 45

	Mothers under 45		Mothers over 45	
Sex of child	First and second children	Third to sixth children	First and second children	Third to sixth children
	Primary			
Male	19.74	24.11	32.14	32.86
Female	19.33	14.08	22.55	32.74
Both sexes	19.53	19.08	27.57	32.81
	Post-primary			
Male	14.81	—	38.10	32.14
Female	1.56	3.33	17.86	21.74
Both sexes	7.63	1.75	26.55	27.45

post-primary schooling. The corresponding female differential is 4.3 months. The median breastfeeding value for male infants of orders 3 to 6 in the case of women with primary schooling (9.7 months) is more than twice the value for women with some advanced schooling (4.1 months). Also female infants of orders 3 to 6 born to mothers under age 45 who are of lower educational status receive 8.9 months breastfeeding, which again is more than twice the corresponding value for children of mothers higher up the educational scale (3.9 months). Put in another form, this signifies that first- and second-order male children of mothers with post-primary schooling are breastfed for a period which is 60% of that for women with only primary schooling. This percentage is somewhat lower for female infants. Similarly, children of orders 3 to 6 born to mothers with secondary schooling are breastfed for a period which is just over 40% of the corresponding value shown for those whose mothers are of a lower educational level.

Many of the foregoing changes indicated by comparing the position of women over age 45 with that of those who are still of childbearing age derive from shifts in the 9-month pattern. Proportions of mothers breastfeeding their infants for 9 months appear in Table 8.8. For those of completed fertility with primary schooling, the proportion of all male infants breastfed for this interval is about one-third. A similar proportion obtains in the case of female infants of orders 3 to 6, but in the case of those of orders 1 and 2 the value for these children is much lower (23%). The proportion of male children of women under age 45 with primary schooling who are breastfed for 9 months drops to one-fifth for those of orders 1 and 2, and to about one-quarter for those of higher birth order. Marked falls in proportions are also in evidence for infants of mothers who have higher education. In the case of mothers with male infants below order 3, 15% are breastfed for 9 months, while the corresponding proportion for female infants is down to 2%. When we turn to children of orders 3 to 6, we see that very few women with some advanced education breastfeed for this length of time. In the case of males there are none, while only 3% of female children are breastfed for such a period.

Notes

1. An analysis of relationships between infant mortality and breastfeeding appears in Ruth Rice Puffer and Carlos V. Serrano, *Patterns of Mortality in Childhood* (Washington: Pan American Health Organisation, 1973), pp. 257 et seq.
2. A comprehensive discussion of the relationship between breastfeeding and reproduction is given in Christopher Tietze, "The Effect of Breastfeeding on the Rate of Conception," *Proceedings International Population Conference, New York, 1961* (London, 1963), pp. 129–135.
3. Puffer and Serrano, *Patterns of Mortality*, p. 258.
4. Several studies have emphasised the declines in periods of breastfeeding in Jamaica; see, for instance, Jacqueline P. Landman and Violet Shaw-Lyon, "Breastfeeding in Decline in Kingston, Jamaica, 1973," *West Indian Medical Journal* 25, no. 1 (March 1976), pp. 43–57.

Chapter 9
Children Living Away From
Their Mothers' Homes

A feature of the West Indian family is the frequency with which women, especially those not formally married, have their children cared for by one of their relatives or by members of some other household. While there are arrangements for institutionalising such situations through adoption and fostering, the shifts of children to households other than their parents' usually take place outside of such institutional forms. The children are, in this context, entrusted to relatives for, in the initial instance, short periods of time, generally with the expectation that at a future date they will return to their families of procreation.

One of the commonest ways in which children are brought up in a home other than their parents' takes the form of the mother establishing a family while still a resident in her parental home and later leaving that home to set up one of her own. If this involves her migrating to some other part of the country she is often unable to take her children with her and leaves them with the grandmother, whose readiness to assume responsibility for them is a central aspect of this pattern of childrearing in the society. It may be intended that the children should spend only a limited period with the grandmother, that is until the mother is satisfactorily settled in her new community. But in most cases the result is that the children remain in the grandmother's home for a very long period. Another way in which children are brought up outside of their parents' home arises when the woman establishes her own family union away from the parental household, and then finds herself unable to support her children. In this case she may resort to the device of asking her own mother or some other relative to take care of the children. Again this may, initially, be taken as a temporary measure, but may become permanent because of the failure of the mother to improve her economic condition sufficiently to resume responsibility for the upkeep of her children.

If the first situation noted above involves the mother moving from a rural to an urban area, the result is that the child is left to be brought up in a rural community and therefore not close to its mother. The same pattern obtains where the children are not born in the home of their grandmother but in the home independently established by the mother. Where the latter establishes herself in an urban area and finds it necessary to send her children to be cared for by their grandparents living in a rural community, these children are once again brought up in a rural setting. Thus a major consequence of sending children to live with relatives is that they tend to be confined to a rural environment in their formative years.

At the outset, two age limits applying to the two sets of data being analysed in this chapter should be noted. One of these is imposed as a feature of the survey, while the second emerges as a consequence of the first. So far as children are concerned, the survey requires that only those under age 15 at the time of the interview should be the subject of questions identifying those living away from their mothers' homes. While no age limit is imposed on mothers to whom such questions are addressed, the fact that a 15-year limit operates in the case of children means that hardly any mothers over age 45 report having children living away from their households. In fact, of the women whose children live away from their households only 2 are over age 45.

Our major concern here is with the conditions under which the children are removed from their parents' homes, with the major characteristics of these children and of their mothers. There are 76 women in the sample who have sent their children to be cared for by relatives or friends, and on the basis of the age distribution of the sample, it is estimated that about 30% of the women of childbearing age have elected to have some of their children brought up in this manner. Many of these 76 women have more than one of their children living away from them; in fact they have 125 children being supported by others, that is, the average number of children per family in this condition is 1.64. And relating the number of children involved in the process to the total number of children ever born to women of childbearing age in the sample, we estimate that about 15% of all children born to women under age 45 in the sample are being cared for by relatives or friends.

The first characteristics of children living away from their parents' home to be considered here are their sex and order of birth, which form the subject of Table 9.1. Of the 125 children involved, 58 or 46% are males and 67 or 54% females. Most of these children are of low-order births. In the case of males, 33 or 57% are first order, while for females there are 23 first order, equivalent to 34% of the total. More females than males appear in the second order, 23 and 9 respectively, so that the proportions under order 3 are not materially different between the sexes, being 72% for males and 69% for females.

When we consider the type of union of the mothers of these children, the outstanding aspects are that the overwhelming majority of children being maintained in this way come from visiting-type unions and that the numbers

Table 9.1 Sex and birth order of children living away from their parents' home

Birth order	Sex of child			%Distribution		
	Male	Female	Total	Male	Female	Total
1	33	23	56	56.9	34.3	44.8
2	9	23	32	15.5	34.3	25.6
3	4	10	14	6.9	14.9	11.2
4	5	6	11	8.6	8.9	8.8
5	3	2	5	5.2	3.0	4.0
6	1	3	4	1.7	4.5	3.2
7 +	3	—	3	5.2	—	2.4
Total	58	67	125	100.0	99.9	100.0

from married unions are negligible. Of the 125 children, 82 or 66% are from visiting-type unions and only 4 from married unions. Consequently the small numbers of children from married unions are combined with those in common-law unions in Table 9.2, which shows the type of union and size of family from which these children are drawn. There does not seem to be any marked concentration in terms of size of family, so far as visiting unions are concerned. But 38% of the children from this type of union are from families of 2 and 3 children. The situation in the case of common-law and married unions is different however. Here there is a marked concentration around families of 4 and 5 children, which together account for 56% of the total in these unions living away from their parents.

The association between the age of the mother at the time of the survey and the sex of the children also calls for examination, and this is the subject of Table 9.3. Comparatively few women under age 20 give out their children to the care of others. And while a slightly larger proportion of those aged 20 to 24 do so, it is not until the age range 25 to 29 that women send away their

Table 9.2 Type of union and size of family from which children are taken

Size of family	Union in which child born			%Distribution		
	Visiting	Common-law and married	Total	Visiting	Common-law and married	Total
1	7	2	9	8.5	4.6	7.2
2	16	4	20	19.5	9.3	16.0
3	15	4	19	18.3	9.3	15.2
4	10	10	20	12.2	23.2	16.0
5	9	14	23	11.0	32.6	18.4
6	6	3	9	7.3	7.0	7.2
7	12	3	15	14.6	7.0	12.0
8 +	7	3	10	8.6	7.0	8.0
Total	82	43	125	100.0	100.0	100.0

Table 9.3 Children living away from their parents' home by sex and age of mother

Age of mother	Sex of child			% Distribution		
	Male	Female	Total	Male	Female	Total
Under 20	3	4	7	5.2	6.0	5.6
20–24	8	10	18	13.8	14.9	14.4
25–29	22	26	48	37.9	38.8	38.4
30–34	9	14	23	15.5	20.9	18.4
35–39	9	7	16	15.5	10.4	12.8
40 +	7	6	13	12.1	9.0	10.4
Total	58	67	125	100.0	100.0	100.0

children on a substantial scale. In the case of male children, 22 or 38% of the total are from families in which the mothers are aged 25 to 29. The same situation is noted for female children, 39% of whom are from families in which the mothers fall within the age range 25 to 29. Despite this appreciable concentration of mothers within this age range, women of all ages are liable to seek the assistance of relatives or others in the maintenance of their children.

The relatives or others to whom children leaving their parents' homes are entrusted are shown in Table 9.4, in association with the type of union in which the child is born. The outstanding characteristic here is the important role played by the grandmother, especially with regard to children born in visiting unions. Of the children of these unions who are not living with their mothers, 62% are under the care of their grandmothers. It is in this context that the term "grandmother" families or households is frequently used in the Caribbean. Whether these grandmothers are heads of households however is not known, although this is suggested by the pattern of relationships within

Table 9.4 Persons caring for children and type of unions in which children living away from their parents' home are born

Person caring for the child	Type of union in which birth occurred				% Distribution		
	Visiting	Common-law	Married	Total	Visiting	Common-law and married	Total
Maternal grandmother	51	16	1	68	62.2	39.5	54.4
Paternal grandmother	7	6	—	13	8.5	13.9	10.4
Father	14	10	—	24	17.1	23.3	19.2
Aunt	5	3	3	11	6.1	14.0	8.8
Other	5	4	—	9	6.1	9.3	7.2
Total	82	39	4	125	100.0	100.0	100.0

households in the country. The second most important individual to whom children from visiting unions are entrusted is the father; 17% of all these children are under the care of their fathers. It is of interest that 9% of these children of visiting unions are entrusted to their paternal grandmothers, and it seems that in many cases these are acting on behalf of their sons, as often this turns out to be a convenient arrangement in so far as the fathers of the children are concerned. It therefore seems plausible to conclude that, directly or indirectly, fathers are responsible for the upkeep of just over one-quarter of the children living away from their mothers. Small proportions of children in visiting unions are under the care of their aunts (6%).

In contrast to children of visiting unions, those in common-law and married unions are less frequently under the care of their maternal grandmothers. The proportion (40%) is much lower than in the case of children born in visiting unions. Of the children born to these types of unions, a substantial proportion (23%) are being cared for by their fathers. This suggests that although at the time of the birth of these children their mothers are in common-law unions, these have been subsequently dissolved, for one reason or another, and that the children have come under the care of their fathers. Two other relatives figure prominently as having responsibilities for these children, paternal grandmothers and aunts, each of these caring for 14% of these children. As in the case of children born in visiting unions, paternal grandmothers may again be acting on behalf of their sons, who, for one reason or another, may have assumed responsibility for the children. Thus we can infer that, directly or indirectly, fathers assume responsibility for 37% of the children of married and common-law unions who do not live with their mothers. It is also to be noted that aunts play a more prominent role among children of married and common-law unions than in the case of visiting unions.

One question put to respondents sought information on the reasons for mothers sending their children to be brought up by relatives or others. From the comprehensive replies given it is clear that in many cases several reasons are operative. And as is to be expected, such shifts of children from one household to another are possible only with some agreement between the mother and the relatives or acquaintance to whose household the child is to be sent. At times, reasons advanced relate only to the mother's situation; at other times only the readiness of the responsible individual at the receiving household to accept the child is considered a sufficient reason. An attempt has been made to determine from the answers given the major reasons advanced for sending children from the mothers' households, and these, in conjunction with the type of union in which the child is born, form the subject of Table 9.5.

Reasons based on economic considerations are important for both types of union. In the case of visiting types, 31% report that their having to go to work necessitates their sending the child away to be maintained by relatives or

Table 9.5 Reason given for children living away from parents' homes and type of union in which they are born

Reason for sending child away	Type of union in which birth occurred			% Distribution		
	Visiting	Common-law and married	Total	Visiting	Common-law and married	Total
Mother had to work	27	14	41	30.7	37.8	32.8
Grandmother wanted child	9	3	12	10.2	8.1	9.6
No support from father	3	—	3	3.5	—	2.4
Better schooling	5	2	7	5.7	5.5	5.6
Financial problem	2	2	4	2.3	5.4	3.2
Taken away by father for support etc.	9	5	14	10.2	13.5	11.2
No space in house	1	3	4	1.1	8.1	3.2
Unable to care for child—sent to father or other relative	12	2	14	13.6	5.4	11.2
Other	20	6	26	22.7	16.2	20.8
Total	88	37	125	100.0	100.0	100.0

others. Other reasons closely linked to this should also be noted. Thus statements that the mother is unable to care for the child are basically economic, as also are reasons to the effect that no support from the father is forthcoming, that financial problems operate, and that the children are taken away by the father for proper support, all essentially are linked to economic conditions of the mother. If therefore we add these to the major one—that the mother has had to go to work—we see that about 60% of these women advanced reasons which are basically economic in form. Of interest are the number of mothers reporting that the child has been sent away because the grandmother wants it. In many other cases this is not put forward as a major reason, but given as a supplementary one. Here also miscellaneous reasons loom large, accounting for 23% of the total.

Similar is the pattern of reasons given with respect to common-law and married mothers. Again economic considerations appear to be of major significance, as in 38% of the cases the mother's necessity to work is stated as the reason. Others that are indirectly at least of an economic nature, such as financial problems, father assuming responsibility for their support, the mother's inability to provide such support, also figure prominently. And when these are added to the reason centering around the mother having to work, we may conclude that economic considerations operate in the case of about 62% of the children, which is very close to the corresponding proportion shown by children of visiting unions. Again there are appreciable numbers of miscellaneous reasons, accounting for 16% of the total.

It is now necessary to place those children sent away from their parents in the context of their families of procreation. Just as in our discussion of infant mortality it proved fruitful to treat losses as events experienced by entire families, as well as separate events without any reference to the families in which they were born, so in the present context it is essential to relate children living away from their parents to the latter's homes. Two aspects of this issue are to be briefly touched on in this discussion. The first involves the numbers of children from each family sent away to be cared for in other households, while the second treats the number of women who entrust their entire families to the care of others.

A considerable number of women have more than one child living away from them with relatives or others. A summary of the numbers of children in each family who are being cared for in this way is as follows:

Number from each family being cared for by relatives or others	*Number of families*
1	44
2	21
3	6
4	3
5	1
6	1
Total	76

While in the majority of cases it is only one child that is maintained by relatives or friends (58%), sizeable numbers of women have placed more than one under such care. Thus 28% have sent away 2 of their children and 8% have sent away 3. In view of this situation, we are again confronted with an issue calling for an analysis of conditions within the family unit which induce the mother to send away one or more of her children.

Another aspect of sending children to relatives or others is that in many cases this takes the form of the mother parting with all her children. This is the case in 18 of the 76 families, that is nearly one-quarter of the total under consideration here. It is true that the majority of these consist of women with only 1 child, but the total number of children involved here (31) is appreciable, accounting for one-quarter of all those in the sample under the care of relatives or others, that is, living outside of their mother's household. The position may be summarised as follows:

Size of entire families being cared for by relatives and others	*Number of families*
1	10
2	6
3	1
6	1
Total	18

Families or Households to Which Children Are Sent

Complementary to the foregoing analysis of size and characteristics of families from which children are sent to be cared for by others would be a picture of families in which such children are placed. And it would be expected that some respondents in the sample would include as members of their households children of relatives or friends under their care. It would seem reasonable to assume that the women reporting the presence of such children would show characteristics in some way complementary to those of respondents reporting that some of their own children are not living with them, but are under the care of relatives or friends. However there is no such conformity. Indeed the numbers reporting the presence of children other than their own is only 20, which is less than one-third of the number of families stating that some of their children are away under the care of relatives or friends. The reasons for this failure of the two sets of data to conform are not clear. It is not believed that the form of sampling contributed materially to this lack of agreement. One possible contributing factor is that interviewers were instructed not to record information on children over 15 years of age. No attempt is made here to account for the lack of conformity between the two sets of data. Consequently the brief analysis of the position is presented with the qualification that it may be definitely biased.

As there are only 20 such women in the sample reporting the presence of children other than their own under their care, not much analysis can be carried out. It is estimated that just under 10% of the women over age 45 in the sample report having children other than their own living with them.

In terms of age distribution, these women are for the most part of advanced age, as the following age grouping shows:

	Number of women
Age group	in age group
Under 40	2
40–44	2
45–49	5
50–54	4
55–59	1
60+	6

The 2 youngest of these women are aged 32 and 38 while the oldest is 64. This suggests that the process of taking over children of other women may be generally done by women who have completed childbearing and whose children have in fact left their households to establish families of their own.

In terms of size of family, these women show wide variation, with 4 having as many as 9 children and 4 being childless. The average size of family for the group of 20 is 2.2. If, however, as seems to be the case, these children are taken under care when the recipient has completed the task of rearing her own children, and may indeed be looking forward to caring for children of others who will provide her with welcome companionship, then the number of children ever born to the women of the receiving family may not affect the issue.

Information has also been sought on the type of union in which the women are involved at the time of their agreeing to care for other women's children. There are a few cases in which the type of union when this responsibility is assumed is not clear, but the overall pattern is that these women to whom children are sent rarely are of the visiting type. The following summarises the picture of their union status:

Type of union	*Number of women*
Visiting	2
Common-law	—
Married	14
Other	4

The complete absence of common-law types and the low representation of the visiting type are the main features of this composition. It is true that at advanced ages the frequency of visiting unions is low, while the proportions married move up sharply, but the pattern of unions shown by these 20 women is atypical from many standpoints.

Another aspect to be considered is the relation between the children and their guardians. This is as follows:

Children's relationship to those caring for them	*Number of children*
No relation	7
Husband's child	5
Niece or nephew	3
Grandchild	3
Husband's niece	2
Cousin's child	1

This pattern of relationship between the children and the women caring for them is at variance with what seems to be the case from an examination of material on the persons assuming responsibility for children who are being cared for outside of their parents' home. The large proportion of these children going to the homes of their grandmothers, according to the latter information, is entirely absent from the picture as obtained from data from households in which such children actually live. Thus, although one section of the information from the sample is in accord with the general picture of children going to live with their grandmothers, another section does not conform to this pattern. Admittedly the very small numbers of women (20) caring for children and the small number of children under such care (21) may be at the root of this discrepancy. But manifestly investigation into this question, both from the standpoint of the family leaving children in the care of others and of families receiving such children, should involve a matching process, so that the extent to which compatible information is received from each can be easily assessed.

Sources of Support for Children Under Age Fifteen

Child support assumes considerable significance in Jamaica because of the presence of visiting and, to a lesser extent, common-law unions. In many cases mothers of the two last-mentioned types have to take legal proceedings against fathers of their children in order to obtain financial help from them. A detailed treatment of the subject is not attempted in this survey; it is intended to cover financial, or any other kind of assistance rendered to ´mothers towards the upkeep of their children. There are several facets of this subject—legal, economic and sociological. An interesting discussion of some of its implications from the standpoint of the abandonment of children is given by Erna Brodber.[1] Moreover the questionnaire sought information on whether support received was enforced through a court order or not, but it is of interest that of all the respondents only 8 report having taken legal action against their partners in order to secure maintenance for their children. Material on the topic analysed here derives from replies to a question on the source of support for each child under age 15, and is regarded mainly of a financial nature, although when the term "self" appears as a source a much less specific concept is implied.

Although in a sense information on source of support complements our earlier analyses in this chapter, a basic difference separates the two forms of data. Whereas in the preceding sections children dealt with lived away from their family of procreation, we are here studying the experience relating to children living within their mothers' households. The following are the sources of support in terms of which the children are described: self, father, both parents, relatives and others. Since these are all children within the mothers' households, the latter are in some measure responsible for their upkeep. Thus, while the appearance of the term "self" signifies that the woman is the main (if not the sole) supporter of her children, the entry of other categories by no means signifies that her role in their upkeep can be ignored. The category "self" is of special relevance in the context of the visiting unions.

Table 9.6 shows the distribution of sources of support for children under

Table 9.6 Proportion (%) distribution of sources of support for children under age 15, by size of family and type of union

| Size of family | Number of children | % Distribution of sources of support for children | | | | | |
		Self	Father	Both parents	Relation of mother	Other	Total
		Visiting					
1–3 children	130	20.76	35.38	25.38	6.15	12.33	100.0
4–5 children	63	19.05	42.86	23.81	3.17	11.11	100.0
6+ children	68	45.59	25.00	19.12	8.82	1.47	100.0
Total	261	26.82	34.48	23.37	6.13	9.20	100.0
		Common-law					
1–3 children	58	10.34	31.03	56.90	—	1.73	100.0
4–5 children	79	8.86	39.24	51.90	—	—	100.0
6+ children	102	13.73	40.20	41.18	0.98	3.91	100.0
Total	239	11.30	37.66	48.54	0.42	2.08	100.0
		Married					
1–3 children	59	10.17	18.64	69.49	1.70	—	100.0
4–5 children	54	9.26	29.63	59.26	1.85	—	100.0
6+ children	68	1.47	25.00	73.53	—	—	100.0
Total	181	6.63	24.31	67.96	1.10	—	100.0
		All family types					
1–3 children	247	15.78	30.36	43.32	3.65	6.89	100.0
4–5 children	196	12.24	37.76	44.90	1.53	3.57	100.0
6+ children	238	19.33	31.51	44.12	2.94	2.10	100.0
Total	681	16.01	32.89	44.05	2.79	4.26	100.0

age 15 by type of union in which they were born and the size of their mothers' families. In the case of visiting relationships, about one-fifth of the children in families with less than 4 children are reported to be maintained by the mother herself. Not much different is the proportion shown for medium-size families (4 to 5 children), but the proportion more than doubles to 46% when families with 6 or more children are examined. This is consistent with the finding that higher up the age scale the proportion of women in visiting unions who are heads of their own households rises appreciably. Support put down to the father alone in a visiting relationship is at a level of 35%, when we consider families of 1 to 3 children. This proportion moves up 43% in the case of medium-size families, but falls appreciably to one-quarter for families with 6 or more children. Support from both parents is recorded for one-quarter of the children from small families, and the proportion for medium-size families is only slightly lower (24%). There is a somewhat lower proportion for women with large families (19%). These data also bring out the extent to which women in visiting relationships rely on assistance from non-family sources in the care of their children. Relatives and friends are responsible for supporting 18% of children in small families; this declines slightly when we turn to families with more than 6 children, but is still 10%.

When we consider common-law types, the evidence is of much less stress on the mother for the upkeep of her children. Proportions of mothers reporting that they are responsible range from 9% for medium-size families to 14% for large families. Support by fathers alone does not differ markedly from that shown in visiting unions, except in the case of large families where it is appreciably higher. Support received from both common-law parents ranges from 57% for small families to 41% for those with 6 or more children. These are in fact twice the corresponding values for visiting parents, which is to be expected in view of the fundamental differences between their structures. Moreover, in contrast to the position shown in visiting relationships, common-law unions exhibit very little child support coming from sources other than the parents. The greatest contribution from extra-parental sources, occurring in the case of large families, is not more than 5%.

As the distinguishing feature of marriage is the sharing of a common household by the parents, we should expect only small proportions of support contributed by mothers alone; these amount to about 10% for families with less than 6 children, while for large families the proportion is less than 2%. By contrast, proportions reflecting contributions by both parents are much larger than is the case with the two other family forms, ranging from 59% to 74%. Upkeep of children coming from fathers alone is somewhat lower than in the case of the other unions, as the contributions here range from 19% to 30%. Once more support from non-parental sources is negligible.

In summary, we may note that for the entire sample, 16% of all children are described as being maintained by their mothers alone and one-third by their fathers alone. Taken together, both parents are responsible for 44% of all children, while the proportion of children coming under support of non-parental sources is about 7%. Thus these data confirm that visiting unions depend most on sources outside the family for aid with their children. It is also of interest that this is most pronounced in smaller families. Indeed the declining dependence on outside resources as size of family rises is consistent with the rise in the proportion of households headed by women at advanced ages of the family cycle who are in visiting unions.

Notes

1. Erna Brodber, *Abandonment of Children in Jamaica* (Kingston: I.S.E.R., University of the West Indies, 1974).

Chapter 10
Large Families

From almost any standpoint, the cardinal facets of fertility in a society center around the experience of women with very large families, sometimes called grande multiparae. In considering the position of such women we are inevitably led to investigate certain questions. Are there any easily identifiable biological or social factors which contribute to the production of these large families? How does heavy childbearing affect the normal life of the mother and what are its effects on other members of the family? A consideration of these in turn directs attention to such topics as age at entry into unions in which they are involved, the duration of such unions, the socio-economic status of women with large families, their religious persuasion, their menstrual histories, their health and the fertility history of their parents.

In a small-scale analysis of the present type, a rigorous, detailed consideration of the above issues is ruled out. What is attempted is a description of certain quantitative aspects of the life and characteristics of women with very large families. The aim is to direct attention to social and biological elements which seem to be paramount in conducing to the production of such families. In view of the very small numbers being treated, tabulation of the data is not feasible. The approach is to give quantitative descriptions of the characteristics; these in effect almost take the form of simple quantitative enumeration of the relevant features of the woman. Although it is inappropriate to produce tabulations for the small numbers of women being studied, the quantitative fertility data on which the descriptions are based appear in Appendix V. The features which the above process reveals can best be illustrated by a few case histories of grande multiparae and 6 of these presented constitute a major portion of the chapter.

For the purpose of this analysis, grande multiparae are defined as women with 10 or more pregnancies or those whose plurality of conceptions yields products totalling 10 or more. Of the 501 women in the sample, 28 or 6% are so classified. Together these are responsible for 316 pregnancies, which is

175

equivalent to 18% of all pregnancies reported by women in the sample. It is the experience of these 28 women with which this chapter is concerned.

It should here be noted that Jamaica has experienced a fall in the proportion of mothers with very large families since 1943. This implies that our sample presents a picture of pressure of numbers within the family which is certainly less acute than anything earlier data would have revealed.

Of the 8 parishes represented in the study all except Portland and St. Ann contribute to the members of large families. It is clear that, in view of the fact that our sampling method was partially purposive, this may very well be an artifact of the methodology. However, it is interesting to note that fertility levels in St. Ann have been dramatically reduced over the past 30 years and it now ranks as the parish with the lowest level of fertility after the entirely urban parish of Kingston and its two adjoining parishes of St. Andrew and St. Thomas. St. Ann, in addition to experiencing marked economic growth over the past 3 decades, has a long history of an active family planning programme.[1] No cases of families in excess of 10 were found in the parish of Portland, which it should be noted, is not a parish with high fertility.

The ages of the women with large families range from 35 to 64 years with the average age being 50. There are 2 women under 40 (aged 35 and 38 respectively) and at the other end one aged 60 and 2 aged 64. In terms of birth cohorts we see that the modal number 9 is that of 1926–30 and the next highest is 6 for women of the 1916-20 cohort. Their general level of education is primary. Women with no schooling number 4, while 1 had only 2 years. It is significant that for the study as a whole only 13 women are recorded as having no schooling and 4 of these are women with large families. In fact 3 of them have the highest and second highest number of pregnancies noted, that is, 16 and 15. The fourth woman without formal schooling has a total of 12 pregnancies. The majority (21) of these women, however, have 5 and more years of primary education and 2 report post-primary levels. The average number of years of schooling stands at just over 6.

Religion, as discussed earlier in Chapter 1, plays an important role in the lives of the people and in particular those of the women. These 28 are fairly evenly divided in terms of their religious persuasions, with 13 professing adherence to the more fundamental sects and another 14 giving the "established" religions as their persuasion. One woman states that she has no religion. In most cases their partners are of similar religious bent.

Marriage

In terms of the established pattern in Jamaica, the majority of these women marry at some point in their lives, usually after initial unions of another type. Thus 22 or 79% are ever married, while their average age at marriage is 27 years. Age at marriage by parity shows that only 5 or 22% of these women marry prior to the commencement of childbearing. Two of the latter are between 15 and 19 at the time of this event, while the other 3 marry in the age interval 20 to 29. Women marrying after having 4 to 9 children number 11, while 2 marry after having 10 to 12 pregnancies.

Since the pattern of marriage, as demonstrated by age and parity at entry into this type, deviates somewhat from the European, it is important to examine some of the reasons given by the women for finally taking this step. As we should expect, the welfare of the children is cited in a fair portion of cases. "It would be very hard for me to leave him and go and take a next man having two children with him"; also this couple felt they could now afford marriage. Another woman "married because I wanted security for my children and felt that if anything happened to B. at work I would not get anything for the children"; she actually asked him to marry her. In the words of another, "they said the life is more honourable," and they felt it would be better for the children.

The concept of respectability is also mentioned, "I would live better, I would able to go to my church regular and the Lord would look upon me more and even our same colour men would have a little more respect for me." In another case, it was felt "that marriage changed my status and made me more respected, and it would help the children."

However, the most interesting aspect of late entry into marriage is the opinion of several women that they are too young for marriage. This rationale is also applied to common-law unions and is generally used when explaining their initial unions, namely visiting, giving rise to their first pregnancies. For example one woman aged 19 at the birth of her first child and whose partner was 28 years old stated that "she saw him and loved him," and he visited her as that was the type of union most convenient for their age group. She broke off the relationship on discovering her pregnancy and said that "even if she had been older at the time she does not think she would have lived with him or married him." She in fact married when she was aged 30 and at parity 8.

Another woman states that "I could not go in another union type as I was too young" (age 19). According to her, in the visiting union there is much freedom, whereas in marriage and common-law there is much violence and unfaithfulness. This woman did in fact get married when she was aged 23 and at parity 4.

The reasoning behind a female of 19 or 20 at parity 1 or 2 claiming that she is too young to live with a man, while obviously having no hesitation in mothering a child or children, is not clear from these data. Cognizance must be taken of the fact that many of these women do have older relatives, often their mothers, to assist them with their childrearing. In view of these attitudes we are led to question the rationale which allows a woman to assume the responsibility for rearing an infant, with its many psychological, physical and social demands, when she possibly feels that because of her young age, she lacks some of the attributes necessary for a meaningful relationship with her partner.

It is quite evident that parents and relatives often play a major role in respect of their unions as in the case of this 19-year-old who said that she and her partner started a visiting union because they loved each other and he asked her father if he could visit her. She did not like the common-law life and her parents would not allow it. They could not marry because "he did not have anything." Her parents did not mind them visiting each other and thought that the common-law union was not right. Another woman stated that they could not enter any other type of union because her relatives would not permit common-law living and her partner did not have enough to marry her, and marriage needs money. She was 14 at the time and had 1 child in this union, which lasted for 2 years. In another case the respondent whose initial union was marriage at age 22 said she did not like her partner as she wasn't ready, but he went to her mother who influenced her to be friendly with him.

Common-Law Unions

As has already been demonstrated, the common-law union is viewed with disapproval by a number of women. However for 4 women, common-law is their most stable type, but of these only 1 remains in this type throughout her life. The other 3 women have 1 or more pregnancies in visiting unions. One woman, who incidentally represents the only pure type, enters this union when both she and her partner are 17, a rather unusual step. The other women enter their unions at ages 23, 30 and 44 respectively. Of the 28 women in this group, 16 or 57% spent some time in common-law unions.

Visiting Unions

In many respects the visiting union is the most challenging to analyse as has been pointed out earlier in this work. Several positive thoughts have been advanced in favour of this type as in the case of the woman who states that she prefers visiting because she "doesn't like living with a man, as they are not worthwhile living with," or the woman who prefers visiting unions as she can leave when she wants. Another woman said that she "liked the visiting union as the men are not stable," and although she is now in a common-law union she does not like it because "it is a sin and you are tied down too much." She likes to be free as she "can't stand worries." As one woman succinctly puts it, "no disadvantage is in that one [the visiting union]."

Union Duration

Union duration, in conjunction with the actual type and the length of time over which a woman has been associated with a given partner, serves to illustrate the degree of stability attributable to a given union. Duration may in fact be examined from several angles. First, we can look at the duration of the most stable union, defined here as the longest duration with any one partner, irrespective of type or types. Since we are here primarily concerned with the degree of the woman's adaptation to a given situation or set of circumstances, the length of time spent in any partnership is important. Secondly, we shall examine the total duration of all the unions in which a woman has been involved and thirdly, we can look at her total duration up to the menopause, which effectively delineates the termination of the childbearing span, or present age if non-menopausal.

In looking at their most stable unions, we note that a total of 623 years are spent in this particular category. This gives an average duration of 22 years per woman. The majority, 16 or 57%, are in unions lasting 20 to 39 years. Only 11% of these women have unions of less than 10 years, while 9 are with 1 partner for periods of 10 to 19 years. Significantly, the woman with the shortest duration, 2 periods of 4 years each, and with 2 partners, is in a pure type visiting union. Our second aspect of stability, total duration of all unions, shows a span of 737 years or an average of 26 years in unions. Over 30 years are spent in unions by 12 women, including one for 41 years. Durations of the other 16 extend over periods of between 10 and 29 years. For the third category of stability indicated, that is up to the menopause or present age, the average length is 25 years. Here 16 women are in unions of 20 years and over, while only 1 stands between 10 and 14 years. Clearly then, unions of long duration are the norm for these women with very large families.

Partners

Following logically from a discussion of the women's duration of union must be an analysis of their partners. There are 73 partners among these 28 women, or an average of 2.6 each. By far the greatest number, 16 or 57%, are associated with only 1 or 2 partners throughout their lives. Thus 2 women have 7 and 8 respectively, while the number of partners of the other 10 range from 3 to 5. It is interesting to note that of the 2 with the greatest number of partners, one has been in a visiting union of 13 years' duration and the other has shifted from common-law to marriage for a total duration of 16 years. Thus multiplicity of partners does not necessarily reduce the potential for relatively long durations of unions.

Of the women with large families, 10 have had only 1 partner during their lives. Of these, 4 are pure types in marriage, another 3 move from common-law to marriage with the same partner, while 2 women move from visiting to married with the same partner. One classical case experiences all three types in a step-wise progression from visiting to common-law to married, with the same partner throughout. All other women have more than 1 partner.

Pregnancies

The major focus of this discussion of large families is the number of pregnancies involved at the individual as well as at the group level. These 28 women together contribute a total of 316 pregnancies, or an average of 11.3 each. The modal number of pregnancies is 10, with 13 women having this number. There is 1 woman with 8 pregnancies and another with 9, while at the other end of the scale there are 3 women reporting 15 pregnancies each and 1 reporting 16. These pregnancies result in 280 livebirths, 30 miscarriages and 13 stillbirths; plurality of conception accounts for the excess of products over pregnancies. The average age at their first pregnancy is 19.8 years and at their last, 40.5 years.

Livebirths account for 89% of the pregnancies or more exactly 87% of the products. The average number of these births is 10 per woman; those having less than 10 livebirths number 10, while 8 have between 11 and 15. It is noteworthy that the woman with the highest number of livebirths (15) has a perfect record, in that these births result from 15 pregnancies. Miscarriages and stillbirths are discussed in connexion with the analysis of foetal loss.

It is well documented that the 3 forms of mating recognised in West Indian societies contribute varying amounts to fertility.[2] It is of interest to consider briefly these contributions, although with only 28 women involved, the results can be no more than suggestive. The visiting, usually taken as the least stable of the 3 union types, contributes 75 pregnancies, consisting of 67 livebirths, 6 miscarriages and 2 stillbirths. The common-law unions give rise to 92 or 29% of all pregnancies, and here early and late foetal loss amounts to 12. Pregnancies to married women total 148, nearly twice that contributed by the visiting type, and equivalent to 47% of all pregnancies. This pattern is not strictly in conformity with the general form of differential by type of union, presented elsewhere in this study, largely because of the relatively large proportion of births attributable to women in common-law unions.

One aspect of the relationship between type of union and level of completed fertility has to be touched on, namely the shifts from initial to terminal union and the level of pregnancy associated with such shifts. Earlier studies have shown that women shifting from a type that is unstable to one of greater stability show higher fertility than shifts from, say, a more stable to a less stable type.[3]

Women whose initial and terminal unions are married contribute 42 or 18% of all pregnancies (233) of ever-married women. No one initially married shifts to common-law or visiting, as a terminal union. One woman with 10 pregnancies who is initially married, however, completes her childbearing period in a single state.

Turning next to those who begin in visiting unions and end in marriage, we see that their pregnancies total 145 or 62% of births to ever-married women;

this is nearly 3½ times the number contributed by women who end in the type of union in which they begin, that is are married throughout. On the other hand, those who, having begun in visiting and end in common-law contribute 20 pregnancies, while those who begin and end in visiting unions have 2 fewer than the preceding group.

Women who begin childbearing in common-law unions and end in marriage have a total of 46 pregnancies, 20% of all pregnancies of those who ultimately marry. Pregnancies contributed by those ending as they begin amount to 24, while 11 are contributed by those who are initially in common-law unions and end as visiting.

Quite clearly then the major shift is from an initial union of the visiting type to that of marriage, and the number of pregnancies to these women (145) is equivalent to 46% of the total of all 316 pregnancies.

The place of delivery and the attendant, if any, are interesting aspects of the study of pregnancies and their outcome. Of the 323 products of these pregnancies, most deliveries, that is 260 or 80%, occur in the home of the woman. Of these, 57% are delivered by nanas, and 79 or 30% by nurses. The 17 deliveries accounted for by the category designated "self" are mainly miscarriages, when in fact the woman does not have assistance. Of the remaining 16 deliveries, 4 are by doctors and 12 by the respondent's mother. Deliveries in hospital total 63, including 1 in a doctor's surgery. These constitute 19% of all products of conception. Nurses deliver 56 (89%), while 6 or 10% are delivered by doctors.

Birth Intervals

An examination of the interval between births shows, as is to be expected, relatively short periods for all birth orders. In the first interval 8 women terminate their second pregnancies less than 1.5 years after the first. For the majority of these women, 11 in all, the interval ranges from 1.5 to 3 years. Only 3 terminate their second pregnancy 4 or more years after the first, while in the case of 6 the interval lies between 3 and 4 years. In the case of the second interval, most of the women (21) show intervals of less than 3 years, while intervals of 3 to 6 years characterise 7 of this category.

The picture is essentially the same for succeeding intervals up to the fourth. There is a slight reduction at the fifth, with only 3 women attaining an interval of 3 or more years. From the sixth onwards, the initial pattern prevails. Thus we note that the average number of years between the first and second births of the 28 women is 2.2 years, that for the second, third and fourth intervals is 2 years and for the fifth, 1.8 years. For the sixth to the ninth interval, the average moves up to between 2.1 and 2.4 years. Higher intervals are omitted as the numbers of births here are very small.

Foetal Loss

In the study of grande multigravidae, examination of the incidence of foetal loss is important since we know that these increase with parity and age. The fact that most of these women also belong to the lower socio-economic groups introduces other factors contributing to increased foetal loss. For example, anaemia may contribute to stillbirths. Because this is a non-medical survey, the usual medical definitions of products of conception in terms of gestational age in weeks and birth weight are not feasible. Most respondents, as well as the interviewers, are familiar with the definitions used here and these are as follows: miscarriage/spontaneous abortion—product of conception of less than 7 months' (28 weeks) duration; stillbirth—the product of conception of more than 7 months (28 weeks) that shows no sign of life at the time of expulsion from the uterus.

Miscarriage/Spontaneous Abortions

As abortion is still illegal in Jamaica and, in addition, generates great moral feelings in some quarters, it was decided not to attempt to differentiate between spontaneous and induced abortions in this survey. However, in respect of this group of women of high fertility, these abortions can be taken to be spontaneous. The number of miscarriages among them is 30, an average of a little over 1 per woman. This total is equivalent to 9.5% of all pregnancies and is therefore within the range estimated for early foetal loss, that is 10% to 20%.

Cognizance must be taken of the problem of recall lapse in discussing relatively short and often traumatic events such as miscarriages. This problem is compounded by the fact that these women are required to recall multiple pregnancies, events which by definition comprise several significant occurrences. For example: was the pregnancy desired, was it trouble free, was the birth "easy," was the sex of the child the preferred one and so on. These and other factors may contribute to no recall or conversely to vivid recall. With these limitations in mind we can proceed to a detailed description of the available data.

These 30 miscarriages are contributed by 14 mothers. The majority (7) experience 1 each, 3 women have between 2 and 3, and for the other 4 the number stands at 4 each. Thus 4 women actually account for the high wastage of 16 pregnancies. Two of these women can be classified as being habitual abortionists, that is having 3 consecutive miscarriages. In 1 woman, these occur in the early months of pregnancy ($1\frac{1}{2}$ to 2 months), at parities 12 to 14, when she is between ages 42 and 43. This particular woman, at age 22 years and at para 1, miscarried male twins at 4 months. In the other woman the miscarriages occur at parities 5 to 7 when she is between the ages of 28 and 34. Most of these miscarriages take place in the fourth month of pregnancy, with 13 or 43% so stated. Only 6 are given as occurring at 2 months or less. This small number is probably accounted for in part by the fact that in the early months of pregnancy a spontaneous abortion may actually be mistaken for a heavy menstrual loss.

Parity assumes importance in the incidence of miscarriages since, as it is a natural complication of pregnancy, the greater the number of conceptions, the greater the risk of miscarriage. Of the 30 abortions, 7 occur at parities 2 and 3 and the largest single group (9) occurs between orders 10 and 12. Between parities 10 and 14, 13 occur, while 17 occur at parities lower than 10. This confirms our earlier point that the incidence of miscarriages increases as the order of parity rises.

So far as age of occurrence of miscarriage is concerned, no firm pattern emerges. Approximately 21 pregnancies terminate either spontaneously or are induced prior to term among women aged 30 and over, thereby substantiating the point that this event rises both with age and parity. Age of mother cross-tabulated by age of father further confirms our argument in respect of age. Highest numbers of miscarriages are recorded for fathers aged 35 to 39 (6) and those 50 to 54 (5). The oldest fathers here are aged 70 to 74, with 2 miscarriages to women aged 40 to 44.

Stillbirths

These 28 women experience in all 13 stillbirths, or an average of 0.5 each, and these amount to 4% of all pregnancies. Actually only 4 women are responsible for these 13 stillbirths; 2 have 1 each, another has 2, while the third contributes 9. The ages of the women at the time of termination range from 24 to 36 years. The youngest father involved is aged 26 and the range for the others span 19 years. For the one woman with 9, details are available for only 4, which include male twins. The sex of 11 is known and of these 10 are male and 1 female. Data are available for only 8 in respect of the number of months of the woman's pregnancy. None of these go to full term; 4 have terms of 7 months, 4 have terms of 8, while 3, including the twins, are of 8.5 months' gestation.

Infant Mortality

Early neonatal and perinatal mortality form important measures of congenital abnormalities, incompatible with the maintenance of vital life functions, or of trauma during or after birth with results similar to the former. Neonatal mortality, while including the first, also embraces some environmental factors, and in the late neonatal period these factors assume even greater dimensions.

Infant mortality among the births to the women under discussion is of particular interest in virtue of their high parities and generally low socio-economic status. There are a total of 25 deaths to infants under 12 months, which is equivalent to a rate of 88 per 1,000 livebirths, a fairly high rate of loss. As is to be expected, the 17 male deaths are a little more than twice that of the females.

Deaths of early neonates equal 10, or 35.84 per 1,000. Unfortunately, causes of death are given for only 3 of these. One is stated as due to respiratory factors and another to prematurity, while the third is allegedly due to the infant falling off a trolley in the hospital. Although the mother states that she is told this by a nurse in the hospital, there is some element of doubt about her account as the infant was only 5 days old. Of these early neonates, 9 are males, thereby conforming to the usual pattern of heavier mortality among this sex. Only 2 deaths occur in the late neonatal period, that is 8 to 28 days, both of these being due to fits or convulsions.

Deaths during the post-neonatal period amount to 13, and it is interesting to note that they are fairly evenly distributed in terms of sex. Here environmental factors assume greater importance. Of the 3 deaths from gastro-enteritis, 2 are males aged 11 and 12 months, while the female succumbs at 6 months. The term used by some women to describe deaths from vomiting and diarrhoea, usually the viral gastro-enteritis of infancy, is "teething water turn down." This description, in addition to being colourful, gives an approximate time of the occurrence of some of these events as infants generally begin teething around the fifth month of age. They are expected to have excessive salivation which overflows from the mouth and results in the baby "dribbling." If, however, the infant is having vomiting and diarrhoea he very quickly becomes dehydrated and obviously salivation will be considerably reduced or cease altogether. Hence the explanation "teething water turn down," a not illogical justification for what is to the mothers an inexplicable phenomenon.

Diseases of the respiratory system are advanced as causes of death in 2 cases. One, a male, died at 6 weeks from pneumonia and the other, a female, died of bronchitis at the age of 12 months, as stated by a doctor. Interestingly enough the mother of the latter had toxaemia of pregnancy when she was carrying this infant. Only 2 other causes of death are given for males, 1 dying at 8 months of malnutrition and the other at 10½ months from convulsions. Causes of death are not stated for the remaining 6 infants.

Twins

The occurrence of multiple births is usually of considerable interest both demographically and medically. In the present context it is of interest to see to what extent multiple births contribute to the formation of large families. In our case the multiple is of 2 only, that is twins.

Several factors influence the propensity for twinning. As has been discussed in Chapter 7, these include advanced age and parity, criteria which these women meet. In addition racial differences in rates are marked, with highest rates recorded being those of African negroes. It is necessary to bear this in mind in considering twinning in Jamaica, which is a predominantly negro society.

Of the 316 pregnancies to the 28 women, 7 sets of liveborn twins are recorded. In addition there is 1 set of stillbirth twins. In respect of pregnancy wastage, 1 set of male twins miscarry at 4 months. In contrast to singleton births, the chances of survival *in utero* is enhanced for twins conceived by mothers of high ages and parities.

The 9 sets of twins are equivalent to a ratio of 1 in 35 pregnancies which is somewhat similar to the rate given by Scheinfeld for African negroes.[4] This is considerably higher than that found in the sample as a whole, where the ratio is 1 in 81 when these 28 women are excluded. These 8 sets (1 set aborted and is therefore excluded) are produced by women of 2 birth cohorts, 4 sets by 2 women of the 1915-19 cohort and 4 by the other 3 of the 1925-29 cohort. Their ages at the time of the births range from 26 to 43 years with 3 occurring in the peak period of 35 to 39 years. Their partners' ages range from 28 to 52 years, but the 1 woman who has 3 consecutive sets is unable to state her partner's age. Their parities, with the exception of the 1 set at para 1, all fall between 5 and 10, a factor which we know increases the chances of twinning.

Twins assume further significance in terms of the sexes produced, that is whether they are 2 boys, 2 girls, or boy/girl, and in addition whether they are identical or fraternal. It is not however possible for us to make any positive identification in terms of 1-egg or 2-egg conceptions, but it is interesting to note that these 8 sets of twins are all of the same sex, that is to say there are no obvious fraternals: 6 sets are boy/boy, including the stillbirths, and 2 are all female. It is therefore quite probable that several of these are in fact 1-egg or identical twins.

All except 2 sets of males are full term. The stillbirths are delivered at 8.5 months and another set of males shows a pregnancy duration of 7 months. These last 2 are borne by the 2 women with the highest parities, the mother of the former being para 9 and the latter para 10.

Mortality among these sets of multiple births is no higher than among similar singletons. One female died at age 12 months of an unstated cause. The other death was of a male who died at 6 years from tetanus.

Intergenerational Data

In view of the possibility that heredity may play a part in the high fertility of these 28 women, some attempt is made to study intergenerational fertility. However, it must be noted that the question designed to elicit this information is, "How many children did your mother have?" This is clarified by indicating whether the figure given is known to be exact or is merely an estimate. It is, however, unlikely that the figure given includes stillbirths and almost certainly does not cover abortions. We have therefore treated these as livebirths and have used the corresponding number of livebirths of the respondents.

Because our respondents are all women with large families their family sizes in terms of livebirths can be listed consecutively from 7 to 15. This is not possible for their mothers and thus their families are grouped in the most convenient manner.

Our respondents' mothers bear a total of 197 children or 28% less than their daughters. A closer look at their respective family sizes shows that whereas the modal number of livebirths for the respondent is 10, their mothers' were heavily concentrated in the 5 to 9 family group, as 17 are recorded as having families of this size. Indeed, while for our respondents there are 17 women with 10 to 15 livebirths, the corresponding approximate family size for their mothers, that is of 10 to 20, is only 4.

Six of the respondents' mothers have 2 to 4 children, as compared with the 3 respondents with the smallest family sizes of 7 and 8. However one of the women with 8 livebirths appears to have achieved a marked reduction of her family size in comparison to that of her mother. Although this respondent has in fact had 16 pregnancies yielding 17 products, her mother is reported to have had 20 children. The average number of children of the respondents' mothers is 7.3, or 2.8 children fewer than the average of the respondents themselves.

Answers to the question on the number of children of mothers of the partners of the respondents may be less reliable, as this information is obtained from the respondent and not from her partner.

Twenty-two respondents have partners at the time of the survey or when they attain age 45 years. As reported, mothers of their partners bear a total of 124 children, or an average of 5.6 each. Of these 22, 6 answered "don't know," that is they knew only of their partners. These cannot be utilised in our analysis. Twelve others are reported as having families of under 10, 3 of 10 to 14 and 1 of 16.

A more realistic comparison of intergenerational fertility can be obtained by looking at the 9 women with only 1 partner. Here we can compare the family size of the women's mothers as well as that of their partners' mothers. Seven of the respondents' mothers have had less than 7 children as compared with the 7 respondents with 9 and 10 children each. In only 2 cases does the number of children of the mother exceed that of the daughter and this by 1 and 2 only. However when we look at the excess of daughters' children over their mothers' we see that this is in the range 3 to 10, a substantial increase. These 9 women have 94 children, that is 39 or 71% more than their mothers. Information is available for the mothers of only 8 partners as 1 partner had died prior to the survey.

Not much can be made of the numbers here as 4 of their mothers are reported as having 1 child. In spite of this, the fact that their sons had almost 3 times the number of children the mothers had cannot be discounted. The excess of the number of children of sons over their mothers amounts to 55, which is significant despite the limitations of the data.

Attitudes to Large Families

In view of the large families of these women an examination of their attitudes to family size is in order. As has been pointed out earlier in this study, there is a marked tendency for these women to take a philosophical attitude to many events in their lives; they are content to ascribe quite a number of these to "the will of God." No definitive evidence is available either in favour of or against these large families. Additionally too it is generally accepted that while a pregnancy may be unwanted, the birth of a child often changes the mother's attitude to one of acceptance.

Nevertheless an indication of their attitudes can be obtained from the question, "How many children do you think a woman should have in her lifetime?" While the response here is an ideal or of a theoretical nature it is significant that for most respondents the stated size is considerably less than their actual family size.

Of these 28 women only 2 failed to respond to this question with a specific number, and it is interesting that they both had 12 livebirths. The total livebirths of the remaining 26 women number 256 while the total of their expressed ideal is 141, about one-half their actual family size. The stated ideal numbers and the women responding can be classified as follows:

No. women responding	Ideal family size
2	2
1	3
8	4
3	5
6	6
1	7
3	8
2	10
Total 26	141

Of the 2 women who state that 10 children is the ideal, 1 did in fact have 10 livebirths, which may indicate either that she had her ideal number or that she is relating the actual to the ideal. In the other case the ideal of 10 is understandable, as this woman had 16 pregnancies including 8 livebirths, but experienced total losses in the form of pregnancy wastage and deaths amounting to 11. A slight preference for girls is the ideal, as the expressed total is 72 as compared with 69 boys.

Data on the fostering of children can also be used as an indicator of attitudes to family size. Of the three women fostering children, one who had 9 livebirths states that she is fostering her cousin's children as her cousin is overseas. She says she has a genuine love for children and they all make a big loving family. Another woman "reared" her niece and nephew, in addition to her own 9 children, as their father had died.

The third woman, who is 47 years old and has 10 livebirths, is fostering 2 children. One, a little boy, is not a relative but his mother is abroad and sends money for his support. The other, a female, is a young cousin of hers and is orphaned. This last addition, although it does present some financial strain on the family, has not prevented her from assuming responsibility for its support.

In view of the very large families of these women the fact that 10% are known to have additions to their families provides justification for concluding that there are no real objections to large families on their part. This is further borne out by the woman who said that some of her children were taken by their father "behind her back." She is very upset as she feels that they will "never come back."

Case Studies

Introduction

The following case studies are presented for two main purposes. The first is to narrow the focus of our discussion on large families in order to see what some of our statistics signify on an individual basis. The second and in many respects the more important is for us to attempt to view these women's lives from their own perspective.

Several points are immediately clear. Undoubtedly there is a distressing lack of information and knowledge regarding the causes of menstruation and pregnancy, two of the most basic biological functions of their bodies. While no claim is made that it is necessary or in fact even desirable that individuals should have detailed knowledge of all aspects of anatomy and physiology, it is quite clear that there are certain areas where some knowledge is desirable, if not vital. This is particularly so in relation to the modern methods of fertility control, nearly all of which interfere with the menstrual cycle in some way. If therefore a woman has no knowledge or an inaccurate concept of what is the cause and function of menstruation, it is highly likely that she is at greater risk, either of delaying the adoption of family planning until a point of near desperation is reached, or of discontinuing a method or methods if all is not as she expects it to be.

The whole question of relationships with a partner or partners is intriguing. In many cases the first relationship hardly qualifies for this term as it is obviously due to a combination of factors resulting in pregnancy but in little more. "We went to school together and I do not know why we became friends. It must have been Satan!" She was "small" (young) and living with her mother. Many of these women are in rural areas with no amenities, no lights and so on. They and their young men, with little to divert their interests, quickly arrive at the point of intercourse where the girls become pregnant. In a number of instances their total bewilderment at this result comes through quite strongly. She said she was sick during the pregnancy (she was aged 19) and had a cold and pains over her body, but she did not go to the doctor as she was very young at the time and was "hiding" her condition from her parents, who only found out about it when she was 8 months pregnant. She in fact "broke off" the relationship when she discovered that she was pregnant.

Their subsequent relationships are more solidly based on emotional, economic or status grounds, often in connexion with their children; "the children play a lot of part." It is interesting to note that the word "love" is not in common usage in referring to men. "I like him, he was loving and kind," or "I really did like him," are typical ways of referring to partners. That is to say, they tend to speak of "liking" a man but "loving" a child.

It is our impression in studying this group that the women appear to expect very little from their partners or children's fathers. Quite clearly there is little bitterness in speaking of the poor treatment often meted out to them by their partners. "The first man didn't treat me good after having the first child. I took a second one and he die. You want some help and I get a next man and he wasn't any good and none of them were any good. All were the same. It was bad luck for me." Any resentment expressed is usually in respect of help for their children denied them. There is also an awareness that many of the men are unable to give more assistance, as in the case of the woman who said that she feels that "C. would give even more support if he could as him have the mind, but not the money." This, however, refers to financial assistance and little reference is made to emotional support of the man for his child. While most women expect to be faithful to their partners and express the view that reciprocity is the ideal, they tend to qualify these statements by admitting that males differ. It appears that while these women demonstrate, both in their durations of unions and in many ways by their family sizes, that men are important, there is an air almost of contempt or possibly mistrust for males in general.

The references made to violence and excessive demands by males, usually given as an explanation for not establishing a household, are noteworthy. "What I was looking for is not what I get." Her husband would drink "and fight me all the time and tear off me clothes." Another woman said her husband was very jealous and used to beat her, while another stated that "the men cannot beat you when visiting, but living together they will beat you." In one case a woman whose only union is marriage says that she has been lucky as she "never know how a man lick stay, thank God." Although most of these women ultimately marry or enter common-law unions, the reasons given for doing so are usually increasing family size, economic or respectability. In several cases, too, the view is expressed that marriage has many disadvantages that have to be borne with fortitude in view of the reasons previously listed.

Although these women are all grande multiparae, it is evident that the deaths of their children affected them profoundly as it did the fathers and the siblings who were old enough to understand. The mother's acceptance of the individuality of each child appears to be borne out by the fact that in most cases no thought is given to replacing the deceased child. The exceptions, both understandable, to this are one woman who lost her first child and therefore desired another and the woman who had several deaths of children and was therefore anxious to replace them. In a number of instances some feeling of guilt is expressed, as in the case of the woman whose young son died of tetanus. She did not apparently take any action when the child told her he had been "stuck" and therefore she feels some guilt over his death. However in most cases a philosophical attitude is taken and, as the friends of one mother pointed out to her, it is better to lose a child than for her to die, as the other children will then be motherless—an irreparable loss. This point is poignantly illustrated in the case of the respondent who was pregnant at the time of the survey and who has since died in childbirth at the age of 35. As this is her fourteenth pregnancy one wonders what effect her death will have on the surviving members of her family.

Respondent 8B80

Louise A. is a 49-year-old married woman living with her 74-year-old husband in a rural, agricultural district. She married him after 4 years of common-law living and in all they have been together for 33 years. Neither of them is at present employed. They both had 8 years of primary schooling and they belong to the Apostolic Church—a fundamentalist religion. Her mother, who was not married to her father, had 3 children while his parents were married and his mother had 5 children. As expected, their respective fathers were both farmers.

At 14 Louise had her first child for a visiting partner—a relationship which ended 9 months after the baby was born. She was working as a shop assistant in a store at which he was a frequent customer and so they became friendly. Before long she got pregnant but they could not think of living together as her grandmother, with whom she grew up, was alive and did not approve of common-law living. Indeed, when she went home to have the baby they "fussed" with her as they thought she was too young to be having a boyfriend at all. If she had waited he would have married her, but she was "a little bit jealous" as a girlfriend had written to tell her that she saw him going to another girl's house. She thereupon wrote him and he came to see her and she told him that she did not want to have anything more to do with him as she heard he was "along with another girl." He protested that it was a lie but in her jealousy she refused to continue seeing him as "I do not want to catch any germs" since he was going with another woman as well as with her. He said that if she did not marry him, he would never get married and "until now he don't married."

Two years later she became friendly with her present partner and suffered a miscarriage almost immediately. She was then living with him and they continued in that union until 2 more children were born. At that stage they decided to get married as she felt "it would be very hard for me to leave him and go and take a next man having 2 children with him." Also they felt he could now afford marriage. They both worked and pooled their resources until they bought the present home they live in.

In all, she has had 12 liveborn children in addition to the miscarriage. They were all delivered at home—the first 2 by a nana, while a trained nurse delivered the rest. She had no complications and apart from the first did not work during any of the pregnancies. She breastfed all her babies for 9 months. She did not use any contraceptives and in fact considered family planning "a sin" at one time "but now I think it is good, so you could give the children better education." She still believes, however, that birth control and abortions are some of the reasons for childlessness as they "upset the workings of the womb." She has heard that a woman can choose the number of children she has now but "in my days I didn't have that knowledge."

Louise thinks that 3 children constitute a small family while 12, like hers, is a large one. Her ideal number, however, is 6—3 boys and 3 girls. She believes that every man and woman should have a child, and she is sorry for the woman who does not have one. She does not think that a woman without a child can be happy as she has no one to help her at home or take care of her when she is sick. At the same time she does not approve of the unmarried woman having children as "keeping themselves from a man—it would be better." Yet she expresses the opinion that it is all right for a woman to have a child for each of her partners because, as long as she is having sex and not using any method of birth control, it is only natural for that to happen, but she does not think that a woman should have two partners at the same time. She thinks that 2 to 3 years apart is good spacing for the children although 5 of hers are only 12 to 16 months apart. She has heard that a nana can tell how many children a woman is going to have by counting the "bumps" on the baby's cord at delivery.

Louise had her first period at age 14 and her last at age 49. She says she has had a "hard time" with the menopause. Her grandmother told her about menstruation and the dangers of "going to a man" after it started, but she does not know the real cause of it. Her periods were regular and at first lasted for 5 days but as she had more children the flow became very heavy and sometimes lasted for as long as 9 days. She went to a doctor who admitted her to hospital and scraped the womb and this checked the "flooding." In addition she sometimes had backache badly and had to stay in bed for a day. During menstruation she was told not to take a cold bath as it would stop her period and cause consumption (tuberculosis). She was also told to keep on a diaper for 9 days after the period stopped to prevent her catching a cold. At the time pads were not available and she had to make her own diapers.

She does not believe that a woman should have sex just before or during her period and she should wait for 9 days after it is finished, but she admits that her husband would not wait that length of time although he did not trouble her while she was actually menstruating. She says that a woman can get pregnant when "the seed from the man go in your womb and your seed—the both of them collide" but it also depends on whether "you and the man come together and get in heat together."

In comparing her two partners she declares she has more affection for her husband as "from the both of us get in friendship, I never find, or hear, or know of him in any way want to keep another woman." She has also been happiest in marriage.

Her mating and reproductive histories are graphically presented in Figure 10.1.

Statistical summary of pregnancy history

Events		Age	Years	Percentages
Age at menarche		14		
Age at menopause		49		
Biological years of potential childbearing	(a)		35	
Age at termination of 1st pregnancy		14		
Age at termination of last pregnancy		36		
Actual years of childbearing	(b)		22	
Years spent in pregnancy	(c)		9.25	
Years spent in breastfeeding	(d)		9.00	
(c) + (d)	(e)		18.25	
Rest of period			3.5	
Total pregnancies		13		
(b) as % (a)				62.9
(c) as % (b)				42.0
(d) as % (b)				40.9
(e) as % (b)				83.0

Average number of years per pregnancy 1.69
(actual years)/(number of pregnancies)

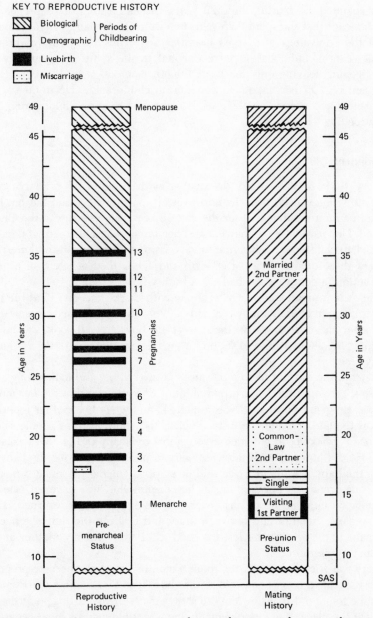

Figure 10.1 Graphic representation of reproductive and mating history of respondent 8B80.

193

Louise had a biological potential of 35 years of childbearing but her actual years spanned 22. During these 22 years, she had a total of 13 pregnancies which meant that she spent 9.25 years in a state of pregnancy. In addition she spent the equivalent of 9 years breastfeeding. Thus 18.3 years of Louise's actual years of childbearing were devoted to the states of pregnancy and breastfeeding, leaving only 3.5 years for other activities. By this we see that she spent 63% of her biological potential in childbearing. Her total years of pregnancy accounted for 42% of her actual years of childbearing, and breastfeeding 41%.

Respondent 2301

Mary S. is a 39-year-old dressmaker with 8 years of primary school education. She was born in the northwestern part of the island but has been living in a metropolitan area for the past 16 years. She belongs to the Church of God. Her parents were married and her father was a railroad worker. She has had 10 children by 3 different unions: visiting, common-law and marriage. Two of these died the day after birth and 1 boy died at age 8 of a bowel obstruction, a condition he had been born with.

Mary's first union was a very brief one with C. She was just 15 at the time. "I was going to church and was afraid of men. My mother used to send me to look after the cows because there were no boys .... It look like he was watching me a long time and set up for me one evening and there was no one at my rescue."

She says she did not like C. because "he was so big and look strong and I was so short and little. I was afraid of him." She was afraid to tell her mother she was pregnant because "I was ashamed" and when her mother found out "it was too late." C. left the district where they both lived as people said he had been "wicked" to get such a young girl pregnant and "he was ashamed too." He did however return occasionally to provide things for the baby but when the baby was about 1 year old he stopped coming for about 4 months. Then one evening as her mother saw him coming she "was so vexed" she shut the door on him and he in turn "was very mad" and never returned. There was no sexual relationship between Mary and C. from the time she became pregnant until the time he left for good as "I was with my mother and he couldn't come there."

Mary was friendly with L. for about 5 months before she became pregnant. At first she liked him as he pretended to be a "good boy" and a Christian but later she found out that he went "to show" every night. At this point she was living at the place of her employment. She was frightened by him because she was in town and her family was not with her. He would say that he didn't love her because she was fat.

She worked through her 8 months of pregnancy and then returned to the country, coming back to Kingston only when the baby was 3 months old. L.

did not provide for her when she was pregnant and it was then, she said, that she started to hate him. When she came back to Kingston he came to see her and gave her money when he saw the baby but she refused to take it. The money dropped to the ground and he went away and never came back. In fact she had no further relationship with him after the baby's birth.

During the 12 months of her visiting union with L. he would come to the place where she lived and worked. They would meet there about twice a week and he would spend the night. There seems to have been no trouble in arranging these meetings. She estimates that they had sex twice a week and met for a total of 24 hours per week. During these meetings they sometimes discussed God and spoke about going to church, but she later found out that he was only pretending to be religious. She expected him to be faithful to her and he expected the same thing.

Mary attributes the end of her relationship to L. to the fact that the man who was to be her third partner kept calling on her "just as a friend" while she was pregnant with L.'s child and that he found out about it. In addition L. had found a "nice looking, slim, girlfriend."

Mary entered her third union with E., a Roman Catholic by religion and a barber by profession, in February 1958 when she was 23 and he was 31. She was not anxious to enter into a permanent union at this time as she was living at her place of employment, liked her work and liked to save money: "I'd be better off if I had stayed there," but E. was anxious to have someone take care of him and wash his clothes so to please him she moved in with him.

They were married on April 1, 1965, 7 months before the birth of their second child. Mary says they were not influenced by anyone to change their union into marriage but that they loved one another and that he feared she was going to leave him. She would have liked to have her 2 sisters, who lived in town, at the wedding but he did not want to have anyone.

Mary's pregnancies all seem to follow the same pattern. All but 2 were full term and there were no complications during pregnancy or after birth. The sixth and seventh children were born after 7 months and died the day after birth. She does not know why and states that during her sixth pregnancy she had "bad feelings" and that there were difficulties in the birth itself.

Her fifth child was born in 1966. She had some "'bad feelings" during this pregnancy but no complications during the birth. She did not breastfeed him because when she tried he brought up everything, so she took him to the hospital where he remained for 10 months with an obstruction in his bowels. In 1974, at the age of 8 he died of this obstruction. His death brought great sadness to the family; the brothers and sisters were upset and missed him and the father lost his appetite and was depressed. Mary's eyes were red and watery as she talked about the child. She said that his death had made her ill and caused her to be emotionally upset. She thinks all her relationships were affected by it and she experienced feelings of guilt. She feels however that the last child has replaced her dead son.

Mary, who was exceptionally articulate and responsive during the whole interview, seems to have had difficulties in answering the questions dealing with assessment of her partner and of her type of union. Her visiting union with L. brought her sexual pleasure but not much affection. She had affection for her third partner while they were in their common-law union but later when they were married, for reasons she did not explain, the relationship brought her much unhappiness. While she lived with him she felt it was a sin to do so. When asked whether she felt any different after marriage, she answered, "I feel I have protection; otherwise it don't make no difference to me, only for the children."

She was frightened when her menses started at age 13 because no one had explained anything about it to her but she had read about it. Her periods are regular and last 7 days and her only problem is a "tired feeling around her waist" while it lasts. She thinks the best time to have sex is before the menses, never during and not for 2 weeks after because "men think you are unclean." She cannot remember where she learned this but she thinks she read it somewhere. Her husband doesn't want to see her when she is menstruating and whenever possible doesn't sleep in the same bed with her during the period. Menstruation, she thinks, is caused by "excess blood." Pregnancy occurs through sexual intercourse but not always, "because the egg don't mature."

Mary started using foam tablets as contraceptives after the birth of her seventh child, and continued until after the birth of the tenth and last child.

Statistical summary of pregnancy history

Events		Age	Years	Percentages
Age at menarche		13		
Age at menopause (still menstruating)		38		
Biological years of potential childbearing	(a)		25	
Age at termination of 1st pregnancy		16		
Age at termination of last pregnancy		37		
Actual years of childbearing	(b)		21	
Years spent in pregnancy	(c)		7.5	
Years spent in breastfeeding	(d)		8.1	
(c) + (d)	(e)		15.6	
Rest of period			5.4	
Total pregnancies		10		
(b) as % (a)				84.0
(c) as % (b)				35.7
(d) as % (b)				38.6
(e) as % (b)				74.3

Average number of years per pregnancy 2.1
(actual years)/(number of pregnancies)

She has heard that drinking boiled senna and salt will get rid of the baby. Also if you drink stout and nutmeg and lie down for an hour, it will get rid of the baby but she herself has never tried it.

She thinks that family planning is good for the country but believes that every man and woman should have children because a childless union "don't make a happy home or marriage." She thinks every woman should choose the number of children she wants.

Her mating and reproductive histories are graphically presented in Figure 10.2.

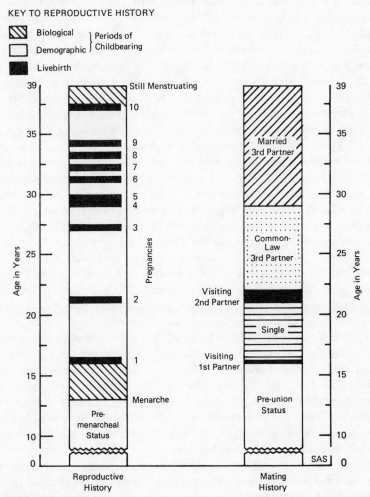

Figure 10.2 Graphic representation of reproductive and mating history of respondent 2301

Mary started menstruating at 13 and is still doing so. Her biological period of potential childbearing is to date 25 years. She had her first child at 16 and her last at 37, which gives an actual childbearing span of 21 years, or we may say that her actual was 84% of her potential. Of her demographic span, 7.5 years or 36% were spent in a state of pregnancy and 8.1 years or 39% were devoted to breastfeeding. Thus of the 21 years, 74% was spent in these two states with a resulting "free" period of only 5.4 years.

Respondent 1071

Miriam S. is a 49-year-old married woman living in a crowded, low-income, urban area. She has been living in this parish for 41 years and took part in a similar study in 1971-72. She started living with her partner, who was 21 years older than she, at the age of 18, and they got married 7 years later. Her mother, who was not married to her father but later married someone else, had 11 children, and in view of the fact that Miriam was born in an agricultural area, it is not surprising that her father was a farmer. She had 8 years of primary schooling but does not know how many years her husband spent in school. He used to be a carpenter but he is not working now as he is 70 years old and in poor health. However he was not at home when the interview took place—"man all over, so long as they are not in bed they doesn't stay home." She herself has never worked. Her husband's parents were married to each other but she does not know how many children his mother had. His father was a preacher in the Jehovah's Witness but both respondent and her husband are members of the Church of God, one of the many fundamentalist churches in the island.

Miriam has 10 children—6 boys and 4 girls—who are all alive and were delivered in the Government Hospital by trained nurses. She was 9 months pregnant with each of them and had no complications during the pregnancies or at the deliveries. She used no contraceptives although there is as much as 4 years difference between the seventh and eighth children. Before she was "saved" she seriously considered tying off her tubes but after she accepted the Lord she saw "where it wasn't right in the sight of the Lord ... so I have out my lot." As a "child of God" she does not believe in family planning—"God is able to take care of the children." She thinks it is important for the development of the country though, as there are those that are "carefree" and just cannot afford to have children. "Responsible people should not use family planning," she declares. She was 19 when she had her first child and 41 when she had her last.

Before she became friendly with her husband, she had another friend with whom she used to have sex. However he was "wild" so she decided to leave him and shortly after started the relationship with her present partner. He visited her for a short while and when she became pregnant she left home and went to live with him as her parents were against the union. It was natural for him to visit at first so that she could get to know him and if she "was not satisfied with him" she would have left him. They got married a year after the fourth child was born because "they said the life is more honourable" and they felt it was better for the children.

In discussing the types of unions she has had, she said "naturally marriage" brought her the most happiness and gave her more status in the community. It is only when her husband does not work that there has been any worry in their marriage.

When they were in a visiting relationship he used to come to her house quite often but she went to his only about once per week, at which time they used to have sex. She remembers him taking her to a garden party once. She says they are both faithful to each other and when asked if she enjoyed having sex with him, she answered, "Must have—with all those children." At present they have sex about 2 or 3 times per month.

Miriam considers her family of 10 children a large one, while one of 2 or 4 children is small in her opinion. She thinks every woman should have a child as they are a help and a blessing in one's old age and people look upon you as barren if you do not have children. Women who do not have children must be lonely and "they must feel like their labour is in vain." She believes they must be always wishing to have one although some are "prejudiced" as they are not married. One of the main reasons every man should have a child is that it ensures that his name does not die with him. She does not think that women have a choice in the number of children they can have, "unless they safeguard themselves." She considers that the best spacing between the children is 2 to 4 years and a good family size is about 4—2 boys and 2 girls.

This lady had her first period at 12 years old and is still menstruating. No one had ever told her about sex or menstruation and she was frightened when she saw her first period. She thinks menstruation is "bad blood" that one needs to get rid of, and although hers is regular and gives her no problem she feels that during that time one should not do "much work." Miriam says that a woman can have sex immediately before menstruation but not during or for at least 3 days after the period ends. She preferred to be menstruating rather than pregnant. She had heard that conception occurred when "some germs moving from the Daddy to the Mummy" came in contact with each other; if there was no contact pregnancy could not take place. She had also heard that some people drink bitters and aloes and others puncture something with a pencil sometimes so as to get rid of their pregnancies.

She loves all her children, but the sixth one—a male—generally "keeps close to her." The others say she loves him most but it is not so—"it is he that loves me most." Her children all call her "Mamma" as she called her mother, although she did "not grow with her."

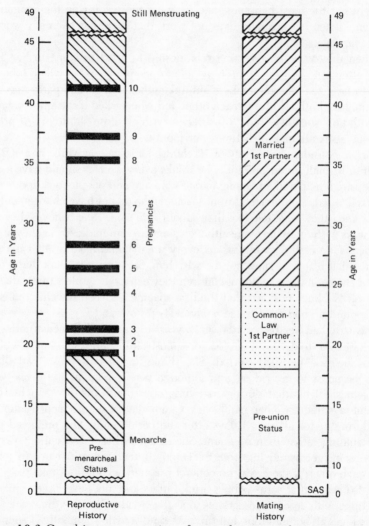

Figure 10.3 Graphic representation of reproductive and mating history of respondent 1071

Statistical summary of pregnancy history

Events		Age	Years	Percentages
Age at menarche		12		
Age at menopause (still menstruating)		49		
Biological years of potential childbearing	(a)		37	
Age at termination of 1st pregnancy		19		
Age at termination of last pregnancy		41		
Actual years of childbearing	(b)		22	
Years spent in pregnancy	(c)		7.5	
Years spent in breastfeeding	(d)		7.5	
(c) + (d)	(e)		15	
Rest of period			7	
Total pregnancies		10		
(b) as % (a)				59.5
(c) as % (b)				34.1
(d) as % (b)				34.1
(e) as % (b)				68.2

Average number of years per pregnancy 2.2
(actual years)/(number of pregnancies)

Her mating and reproductive histories are graphically presented in Figure 10.3.

Miriam's biological years of potential childbearing are to date 37 years and of these she has, by having her first child at age 19 and last at 41, achieved a demographic span of childbearing of 22 years. She has therefore spent 60% of her biological potential in actual childbearing.

Of those 22 years, 7.5 or 34% were devoted to the actual state of pregnancy. If we add to this another 7.5 years occupied in breastfeeding her 10 children we see that Miriam in fact spent 68% of her (demographic) childbearing span in pregnancy and breastfeeding.

The above profile of a life largely devoted to the bearing and rearing of children raises the question of the time or indeed the energy available for the development of other aspects of her life. Clearly this lady has during the 31 years of her relationship, which commenced as common-law and led into marriage, had a satisfactory life with her only partner. However her statement that she considers a good family size as 4 seems to validate our original question concerning the lack of total development of this woman, for which her heavy involvement in childbearing is responsible.

Respondent 6874

Mabel W. is a 48-year-old housewife living in a hilly, rural district. The village is comprised of small holdings usually inherited by the people who work on the adjoining estates or in the nearby city. She has been married for 27 years. Her husband, who is 17 years older than she, used to be a ranger on a property but he has not worked for some time as he has been ill—"his nerves cause him to go to Bellevue" (a mental hospital). She had 5 years of primary schooling but does not know how many years her husband spent in school. In neither case were their respective mothers married to their fathers. Her mother had 5 children and she thinks his mother had 6. Her father was a road headman and she lived with him "and my father wife who I grow with." When she and her husband fell in love she told him he would have to speak to her "mother"—in reality her stepmother—who said that "we couldn't live that life" and they would have to get married. "We read about in the Bible that marriage life is really living up to God's requirements" while the other types of unions are not so good because they are "a lawlessness type of living." Respondent is a Jehovah's Witness, although her stepmother who seemed to have had a great deal of influence over her was a Baptist and her husband does not belong to any church. Her church does not approve of common-law living and if a member goes into it, the church will "disfellowship" the person. If a girl gets pregnant out of wedlock, the church "disfellowships" her too but if after having the baby she realises that she has done "something wrong in the sight of Jehovah God," she may come back and be reinstated as a Witness.

After a late start she had 9 pregnancies, 2 of which resulted in twin births while a third was a miscarriage. She was already 28 years old and 7 years married before she had her first pregnancy, which produced male twins who were delivered at home by a trained nurse. She had a lot of vomiting during this pregnancy but there were no complications in her subsequent pregnancies. Apart from the third child, born 2 years after the twins, which she breastfed for 6 months, all her others were breastfed for approximately 3 months. She used no contraceptives and worked for a short while during the first 3 pregnancies. Her fourth child was the only one delivered by a nana and like the others, its birth presented no problems. Her sixth pregnancy also resulted in male twins—one of whom died at 6 years of age from tetanus. The year after the twins were born she suffered a miscarriage when she was 4 months pregnant and was attended to by a doctor because she continued to pass blood. The respondent remembered all the children but was confused by the order in which they came. The interviewer was greatly assisted by having the birth certificates for most of them.

She thinks 10 children can be considered a large family while 1 to 4 children constitute a small one and in fact she chose the latter number—2 boys and 2 girls—when asked how many children a woman should have in her lifetime. Every man and woman should have a child so "that they can take care of you when you are older." She thought childlessness may be the result of the partners "not matching" or the woman may be "ill" but whatever the reasons the woman who had no children "must feel embarrassment." Mabel feels that a married woman can take family planning and so decide how many children she wants to have. She should consult with her husband "because he is the head" of the household. Jehovah's Witnesses are not against family planning for married people: "I am not speaking of an unmarried person because they do not have the knowledge to know that they shouldn't go about and have the children like that." She thinks it is a sin to have children and not take care of them. When she was having her children times were not as hard as they are now for people having young babies—"even the baby's feed is expensive." She says when families are large the parents are unable to help the children as they should, so family planning is important for the development of the country. She has never heard that a woman should have a certain number of children but she knows that one can choose the amount she wants by using family planning.

Before she had any, she and her husband used to discuss the question of having children. She thought the best spacing between each child was about a year and in fact 4 of her pregnancies are about 16 months apart. She had her last child nearly 7 years ago but she has not seen her period for 2 months and she wonders, "I don't know if . . . what happen to it." In fact, she has not had sex with her husband for about a year. They love each other still but not as much as when they were younger and since coming back from the hospital "is not that way as before." She says they have both been faithful to each other and when they used to have sex about 6 times a month, she enjoyed it.

Mabel was 16 when she had her first period but still does not know what causes it, apart from "when a girl reach a certain age they are supposed to see their menses." Her periods were regular and lasted 6 days and there were no complications, although as a rule it was heavy on the second day and she had to remain at home, though not in bed. Her stepmother had told her about menstruation and sex but she does not know how a woman gets pregnant either, apart from having sex with a man. She thinks a woman can have sexual intercourse before her period but not during nor up to 14 days after and she uses lukewarm water to bathe in at that time. She has heard that one can go to a doctor to get rid of a baby.

In discussing her children, who all called her "Mamma," she mentioned that she had a special feeling for one of the first set of twins, just because he is more affectionate and knows "how to handle a mother." He is the only one not living at home at present. She said she was "very, very much sorry" at the death of her son and it took her a long time to recover. She felt that if she had taken him to the doctor the moment he got "stuck" he may not have died.

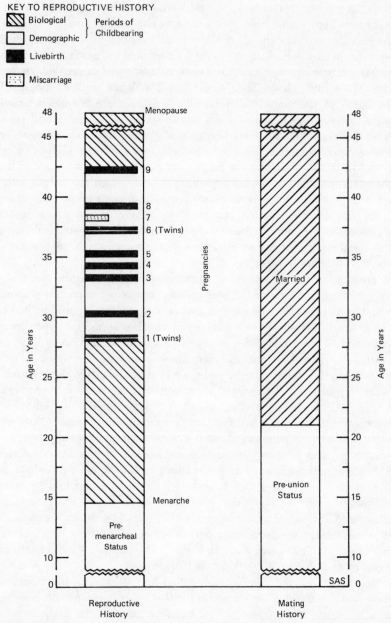

Figure 10.4 Graphic representation of reproductive and mating history of respondent 6874

The father as well as the rest of the family were very sorry too as they "did really love him."

She is a very pleasant, cooperative woman with a strong moralistic streak in her. She stated "it would not be a good life" to have children for different partners. She did not participate in a similar study in 1971–72.

Her mating and reproductive histories are graphically presented in Figure 10.4.

Mabel started to menstruate at age 16 and continued for 32 years, a period which constitutes her biological years of potential childbearing. She was 28 years old when she had her first pregnancy and 42 at her last. Thus her actual years of childbearing extend over a period of 14 years during which she had a total of 9 pregnancies. Looking at the time actually spent in a state of pregnancy we see that this is equivalent to 6.3 years. Mabel did not however spend much time on breastfeeding, as the total period here amounts to 2.5 years. In summary we note that, out of a childbeaing span of 14 years, Mabel spent 9 years or 63% either carrying a pregnancy or breastfeeding. Since the 14-year span of her childbearing period is equivalent to 44% of her potential we are left with the impression that in view of the extended period of time spent directly in bearing and childrearing, the opportunities for her social development have been noticeably affected.

Statistical summary of pregnancy history

Events		Age	Years	Percentages
Age at menarche		16		
Age at menopause		48		
Biological years of potential childbearing	(a)		32	
Age at termination of 1st pregnancy		28		
Age at termination of last pregnancy		42		
Actual years of childbearing	(b)		14	
Years spent in pregnancy	(c)		6.3	
Years spent in breastfeeding	(d)		2.5	
(c) + (d)	(e)		8.8	
Rest of period			5.2	
Total pregnancies	9			
(b) as % (a)				43.8
(c) as % (b)				45.0
(d) as % (b)				17.9
(e) as % (b)				62.9

Average number of years per pregnancy 1.6
(actual years)/(number of pregnancies)

Respondent 2158

Carol P. is a 57-year-old unemployed married woman living in the country. She has had 11 years of primary education and some post-primary. She is a Roman Catholic and daughter of a station agent. Her parents were not married and she was not brought up by her mother.

All of her 12 children were fathered by one partner, B., an Anglican who is now 54 years old and a machine operator. The initial union with him was a visiting one which started in 1943 when she was 26 and he was 23. Carol was living with an elderly lady and B. was living nearby. She does not recall clearly the period when she was in a visiting relationship as it was a very long time ago. She thinks they had sex about 12 times a month and discussed things together. He once gave her a medal and said it was to be for their first child.

Carol feels there are no special advantages to the visiting unions. They entered into a common-law union because "I consider that I don't have any mother, my father died, my grandmother died, so I would like a companion for myself and I was living with a stranger though they treat me nice." She informed the lady she was living with of the change of arrangements and she agreed to it. Their first child was born in October 1944, but this did not influence them to enter the common-law union. The pregnancy was not planned, though desired, and the child had no effect on their sexual relationship, but did help to stabilise the union; "the children play a lot of part."

Their common-law union lasted from 1943 to November 1950, during which time they had 5 children. In November 1950 Carol and B. were married. This step was taken because she wanted security for her children and felt that if anything happened to B. at work she would not get anything for the children. The nurse who delivered her children encouraged her to get married and she took the initiative and asked him to marry her.

Carol has 12 children (11 pregnancies with 1 set of twins). Ten of the children are living while 2, the fourth and the twelfth, both died at the age of 11 months. Her pregnancies were normal, except for the twins who were born at 7 months. They were weak and had to be bottle fed. Her first 3 children were delivered by a doctor at the hospital and the others by a nurse at her home. There were no complications during the pregnancies, during or after the births. There was great sadness when the children died and she still thinks about them and wonders how they would be, had they lived. The death from diarrhoea of the last child is particularly sad and she states that the doctor told her the diarrhoea was caused by the "teething water." Carol was ill and lost weight and their father was also upset, "since we both love our children." She was consoled by her friends who told her that it was better that the baby died and she remained because she had to take care of the other

children: "you can get another baby, but a baby cannot get another mother."
She did not feel guilty about the deaths because she took them to the doctor
and got medicine for them.

She has heard people say one should have a certain number of children, but
doesn't know how this number can be determined. Two children constitute a
small family for her and 10 a large one. Every woman should have a child, if
not it shows she is cursed and to be pitied. "Children are like an old age
pension; they can look after you when you get old because money is not all."
The cause of childlessness "is a part of God's work. They say that there is a
bearing fruit tree and a barren fig tree and I don't know if God has built some
women off the barren fig tree."

Carol has no favourites among her children who call her "Mummy." As she
did not grow with her mother she called her by her Christian name as she
heard other people calling her that.

She feels that family planning is good and if she had heard of it in "my
days" she would not have had so many children. She thinks it is good for the
country because "we would have less children, especially those people who
can't afford it." Carol has heard of no way to get rid of a baby and became
quite upset at being asked this question, saying she would not discuss this
with anyone because even to talk about it she feels her "bones shiver." She
further stated that she does not listen to "any talk about that" as she doesn't
like it.

Her menses began when she was aged 15 and stopped at age 55. Her
grandmother had explained menstruation to her, but no one had explained
sex. Her periods were regular, lasted for 6 to 7 days and she felt slight
discomfort in her back during them. A woman, she thinks, should have no
sexual intercourse just before or during the menses and should wait 3 to 4
days after the period. When she was menstruating her husband changed
position in their bed and they slept in opposite directions with his head at her
feet. Menstruation is caused by "waste matter of the blood that you have in
your body." When asked if she preferred menstruating to being pregnant she
answered, "if you have someone standing by you it's not bad being pregnant."
When asked again which she preferred, Carol said, "I prefer the two of
them." She does not know how one gets pregnant. She has heard that while
menstruating one should not touch a "young baby" and if you are boiling
sugar or guava jelly you should not look into it.

In assessing her partner Carol feels her husband is very responsive
in his economic support of her and the children, in the affection he gives
her, as a sexual partner and as a father. In assessing the different stages
of her union, the common-law and marriage seem to have brought her
equal satisfaction.

Carol did not participate in the previous study of 1971–72 as she was not in
the area, although she has lived in this parish for 35 years.

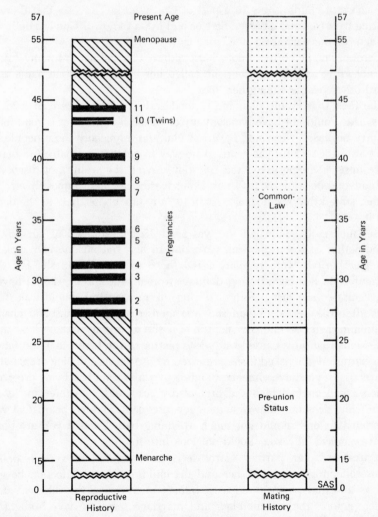

Figure 10.5 Graphic representation of reproductive and mating history of respondent 2158

Statistical summary of pregnancy history

Events		Age	Years	Percentages
Age at menarche		15		
Age at menopause		55		
Biological years of potential childbearing	(a)		40	
Age at termination of 1st pregnancy		27		
Age at termination of last pregnancy		44		
Actual years of childbearing	(b)		17	
Years spent in pregnancy	(c)		8.1	
Years spent in breastfeeding	(d)		8.8	
(c) + (d)	(e)		16.9	
Rest of period			0.1	
Total pregnancies		11		
(b) as % (a)				42.5
(c) as % (b)				47.6
(d) as % (b)				51.8
(e) as % (b)				99.4

Average number of years per pregnancy 1.5
(actual years)/(number of pregnancies)

Her mating and reproductive histories are graphically presented in Figure 10.5.

Carol had her first menses at age 15 and her last when she was age 55, a span of 40 years. With her first pregnancy at age 27 and her last at 44, her actual years of childbearing cover 17 years or 43% of her biological potential. She spends the equivalent of a total of 8 years in pregnancy and another 9 years in breastfeeding, thus the total of these two series of events amounts to 99% of her actual years of childbearing.

Carol's account of her life shows a long and clearly satisfactory relationship with her only partner and husband and a demonstrable love for her children and their well-being. However her comment that had family planning been available in "my days" she would not have had as many children raises the question as to whether she feels that some aspect of her life has been sacrificed at the expense of extended childbearing and childrearing.

Respondent 6708

Agnes F. is an unemployed married woman aged 45 who has been separated from her husband for 3 years. She have lived all her life in one parish but did not participate in a similar study in 1971–72 as she was not in the area. She had no schooling as she always suffered from an ulcer on her leg which prevented her from attending classes. She has had 17 pregnancies, following in the footsteps of her mother who had 20 children and her husband's mother who had 16. Only 4 of her children have survived however. Her mother was not married to her father, who was a policeman, but her husband's parents were married. Her husband, who is now 50 years old, had 8 years of primary schooling. They are both Baptists.

She was "romping in the moonshine" with her sisters and brothers when they went home without calling her and told her mother that they did not know where she was, so her mother locked her out and she went and slept with her first partner. This was the beginning of the friendship but as his father and her mother were very strict, they had to "t'ief pass" to be able to see each other. Nearly 2 years later, when she was 21 and he 18, she had her first child but because they were "so young," his stepmother and her mother took the money he provided and bought the things she would need for the baby. She had a difficult labour, culminating in her having fits so that the doctor had to come to her home to deliver her. Further problems arose when she "got a tear" and he had to visit her every other day for 2 weeks. She had not expected to have a baby as she really knew nothing about sex and the complications of the delivery made her a little afraid of having sexual relations for a while after that. However, she says repeatedly they love each other "until now." Paradoxically they broke up because she didn't want to marry him and they both left the district for different parts of the island.

About a year later, she entered into a common-law union with her second partner as she thought it would be a better life, but she says when she is "in friendship with anyone and she becomes pregnant, she finds that they want to handle me bad and me leave them whether me have the baby or not, me just leave them." Nine days after their child was born without any complications, she left and went home and when she returned a month later she found that he had another girlfriend. In retrospect she says she did not love him at all. The baby was breastfed for 4 months and died at 8 months from malnutrition because "me have to leave him to go work and they never feed him meantime."

She entered into a common-law union with her third partner, 3 years later, and had another child, but 3 months after the baby was born, they had a fuss and "he fight me and I move out of his house." Although they were no longer living together, he still visited her and she had 4 more children for him, none of which survived. The first of these died at 20 months from gastro-enteritis, the second lived for only a few hours, and the third and fourth were stillbirths. She had no complications during these 5 pregnancies or at delivery, but a month before the first stillbirth she had slipped while working in the banana walk after a rainfall and the second stillbirth was 2 weeks premature.

Her fourth partner was the man she eventually married. Their first child was born in the visiting union and died at 10½ months from convulsions. The following year, when she had been married for just a month, she slipped on the floor after her husband had cleaned it, and was just able to make it to the hospital where the doctor delivered twin stillbirths. After that she had to go to him for further treatment as he said her "nerves was getting bad." She afterwards had 2 female children for her husband who are alive and well. She had high blood pressure during the penultimate pregnancy and a long labour, lasting 7 days. The doctor said "me eat too much ice and the baby will come cold." That child would not take the breast at all.

After the last child was born, she had a tubal ligation. She is very glad about it as she feels if she hadn't been stopped "you wouldn't see me alive." She is enthusiastic about family planning and says she can recommend it because it has not only helped her very much but "thousands of us" as well. On the other hand she says "anytime God bless you, you suppose to bring forth," and deems it foolishness for people to be boiling different bushes to procure an abortion.

She decided to get married "because I would live better, I would be able to go to my Church more regular and the Lord would look upon me more and even our same colour men would have a little more respect for me." Unfortunately, "what I was looking for is not what I get." Her husband used to go out drinking with his sister and he would come home and destroy her things "and fight me all the time and tear off me clothes." One day she had to go to the Probation Officer to show him how he had torn off her dress and she also went to the police another time because of "how him handle me," so when she could stand it no longer, she left him. His mother and his sister also started "to live bad" with her because her husband had bought a house and his mother said "that we cannot live in house and she live in rent house" so one day when she came home after work she discovered that her husband had moved his mother into their home and she was very angry, "I cuss some word ... and go on bad." She does not know how she married him as she "don't love him to that." He has no ambition and all he wants to do is to "drink rum and lay down." She says he still loves her, and supports his children as best as he can. In fact the children see him every day now as they stop at his home going and coming from school and sometimes they spend a week at a time at his house.

This woman is quite certain that she has had 17 pregnancies, 11 of which were either stillbirths or died shortly after birth. Apart from the first, they were all delivered in hospital and "the Government" took care of the disposal of these children, "10 boys and 1 girl me bury." This includes her fifth, sixth, seventh and ninth pregnancies (twins) which were mentioned earlier. She could account for only 11 pregnancies however and said "me lose them so fast me don't even remember." Three, her second, fourth and eighth children, died at 8, 20 and 10½ months respectively. Four children are alive and well—first, third, tenth and eleventh.

She felt very sad about the deaths of the children—to know that she carried them so long and felt the pain and then to have them die. She remained upset for as long as 9 months to a year when she thought of all the other women who had their children while hers were dead and she didn't have them to hold and play with. Her husband took it very badly when his children died but she does not know about the other fathers. As a result of all this her sexual relations increased as she "wanted a baby to hold."

Agnes seems to be very conscious of pain associated with childbirth. She mentions it when talking about the children's deaths and she says she feels better when she is not pregnant because she does not feel any pain then. Again, she thought every woman should have a child so that she can feel the pain and not "ill-buse" children as she will remember the pain she felt in having one.

She thinks that a family of 16 or more children can be considered large, while one of 10 is small, but ideally a woman should not have more than 10—4 boys and 6 girls. She shows her partiality to girls by declaring that she has a special feeling for her second to last child, as it was the first girl she "raised." The child is very delicate and inclined to get colds easily so she makes her wear a merino (vest) all the time. She is also quiet in contrast to her younger sister, who is rough.

Agnes believes that a childless woman must feel embarrassed to hear other people being called "Mamma" and she cannot be, but some women are "not born to have" while "some receive and they destroy it." Her children call her "Mamma" but she called her mother "Miss Rose" as everyone called her that. She thinks that every man should have a child so that he has someone to work for at all times, and it is right for a woman to have a child for each of her partners as she did. The best spacing for the children would be "a good jump"—2 years apart, but she had hers "fast"—1 to 1½ years apart.

She was 13 when she started menstruating and has not stopped yet. Her mother told her to expect it but she has no idea of the cause of it and feels "it is the good Lord work out that." Her periods were regular and lasted 6 days. She definitely prefers to be menstruating rather than pregnant as she had no problems with the former. She feels that a woman gets pregnant when she has sex too quickly after menstruating and there is nothing wrong with her having sex just before her menstruation but not during nor up to 5 days after it is finished.

Agnes expected that she and her partners would be faithful to each other. She enjoyed having sex with them 2 or 3 times per week but she has felt "very, very much despair" in all the unions she has been in.

Her mating and reproductive histories are graphically presented in Figure 10.6.

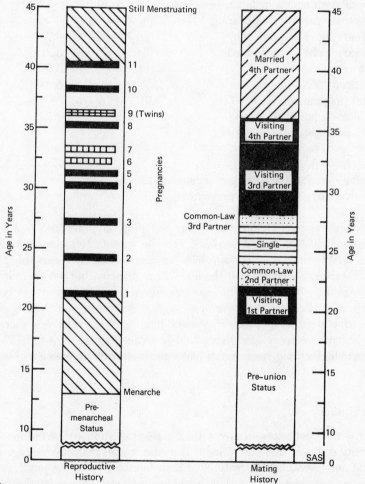

Note: Five pregnancies are not depicted due to the respondent's inability to recall their dates of occurrences.

Figure 10.6 Graphic representation of reproductive and mating history of respondent 6708

213

Statistical summary of pregnancy history

Events		Age	Years	Percentages
Age at menarche		13		
Age at menopause (still menstruating)		45		
Biological years of potential childbearing	(a)		32	
Age at termination of 1st pregnancy		21		
Age at termination of last pregnancy		40		
Actual years of childbearing	(b)		19	
Years spent in pregnancy	(c)		10.7	
Years spent in breastfeeding	(d)		3.2	
(c) + (d)	(e)		13.9	
Rest of period			5.3	
Total pregnancies		16		
(b) as % (a)				59.4
(c) as % (b)				56.6
(d) as % (b)				16.6
(e) as % (b)				73.2

Average number of years per pregnancy 1.2
(actual years)/(number of pregnancies)

Agnes has been menstruating for the past 32 years and had her first pregnancy at age 21 and her last when she was 40. Her actual childbearing span (19 years) is therefore 59% of her biological years of potential childbearing. She states that she had 17 pregnancies, but we are only able to account for 16 statistically. She spends the equivalent of 11 years in pregnancy, but because she has so few livebirths her total period of breastfeeding amounts to only 3 years. In spite of the relatively short period of the latter activity, pregnancy and breastfeeding account for 73% of her actual childbearing span. Agnes had a pregnancy on an average of every 1.2 years.

Conclusion

It is now necessary to give a brief statistical summary of the mating and fertility status of these 28 women. The case studies that have been presented bring out several salient features of their families, while the problems facing them as a consequence of their having to raise these large families are from time to time mentioned. What seems unexpected is that in no case is there any serious complaint of being overwhelmed by problems stemming from the size of their families. There are indeed complaints made by some of the treatment meted out to them by their partners, but these do not give the impression of presenting insuperable hardships. There are also hints of economic difficulties some mothers face as a result of their having to contend with so many children, but once more the general impression is that these mothers are able to overcome these in some way. Of relevance here is the fact that with the exception of one respondent who had a tubal ligation, no case of effective use of contraception is recorded by these women, although they admit at this stage that resort to such measures should be good for the country as a whole.

While none of these women appears to be overwhelmed by problems stemming from large families, it is difficult to resist the conclusion that the lengthy periods spent in pregnancy and in caring for large numbers of children must have to some degree curtailed appreciably the quality of their lives.

Measured in strict biological terms, that is in terms of the difference between the age at menarche and the age at menopause, the biological potential period of childbearing of this group of women amounts to 31.5 years. If this is calculated only on the basis of women who have attained their menopause, the duration amounts to 33.2 years. Not all of this represents a span of years during which the woman has been at risk of childbearing. The latter can be effectively assessed only if we exclude periods in which she is not in a union. When this correction is made, that is when we take into account only the years which these 28 women spend in marriage, common-law or visiting unions, then the average period at risk is brought down to 26.3 years. A further adjustment can be made by terminating the period at risk at the age at menopause, and when this is done it is reduced to 24.7 years. Thus we can conclude that the years of involvement in a union within the childbearing span amount to about 74.4% of the total biological period of childbearing. Another useful interval from the standpoint of childbearing can be identified; this covers the time between the average age at birth of the first child (19.8 years) and the average age at the birth of the last child (40.5 years). Thus an even shorter period of 20.7 years is obtained.

Let us next look at the average time spent by women in two important components of childbearing. The first is the total months of pregnancy. Since we are here dealing with all types of pregnancy, the overall average will be somewhat less than 9 months; in fact it amounts to 8.4 months per pregnancy. Taking into account the total number of pregnancies in which the woman is involved, we can arrive at an estimate of the average number of years each one spends in pregnancy in producing her liveborn, stillborn children as well as miscarriages. This stands at 7.89 years, and is equivalent to 32% of the total period of 24.7 years, which we have taken as the childbearing span extending from the entry into a family union up to the menopause. If we use as the period of childbearing the years between the birth of the first child and that of the last (20.75 years), then we can say that the period spent in pregnancy by the average mother takes up 38% of her total childbearing span.

The second important commitment of the mother is to breastfeeding of her children. The average period spent breastfeeding the 280 liveborn children these 28 women have is 7.9 months. And when the total time each woman spends breastfeeding her entire family is considered, the average time passed in this activity totals 6.71 years. This is equivalent to 27% of the childbearing span of 24.71 years, or to 32% of the shorter span of 20.75 years.

When we combine the periods spent by the average mother in the state of pregnancy and in breastfeeding, a total of 14.60 years per woman is obtained. Thus the average mother passes 59% of her span of 24.71 years in these essentially biological processes of childbearing. The proportion is much higher (70%) if these periods of biological commitment are related to the shorter span of 20.75 years. We can therefore conclude that on the average the mother is, over the whole of her childbearing lifetime, free of these commitments for a period of between 10 and 6 years, depending on how we assess the total childbearing span.

Two qualifications have to be made to the above argument. In the first place child care does not end at age 45 or at the menopause, but goes on much further, so that restricting it either to the present age of the mother or to her age at menopause is not justified. In fact rearing her complete family probably extends some 15 years beyond either of these ages. Again we must emphasise that during the childbearing period the mother is faced with caring for several children at the same time.

One way of illustrating the implications of the growing family for the mother and the strain of childbearing and child care involved is to trace the expansion and subsequent decline in family size. When these processes are traced through the family cycle we see how the demands on the mother increase with the number of children living in the household. Then after the maximum size is attained and the elder children cease to be her responsibility, the numbers in the household decline and with this the demands of the family on her time and energy are reduced, until there comes a time when she is free of such responsibilities.

This process can be illustrated by considering the position of the "average" woman of the group of 28 being studied in this chapter. Here we take as the starting point of the calculation the average age at birth of the first child, which is about 20 years, and the average number of liveborn children for the group, which is 10. Then we calculate the average intervals between successive livebirths for these 28 women. And by adding these average intervals successively to the average age at birth of first child we secure estimates of the ages at which this "average" mother bears her 10 children. These can be used to trace the build-up of the family. Here it must be noted that 2 simplifying assumptions are introduced into the argument. In the first place, it is assumed that each child remains under the mother's direct care until it attains age 15, when it leaves her home. The second assumption is that none of the children dies during the course of the family cycle.

The position as determined from the experience of the 28 women is as follows:

Age of mother	Number of children ever born to stated age	Number of children attaining age 15 at mother's stated age	Number of children under direct care of mother
20	1	—	1
25	3	—	3
30	6	—	6
35	7	1	6
39	10	2	8
40	10	3	7
45	10	5	5
50	10	7	3
54	10	10	—

These show how many children are directly under the mother's care at the several ages. Thus by age 30 she is looking after 6 children and it is not until age 35 that there begins to be some withdrawal of children from the family and a lightening of the mother's burden of child care. The maximum number under her care is attained at age 39, after which increasing numbers attain age 15 and therefore withdraw from the family. By age 54 all children have passed age 15 and therefore cease to be a responsibility for the woman. In summary it can be said that the maximum number of children in the household (8) is attained by age 39 and that up to age 45 there are still 5 children under her care, and it is not until age 54 that she is entirely free of the burden of child care.

Notes

1. See Sonja A. Sinclair, "A Fertility Analysis of Jamaica: Recent Trends with Reference to the Parish of St. Ann," *Social and Economic Studies* 23, no. 4 (December 1974).
2. G. W. Roberts, *Fertility and Mating in Four West Indian Populations* (Kingston: I.S.E.R., University of the West Indies, 1975).
3. Loc. cit.
4. Amram Scheinfeld, *Twins and Supertwins* (New York: Penguin, 1973).

Chapter 11
Small Families

In contrast to women with large families, that is those with more than 10 pregnancies, are those who have 3 or less. And here again we have designated as small families only women who from the standpoint of age or menstrual history have completed their childbearing span. The 70 women classified as having small families have been subdivided into 3 distinct groups: primiparae, and multiparae at parities 2 and 3. The first 2 categories will be discussed in detail while the third, which differs very little from the second, will be introduced for comparative purposes. These 3 groups constitute 14% of the total respondents in the sample and are analysed in order to show how small family patterns contrast with the position of the large families, which have already been dealt with.

Again, in view of the very small numbers with which we are dealing, it is inappropriate to try to present tabulations. The procedure will be the same as that followed in the discussion of large families, that is a simple description of the quantitative material illustrating the features of these women.

Primiparae

General Characteristics

The number of women with 1 pregnancy amounts to 26 and these are located in all but 1 of the 8 parishes from which this sample is drawn. The exception is St. Elizabeth, one of the island's high fertility parishes. Significantly, St. Ann and Portland, both areas in which some reductions in fertility have been noted, are represented here, but are not represented in the group comprising large families.

Women with a single pregnancy account for 5% of all women in the sample and 37% of the group with less than 4 pregnancies. Their ages range from 40 to 64 years, with an average of 53. In respect of their religious persuasion we observe that the majority belong to denominations considered as "established." Thus 18 or 69% are so classified, while 8 profess adherence to the more fundamental types and other sects. Of these 26 women, 5 have post-primary schooling, and among the 21 who have only primary-level education, 3 have 5 years or less, while the remaining 18 have 6 to 8 years.

Union Types and Partners

Since we are dealing with primigravidae, the union types in which these women are involved assume greater importance as measures of exposure to the risk of childbearing than is the case with women with larger families. A fairly high proportion (65%) have at some stage of their reproductive life been married. Of these 17 ever-married women, 6 remain married throughout their childbearing span. At the time of the interview, 13 of these women are married, and 3 are widowed. The average age at marriage among these women is 30 years, while only in the case of 6 of them have their pregnancies occurred when married. The common-law type is not strongly represented here, as only 19% have ever lived in this type of union and in all cases they participated in other types as well. No pregnancies take place when any of these women are in common-law union.s As we should expect, with the exception of the 6 women who have always been in married unions, the remaining 20 all have initial unions of the visiting type.

An examination of the unions in which their single pregnancies occur shows that 20 or 77% are in visiting unions, that is all women with the exception of 6 who remain married throughout their reproductive life. Of the 26 pregnancies produced, 24 occur in their first or only union.

Together, these women have been associated with 47 partners, that is an average of 1.81 each. The modal number of partners is 1, with 12 women reporting this number. Seven report having 2 partners; 5 have 3 partners, and the highest number of partners is 5, reported by 1 woman.

Union Duration

As in the case of the large families, 3 aspects of union duration will be discussed: in terms of most stable union, total of all unions and total of all unions up to the menopause or present age. Durations of their most stable unions are available for 23 women, while for 2 of them durations of all their unions are unknown and we have therefore used the longest available. In the third case no durations are given and this woman is omitted. The 25 women analysed in respect of their most stable union show an average of 15 years and range from less than 1 year to 44 years with bi-modal peaking at 5 to 9 years and 20 to 24. It is noteworthy that the 3 women with durations of less than 5 years are each in a single visiting union lasting 9 months, 1 year and 2 years respectively. They subsequently spend their remaining lives of 41, 34 and 37 years in single states.

Total duration of all unions is examined for 24 women, the remaining 2 being incomplete. This totals 458 years or an average of 19 years each. Again the peaking of the distribution is bi-modal, with 6 women each having durations of 10 to 14 and 20 to 24 years. Those with durations below 10 years number 6 and those between 15 and 44 years number 5.

Four women are still menstruating, but in view of the fact that they have their only pregnancy in their first or early in their only union they can justifiably be taken as having completed their childbearing. On this basis, 24 women are analysed in respect of the total duration of all their unions up to the menopause. The average duration is 15 years with a distribution essentially the same as that of the category previously discussed.

In summarising the durations of these women we note that the average duration of their most stable unions and their total duration to menopause is the same, 15 years, while the average for the total duration of all their unions is only 4 years more. These are all considerably below those of the women with large families where the corresponding averages are 22, 27 and 25 years respectively.

Relevant to this discussion is an examination of the single periods experienced by these women. Not all are involved, in fact 9 women remain in unions throughout their childbearing span, while for another 2 the exact single periods are unknown. The majority (9) of the 15 women who remain single, and therefore not at risk of pregnancy, do so for periods ranging from 10 to 41 years, and interestingly those with the longest durations of 34, 37 and 41 years respectively have each been in only one visiting union of 2 years or less. Another 3 have single periods of 21, 23 and 24 years, but here the first has 2 periods between visiting unions totalling 21 years, while in the latter case both these women are widows.

Of the 6 women whose single states total 10 years or less, 3 show very short durations in this state—2 years each—while for the other 3 the periods spent in this state are 4, 8 and 9 years respectively. The average number of years single for all 26 women is 16.

The total number of years single up to the menopause shows much shorter durations, as expected. Eight women are single for periods extending from 2 to 9 years. Only 2 women have durations of 25 to 29 years and the remaining 5 have between 10 and 24 years. The average number of years here is therefore 12. These very long periods in which so many women are not at risk of pregnancy can be considered as one of the sociological factors contributing to their very low fertility.

Menstrual and Reproductive Histories

The menstrual history of these women assumes importance in view of their low fertility and may to some degree suggest departures from normalcy in terms of reproduction. Their ages at menarche range from 11 to 19 years. The modal age is 15 years with 11 women having their first menstruation at this time. Another 5 state that menarche occurs between the ages of 15 and 19 years while the other 7 start between 11 and 14 years of age. Interestingly 1 woman did not have her first period until after the birth of her child when she was age 13. The average age at menarche is also 15 years.

All but 4 women are past the menopause which they experienced at an average age of 46 years, thus the years between menarche and menopause average 31 for those who have actually passed the menopause. For those who are non-menopausal the average number of years between menarche and their present age is 28. Their average age is 42 years.

In view of the very low fertility of the women under discussion reasons must be sought from an examination of their menstrual and pregnancy histories. Most women report that their periods were regular and lasted an average of 5 days. Only 1 woman reports irregular periods.

Their pregnancy histories show that a number of them have had complications of the type that might have contributed to sub-fertility. For example, 2 had prolonged labour, a condition indicating uterine dysfunction or some possible foetal cause such as a breech presentation or an abnormally large foetus. In another case the woman reports vomiting and hypertension during the pregnancy and post-partum hypotension. This is highly suggestive of a pre-eclamptic episode, which when taken in conjunction with her relatively high age (29 years) at this her first pregnancy probably militates against future conceptions. Another woman reports post-partum hypertension. Hyperemesis in pregnancy is reported in 2 cases, one being an elderly primigravida. In the other case the woman states that she had pains in her hip during menstruation and had a post-partum oophorectomy, thus reducing by 50% her future chances of conception.

One ectopic gestation which aborted at 3 months when the woman was aged 18 is reported, and here again there is a suggestion of underlying abnormal pathology. These 6 women therefore all had conditions which may have contributed to their low fertility.

Nearly one-third (31%) of this group of women experience premature cessation of menstruation, the so-called artificial menopause, as a result of surgery on their reproductive systems. While in most cases the surgery is performed several years after their single pregnancy, it is safe to assume that the pre-surgical conditions probably existed for some years prior to the actual operation and therefore played some part in their low fertility. Their ages at the time of surgery range from 33 to 50 years and the average is 43 years. Only 2 women cite problems of menstruation; one states that she had a heavy flow and started to have pains a few years after menarche. The other had irregular periods with dysmenorrhoea and vomiting. She was told by a doctor that she had an ovarian cyst. All but 2 women have complications—during pregnancy, in labour or post-partum.

Thus we see that the same woman who reports menorrhagia and dysmenorrhoea has, at age 33, a Caesarean section performed because of uterine inertia, and this was followed by oophorectomy and hysterectomy for post-partum haemorrhage. The woman with the ovarian cyst delivered a livebirth at age 19 but was in labour for 5 days during which time she was on medication prescribed by a physician. At birth the umbilical cord encircled the infant's neck and initial inspiration was delayed. Oophorectory was performed when she was age 40.

The only woman of this group who did not have a livebirth had a spontaneous abortion when she was 2 months pregnant at age 39. This was accompanied or caused by heavy bleeding, but medical assistance was not sought. Surgery of an unspecified nature was performed 2 years later and menstruation ceased. Another woman who had a livebirth without any complications reports that she consulted a doctor prior to this pregnancy. This is highly suggestive of some problem in conception. She used a contraceptive pill for an undetermined time after the birth, but again the reason for her later surgery is not stated. The fifth case haemorrhaged during labour and had a hysterectomy several years later when she was 46. Yet another woman who states that she had the same operation for a growth when she was age 47 had a poor pregnancy history. She had kidney problems with oedema of the legs during pregnancy and had post-partum convulsions, thus indicating that she had a severe case of pre-eclamptic toxaemia culminating in eclampsia. In the eighth case the birth was 2 months premature due to a fall. This woman also had a growth removed at age 55.

As it is well documented that the incidence of fibromyomata (fibroids) is high in negro women, it is safe to assume that the growths referred to fall into this category of uterine tumours. Fibromyomata are of unknown aetiology but, as Pinkerton and Stewart have argued, the factor(s) predisposing to their formation may also predispose to the high incidence of infertility and sub-fertility among negro women in general and our group in particular.[1] In summary we note that of the 26 women under discussion 14 or 54% have medical conditions which may contribute to their very low fertility.

Pregnancy, Foetal Loss and Infant Mortality

The average age of these women at their only pregnancy is 23 years and their 26 pregnancies result in 21 livebirths, 4 miscarriages and 1 stillbirth. Their livebirths are breastfed for an average of 9 months each.

Four women had miscarriages at between 2 and 4 months of pregnancy. Two of these were age 18 and 19 at the time of the occurrence and the other 2 were 39 and 41 years respectively. One woman delivered a stillborn female at age 18.

There were 2 infant deaths which occurred at ages 6 and 9 months. The cause of death of the former is not stated and the latter died of an "upset stomach." The only other death is of a 2-year-old who died of fever.

While the losses here are not large in terms of numbers they do constitute real trauma as they are the only pregnancies of these women. This is well demonstrated by the mother of the 9-month-old who died of an upset stomach in 1934 and who said that she cried and was very sad because "it was just as if I knew I was not going to have any more." She states that she still feels sad about the death. Another woman admits that she feels jealous of her sister who has 7 children.

Intergenerational Data

All, except one woman, are aware of the number of children borne by their mothers and these average 6.4 each. Only 3 of the respondents' mothers have the same family size as their daughters, while another 3 exceed our respondents by one child.

Since the average family size of the respondents' mothers is so much greater than our respondents', we may conclude that this survey provides no evidence that the low fertility levels of these women is inherited from their mothers. Data on the number of children of their partners' mothers are not meaningful as in only 9 cases did the woman have her single pregnancy for her present partner.

Conclusion

This brief analysis of various aspects of the lives of sub-fertile women demonstrates that there are two major contributing factors, the sociological and the medical.

Their periods at risk, as shown by their union durations, bring out two main points. The first is the often short and casual nature of the initial visiting union which terminates at the occurrence of pregnancy; in addition several of these women spend very long periods outside of any union and therefore their time at risk of childbearing is considerably reduced. While these points would seem to indicate a conscious desire to limit family size, their statements in respect of children do not bear this out. In fact the evidence is that most of these women expected and wanted more children.

The second major factor is medical, as brought out in the discussion on their menstrual and reproductive histories. The contribution of the causal factors of fibroids to infertility and sub-fertility is undoubtedly an important one. It must be noted here that these are older women, average age 53 years. There has been a marked redress in infertility and sub-fertility among younger women due to the many improvements which have been effected in general health care and in obstetrics and gynaecology in particular.[2]

The case studies at the end of the chapter set out in detail the lives of some of these women with small families and illustrate vividly several aspects of our discussion. One of the most significant features is that in 3 of the 4 cases presented their single pregnancy is as a result of a casual relationship.

Parity Two

General Characteristics

Women with only 2 pregnancies number 19 or 3.8% of all women with small families. They are drawn from 6 of the 8 parishes represented in the sample, the parishes in which they do not appear being Portland and the high fertility parish of St. Elizabeth. As in the case of the primiparae, their average age is 53 years with the range being from 45 to 63 years. The majority (14) of these women belong to the "established" churches and they had an average of 6 years of primary schooling.

Union Types and Partners

A marked variety of union types characterises these women, only 4 of whom are pure types. Of these 4, marriage accounts for the only union in 3 cases, while the fourth is a common-law union. As our previous discussions, in accordance with the family forms depicted, have shown, most first unions are of the visiting type while, by the end of the childbearing span, 11 or 58% have contracted marriages. The multiplicity of unions demonstrated is matched by a variety of partners. Between them these women have 42 partners or an average of 2.2 each. The maximum number of partners is 5.

Union Duration

We next examine union duration in terms of the three measures already indicated. Duration of the most stable union, irrespective of type, is analysed for 18 women, as all dates are not available for the nineteenth woman. This category of duration ranges from 5 years to 38 years with an average of 16.1 years. Only 3 women were in their most stable union for periods of less than 10 years. Total duration of all unions is examined for 17 women in view of the fact that all the relevant information is not available for 2 women. Here the range is for 5 years to 43 years, with an average of 22.1 years.

Total duration of all unions up to the menopause, or present age if non-menopausal, gives an average only slightly below that of the previous category, that is 19 years.

It is evident that for all 3 aspects of union duration the average spans are relatively long, thus providing a considerable period of exposure to risk of childbearing. The years spent in single states average only 5. Yet these women have no more than 2 pregnancies each.

Menstrual and Reproductive Histories

Menarche, signalling the biological commencement of the potential period of childbearing, begins at a mean age of 14.7 years.

With 12 menopausal women the average age of this event is 49 years. Of these 12 women, 3 experienced the menopause artificially, through medical intervention, which took place on the average at age 46. Surgery was performed on 2 of these women while the third woman was given an injection after developing diabetes mellitus. This woman reports that menstruation ceased after this injection.

Pregnancy, Foetal Loss and Infant Mortality

Of the 19 first pregnancies of these women, 16 are livebirths, 2 stillbirths and 1 a miscarriage. The youngest mother is 16 years, the oldest 37 and the average age of the group is 24 years. One neonatal death, that of a 1-month-old female infant, is recorded.

The second pregnancies of these women terminated on an average of 5.21 years after their first. Here again there are 16 livebirths and the 3 losses are in the form of miscarriages. The single neonatal death is of a male, delivered by Caeserian section but who succumbed to a cerebral haemorrhage after 24 hours.

Contraception does not contribute much to the low · fertility of these women as only 3 report ever having used a method. One woman used the diaphragm but only after her first pregnancy, another reports that her partner used the condom in the first interpregnancy interval while she took the pill after her second pregnancy. In the third case the condom was the method of choice prior to and after her first pregnancy.

The time of the occurrence of these pregnancies is interesting as all but 1 woman had at least 1 conception in her first union. Thus 27 of these 38 pregnancies occurred in the first union, which for 4 women is their only union. Nearly one-half of these women had both of their pregnancies by 2 different fathers. The lengths of their interpregnancy intervals range from 1 year to 21 years with an average of 4 years. The average number of years between the termination of the last pregnancy and the menopause is 19 years.

An examination of breastfeeding patterns practised by these women shows that the first-born infants are fed for an average period of 6 months while the later born are weaned at 7 months. Only in 2 cases were livebirths not breastfed.

In summarising these pregnancy histories it is evident that there are no significant problems or techniques employed which can in any way contribute to their low fertility.

Intergenerational Data

All these women are able to report on the number of siblings they have and as in our discussion of primiparae these are all assumed to be livebirths. The family size of the mothers of our respondents range from 2 to 12, but the majority were of high parity as only 3 had less than 4 children. Their total livebirths, 121, amount to 3.8 times the average number of their daughters'. This gives an average family size of 6 as compared with the 1.7 livebirths of their daughters. Clearly the question of heredity throws no light on the subject.

Conclusion

Unlike the analysis of women with 1 pregnancy, no clear evidence is available to account for the fact that these 19 women have only 2 pregnancies. As the examination of union duration has shown, relatively long periods are spent during which it is assumed that the woman is at risk of childbearing. As was pointed out earlier only 5 years on an average are spent outside of any union.

Their concept of the ideal number of children a woman should have in her lifetime indicates that a larger family than that achieved is the ideal, as the sizes given average 4 per woman. The examination of the reproductive and pregnancy histories also does not provide any clear evidence to suggest underlying bio-medical causes for these small families.

In view of the fact that these are older women of only moderate educational attainment the reasons for and the methods of attaining these small families remain inconclusive.

Comparison of Women With Large and Small Families

In order to identify areas of similarity and of difference between women with very large families and those with small families, a comparative examination of their experiences is in order. The numbers of women in the various family size categories are as follows:

Family size	Numbers in group	% of whole sample	% of total of small families
Small families			
Parity 1	26	5.2	37.14
Parity 2	19	3.8	27.14
Parity 3	25	5.0	35.71
Total	70	14.0	99.99
Large families	28	6.0	—

General Characteristics

The average ages of the parity 1 and 2 women is 53 years while those of parity 3 is 1 year lower. The grande multiparae are on an average 3 years younger than the women with 1 and 2 pregnancies. Thus the differences in respect of age are not great.

The overall standard of education for these 4 groups of women is similar as all have an average of at least 6 years of primary level education. The number of women with post-primary education constitutes a small proportion of all groups but is highest for those with 3 pregnancies.

The overwhelming majority of these 98 women profess adherence to some religious denomination or sect and these may conveniently be classified as either "established" or fundamentalist. Thus we see that the proportions of women of parity 1 and 3 are similar for those of the "established" churches, 69% and 68% respectively. Women with 2 pregnancies show a higher proportion in this category, 74%. However, the real difference is between these 3 groups and the mothers of large families where only one-half belong to the more formal religions.

While no firm evidence is available in respect of the link between religious belief and fertility patterns it is significant that a greater proportion of the grande multiparae profess adherence to the fundamental sects, so that these women with large families are classified as 46% fundamentalist, 4% no religion and 50% "established" churches.

Union Types and Partners

Since we are concerned with the two extremes of fertility, the very high and the low, the types of unions in which the women are involved and durations in each type are of marked importance. A considerable proportion of all the women under examination are at some point involved in a visiting union, 64 or 65% of these 98 women. The percentage of primiparae is 77%, the highest for all 4 groups, and this supports the findings that this type of union serves as a curb to fertility.

Women of parity 2 have a lower participation at 63% and for those at parity 3, just over one-half are involved in visiting unions. Women with large families participate in many unions and therefore the relatively high percentage of 71 who spend some time in visiting unions is understandable.

As has been brought out in our previous discussions, common-law unions are the lowest on the scale of ranking from several perspectives. The proportions of women who have ever been involved in this type of union are markedly lower than for the visiting type. Again women with a single pregnancy have the lowest percentage in this type, 19% as compared with the 58% for women of parity 2 and the 57% for women with large families. Common-law unions are participated in by 36% of women of parity 3.

In accord with our knowledge of the contribution of the various unions to fertility it is not surprising that for women with 1 pregnancy only 65% have ever been married. Rates for parity 2 women are even lower at 58%. However because of the high proportion of these women who are in common-law unions these percentages are fairly significant since we know that cohabitation is associated with relatively high fertility performance.

Women of parity 3 show a marked increase over the 2 previous groups as here 72% of all women are married. As expected the grande multiparae show the greatest proportions as married, 79%. Thus it is clearly demonstrated that marriage is, for a considerable proportion of women in these groups, the norm.

The average age at marriage is similar for women of the 2 lowest parities, 30 and 31 years, while those of parity 3 marry at a mean age of 28 years. Those women with large families marry on an average of 3 years earlier than the primiparae. The lack of legal ties in 2 of the 3 types of unions under discussion facilitates the movements of partners both in and out of any given union. Therefore it is necessary to see if this is reflected in the numbers of partners these women have.

Both the parity 1 and parity 3 women have an average of 1.8 partners each. Those of parity 2 have 2.2 and women with large families have 2.6 partners each, which is in accord with their multiple unions.

Union Duration

As our previous discussion has shown, union duration assumes importance as it partly determines degree of exposure to risk of childbearing. This is of major significance in any comparison of differing family sizes.

The most stable union, that of the longest unbroken duration irrespective of type, increases in linear progression from primiparae to grande multiparae. Thus the first group averages 15 years and rises to 17 years for the third while women with large families spend an average of 22 years in their most stable union.

Another approach to the examination of union duration is to take the total of all unions in which the woman has been involved. Again the increase is wholly linear in terms of the 4 groups. Parity 1 women spend a mean total of 19 years in unions and those of parities 2 and 3 spend an average of 22 years each in all their unions. The grande multiparae are in unions for an average of 26 years.

The third category of union duration is the total of all unions of these women up to their menopause. These averages commence at 15 years for the sub-fertile women and rise to 19 and 20 years for the 2 succeeding groups. Women with large families have spent an average of 25 years in unions by the time they reach the menopause.

Following from this discussion on the average number of years spent in the various categories of union is an examination of the number of years during which these women are not involved in any union, that is their single periods. These single periods are a major feature of women with only 1 pregnancy since they represent periods when the woman is not at risk of conception. Thus the 16 years that these women spend on average without a partner assumes marked significance when we note that this is more than 3 times that for women of parities 2 and 3 and the grande multiparae.

Menstrual and Reproductive Histories

The onset of menstruation is important for several reasons—the prime one being its significance as the biological commencement of the childbearing period. For all 4 groups of women the average age at menarche is 15 years.

Menopause, or the cessation of menstruation, signifies, among other changes, , the biological termination of the childbearing span. Unlike menarche some variation in the mean age at menopause is evident. Women of parity 1 experience this event at an average of 46 years of age, while that for those of parity 2 occurs 3 years later. Parity 3 women are menopausal 1 year earlier than those of parity 1, and women with large families are on an average 48 years of age at the time of the occurrence of this event.

The intervening years between these 2 events, the biological period of childbearing, can be examined for women who are post-menopausal. The greatest period is for women of parity 2 who have a mean of 34 years. For those of parities of 1 and 3 the period is 31 years, and women with large families average 32 years. Thus average family size is not closely linked to age at menarche and menopause.

One of the major features emerging from the data of these varying size families is the extent to which women are artificially brought to the menopause. Of the 66 women who are menopausal, 27% experienced this event through surgical intervention.

Since surgery of the reproductive system is, at older ages, usually of an elective nature it implies that the pre-surgical condition will have existed for some time prior to the actual operation. In addition it is known that the majority of these operations are performed for the removal of intra-uterine growths (often fibroids) and the implication is that these tumours may pre-dispose to either sub-fertility or infertility. This assumption is strengthened by a comparison of the proportions of women in large and small families experiencing an artificial menopause.

For women with a single pregnancy this is 36%, while for those with 2 pregnancies it is 25%. Only 21% of grande multiparae were subjected to surgery and 22% of those of parity 3. Thus the difference between the primiparae and the grande multiparae is highly significant as the latter are 59% less than the former.

The total pregnancies of the 70 women with small families is 44% less than that of the 28 women with large families. Mean pregnancies for women with fewer than 4 pregnancies is 2 each as compared with the 11.3 of the grande multiparae.

In view of the reversal of the order of childbearing in relation to marriage it is interesting to note the proportions of women who marry prior to childbearing. Women of parity 3 have the highest rates with 32% marrying before commencing childbearing. For parity 2 the rate is 26% and for parity 1, 23%. Only 18% of the women with large families are married before commencing their family building.

In conclusion we reiterate that there are many areas of real difference within the 3 groups of women comprising the small families on the one hand and between them and the women with large families on the other.

Case Studies

Respondent 8A62

Norma S. is a 60-year-old married woman living in a parish capital near the center of the island. There are many similarities between her husband and herself: they are the same age, they both attended primary school for approximately 6 years each, their parents were married and they are members of the Missionary Association Church, a fundamentalist religion. She is not working now, but used to be a ward maid at the Government Hospital. Her husband is self-employed as a contractor and builder. Her father was a cultivator and her mother had 14 children, including 3 sets of twins, while his father was headman on a property and his mother had 6 children.

Norma had a male child when she was 19, which was delivered by a nana, prematurely, after she had a fall. Apart from that, there were no complications, and she worked in the house as usual, during the pregnancy. She breastfed the baby for a year because "in those days parents told you that the baby must nurse for a year." Norma had known the baby's father throughout their school days, and as they were in the same classes, he was about the same age as she. She states quite clearly that she liked him, but it was not a "love relationship." She had been sent by her father to a tailor to get "a pair of pants." The tailor was a "rummer" and had gone to the shop to drink rum. "It so happen, rain started to pour, and we as two little teenagers fool, until we start to play with each other until this thing happen and that's all about it . . . . It was strange to me when my mother tell me I was making a baby. I couldn't understand what she was talking about." This is why she believes one should be "outspoken" to children at an early age. After she had the baby, her father sent her out of the district, so that she and the young man could not come in contact with each other again. This was her only pregnancy.

Her second partner was the man she really loved. He visited her for 5 years but they broke up because his mother was not nice to her. He cultivated bananas and cane and gave her presents but no regular support. She did not mind this as she had a regular job then. She was happiest with this partner.

When she met her third partner, whom she later married, he visited her for a while and then went away. While he was abroad, she was told by a jeweller that he had an engagement ring for her from him. Eighteen months later he returned and they married 3 months after that.

She enjoyed having sex with him, but "he is a very sexy man and July coming one year, he doesn't say anything to me." She did not know the reason for this, and one night she was feeling bad about it and went to sleep in another room. He asked her why she had gone and said, "You think now is the days when I am going to run after you again . . . that is over, in fact everything is over." At first, she did not believe he was serious, but as time passed, he stayed out late and she "fussed" about it, until she realised that since "he is not worrying about me, why should I worry about him, and then I just asked the Lord to . . . ." At this stage Norma was overcome with emotion and cried. However, she continued, saying she spoke to him about it and he tried to make an excuse. She "did sort of believe him" as at one time a doctor had told him that "as he was a bit excited some times during sex and he used to have a little bleeding, he was to keep away for a time." They were both worried however, so he went to the city to consult a specialist, but that doctor told him "it wasn't anything, it was just excited," as it only happened when they had sex. Again she broke down crying and said she thought that was the reason for his keeping away from her but she is obviously not sure of this as she describes him as a "wild" man and he "shares the affection" and this has brought difficulties in the past. She however, has always been faithful to him. "If anyone tell him anything about me, he would push a fist in their mouth."

Norma loves children and she explained that the reason she said 5 children were a small family was that her husband had 4 and together with her own, they "used to live such a happy life" when the children were at school, but of course they have now all grown up and are on their own. It appears that those 4 did not actually live with her, because she mentions a child she fostered, whom her husband later acknowledged as his, although "he did not give it to her on the strength of that." This child made their family life even happier. She says she never thinks of fewer than 10 children as a large family and if you have the right partner 8 is a "good number"—4 boys and 4 girls. She believes that every woman should have a child and those who have none cannot have love and affection for other women's children. She thinks that the reasons for childlessness may be that some women do not start having children early and when they are "over mature," they are "timid" to have one, while some young women prevent themselves having one and regret it at "coming of age." She is totally against family planning, "I am not in this world nor the world to come, come to that." She feels that if everybody would get down and work to support the children, it would be the happiest thing to have them, but many of the people are too lazy.

She has heard that a nurse can tell a woman how many children she is going to have, as it shows at delivery, but now women are choosing the number of children they want. She was quite shocked to think of a woman having a child for each of her partners and declared that 15- and 16-year-olds should not be having them.

Norma started menstruating at 17 and stopped at 54 when she had a tumour removed. To her, menstruation is a natural function of a woman "as it is a thing that your parents always warn you to expect." They did not explain about sex to her, however, which was the reason she was so surprised at age 19 to find herself pregnant. She still thinks that a woman gets pregnant "when you both love each other, and you both get together, and you both have the same inclination for each other" and she does not know why it happens only at certain times.

Norma is a very pleasant, warm-hearted person, who is at present in an unhappy situation and is confused by it.

Respondent 2150

Sybil E. is a 62-year-old married woman living in a middle-class suburb. She and her husband are both retired teachers but he is now involved in the wider aspects of education at government level. Their fathers were teachers also and their parents were married to each other. Sybil is a Baptist and her husband is Anglican but in this society this difference between recognised religions is not important as a rule.

Although her mother had 8 children, only 3 of her siblings have had children of their own, while in her husband's family of 12, he and another brother have had none. Sybil has been pregnant only once and this resulted in a miscarriage at 2 months. The incident took place on Easter Sunday while she was playing the organ at church, 2 years before they got married. She said it had been a long function and she had to use a foot pedal while playing, when she felt her clothes saturated and discovered she was bleeding. Perhaps because they were two "stupid people," she did not seek any medical attention. They "felt ashamed about the whole thing," and she knew he would not have wanted her to tell even a nurse, as he considered it "too private." They decided to get married eventually as they were both "getting on in age"—they were 40 years old at that time—and he felt the time had come for him to do so and she agreed. They also wanted to have children but never discussed this at any length as "they took it for granted" that they would have. She is not absolutely sure of the date but she thinks it was about a year later that she had an "operation" on her doctor's advice, because of heavy bleeding. She stopped menstruating after that.

The interviewer found her very shy and "fearful" and on many occasions had to stress the confidentiality of the interview, but for a woman of her age and background, she has been very frank in discussing events in her past, which she could easily have hidden. She had her first boyfriend in the days when one had to be "as circumspect as possible," and she did not want her parents even to know about him. They had sex occasionally but in retrospect she does not think that she had any special love for him, but because other girls she knew had boyfriends, she thought she would like to have one too. She decided to end the relationship because he was fair complexioned and one of his sisters objected to "her fair skin brother being friendly with a dark skin girl."

She was living alone when she met her second partner. He had a farm and she bought a cow which he kept for her and they would often discuss this when he visited. They had sex about once per week at her house as living on her own she felt more relaxed there and there was no difficulty in arranging this.

After this broke up she met the man who was to become her husband. He was able to visit her only during the holidays as they lived in different parishes far away from each other. She says she enjoys having sex with him and they have expected each to be faithful to the other. She has been very happy in this marriage.

Sybil started menstruating at 12. Her mother explained it to her and she thinks of it as "just the natural make-up of women." In her youth her periods were regular and lasted 5 days and did not affect her normal activities in any way but as she grew older, the bleeding became heavy and she did not exercise much at that time. When she was growing up she had been told that she should not bathe at that time but should just "wash up" with warm water and also that she "should not burn her diaper" but she never did believe in those things.

No one explained sex to Sybil, however, and she remembers when she was young, a schoolmate of hers had a baby and she could not understand how she could know who was the father of the child as she was not married. She knows a woman gets pregnant by having sexual intercourse and she has been hearing that if one has sex a certain number of days before menstruation one can get pregnant but she never "checked it out" as she was "past that time." Sybil sees nothing wrong in having sex just before and after menstruation but not during it and her partner would abstain at that time.

Sybil believes that every woman should have a child as everybody likes to "reproduce yourself," and when a childless woman sees other people's children she feels as if she would like to have one like that. Some women are "not born to have" while sometimes "it is the husband not born to have." She has heard "by the way" that every woman should have a certain amount of children but she does not believe this, as in these modern days a woman can use family planning to limit her family. As long as a man can maintain his child, he should have one, but she does not think a woman should have a child for each of her partners.

When she thinks of the size of the families that she and her husband come from (8 and 12 respectively) she feels that 8 children constitute a large family, while one of 3—2 boys and a girl—is ideal and may be considered small.

Because of the high cost of living she thinks that family planning is a very good thing. The Government cannot cope with the large population and "education will never able to catch up." When asked about abortion she laughingly said she kept far away from those things although she had heard about boiling bush tea and taking Epsom salts.

Respondent 6710

Kathleen A. is a 44-year-old married woman who was in a common-law union with her partner for 4 years prior to marriage, which took place 6 years ago. She has lived in the same parish all her life but was not asked to participate in a similar study in 1971-72. She is not employed at present but her husband rents an acre of land which he cultivates for himself. Her father was also a farmer but she does not know the occupation of her husband's father. Her mother, who was not married to her father, had 9 children, while his parents were married and his mother had 5 children. Both Kathleen and her husband had many years of primary schooling, she for 7 years and he for 8. They are members of the Pilgrim Holiness Church, one of the many fundamentalist religions in the island.

Kathleen has had only one pregnancy, which resulted in a male child, when she was 17. She was perfectly well during the pregnancy and washed and cleaned as usual in the home. In fact she says that she "felt good" during that time. The baby was delivered by a nana and she breastfed the child for 9 months. She used to live with a lady who would ask her to take messages to a policeman at the station. There she met her baby's father, who was a "big man" about 33 years old. He visited her a few times at her home and she got pregnant almost immediately. They were not really "friends" and when he was told that she was expecting a baby "he keeps away." Before she had the baby she found out that he was married and then she also kept away from him. Actually they had nothing to do with each other from the time she was about 3 months pregnant, and she got no support from him until the child started "to ups and down." At the time she "liked" him but since she "get to be a big woman" she feels "love" for him as "if it were not for him I may not have had a child."

After she had the baby her mother told her, "I'm not to talk to anybody because the child's foot will break, so I used to get scared." It is said that "if you had a baby and you had a next person, and that person is not the baby's father, and you move with that person, after a time the baby get backward, take long to walk, and all that."

Three or four years later she met "a next gentleman" and was in a common-law union with him for about 3 years. He used to gamble and she did not like it and when she spoke to him "it bring a fuss" so she gradually ended the relationship.

She and her third partner were also in a common-law union for 3 years. "As I and them live together and things is not to my suit, I just leave and I just live for myself. The majority of times I live for myself." She says she works hard and does not like to see how many men "take disadvantage" of women so she likes to depend upon herself. She was single "for a good period of time" after that friendship broke up.

Another man visited her for some time between her third partner and her husband, but she cannot remember the dates of this visiting union, nor was she able to give any information on this, her fourth union.

Her husband lived with her for 4 years and she decided that "to live in sin, it don't pay" so they started going to church and "accept the Lord as our personal saviour and Lord." People said "if we are going to church we cannot live that common-law life any more," so they decided to get married, "and although we haven't got anything but still we thank God we are living a happy life." She loves her husband "because he is so dear to me." She has no children for him but he had with other partners prior to this relationship. Her husband lives away and comes home on weekends only, so on the average they have sex about once per week. She does not enjoy it so much now, but nevertheless they are both faithful to each other.

Kathleen thinks that the common-law union is better than visiting, from the point of view of security, "if you are sick you have somebody to help, and when you are not working you have someone to give financial help." It is also better to settle down with one person than to be running "ups and down." Marriage is the best of all for her and she is extremely happy in this union.

She thinks that a family with 3 children is small, while one with 6 is large. Her ideal number however is 4—2 boys and 2 girls. She also says she would have been very happy if she had had a girl rather than a boy "still I am glad for him." It is important for every woman to have a child because "the Bible says a woman's womb is blessed by having children" and a woman who has none is "barren." "A tree should be cut down, if it is a bearing fruit tree and it don't bear, it should be hewn down." Nevertheless some women "don't born to have a child" while others may have had "appendix or they had a growth and they cut it" and this has prevented their having children. Every man should have a child also as "children is a part of your life when you become old" and many people die from want because they have nobody to take care of them.

Kathleen was 15 when she started menstruating and she has not stopped yet. Her mother had told her to expect it and she feels "if you are a healthy person, it is just the time when something should leave your body" so she was not frightened when she saw it. Her periods are regular and last 4 days but in the last year she has had a "low pain in her belly" and she has to relax at that time. She feels that a woman can have sexual intercourse just before her period but not during nor up to 7 days after it is finished. She has no idea of the causes of pregnancy.

Kathleen felt that family planning was not good and she had heard a lot of people say that they became sick after putting in the coil. She had also heard it was put in free but it "costs a lot to get it out back." She said she would never take it and cannot see how it can help in the development of the country. Her mating and reproductive histories are graphically presented in Figure 11.1.

Respondent 6830

Maisie R. is 57 years old and describes herself as a housewife although she has never been in a "regular" union, and her only child died when it was 9 months old, 40 years ago. Her mother, who was not married to her father, had 2 children. Maisie had 7 years primary schooling and is a member of the Anglican Church.

She met the baby's father when she used to go out in the evenings with a girlfriend for walks, and this man "talk up to this other woman and she kind of force me on to him." He was "a very big man"—meaning he was older than she—"You know some big men just love to fool around and spoil little young girls." At first she liked him very much and as she was hiding the relationship from her mother, they used to meet on weekends, when he would take her to his mother's home in the country. His mother had rented the home but he "as a son" could go there and "carry on his rackets" although someone else was living there. They would have sex, although "when a girl first having sex, it's not very much enjoyable," then he would bring her home early. They had been friendly just 3 months when she became pregnant—a condition which she had told him she was afraid of.

She had a "weak stomach" during her pregnancy and vomited a great deal, but there were no complications after the baby was delivered by a nana at home. When the child was born "she wasn't so very strong, she never looked so very healthy," but Maisie breastfed her for 7 months. By this time, Maisie had already broken off the relationship with the baby's father when she was

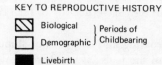

Figure 11.1 Graphic representation of reproductive and mating history of respondent 6710

238

about 6 months pregnant. She had discovered he was married and although she did not want to be mixed up with him any more, she expected him to take care of the child. He had never supported her—"only a little pocket money"—and after the child was born and her mother had paid the midwife and provided everything else she wrote him a letter. In reply he sent her 40 shillings and that is all she ever got from him. Her mother did not "nag" her about getting pregnant even though she "shouldered all of the responsibility" up to the death of the child when again her mother and aunt stood the cost of the burial. She was very disappointed in him and became afraid of getting pregnant again and "don't get any care." She says she has never been in any other union since, although she has had one or two casual boyfriends.

The death of the baby made her very sad and she cried, "just as if I know I wasn't going to have any more." She was "break down" from "fretration." The baby had had an upset stomach for 3 days and brought up everything she drank. Maisie's aunt took her to the doctor, who gave her a bottle with some medicine which smelled like magnesia and as she gave her the first dose, she died. "All now I still feel sad about it," when she sees that she has not had any more children and that there is no one to take care of her if she should live to be her mother's age. She had no feeling of guilt about the tragedy as she had always taken care of her, nor did she consider replacing the child unless she was married. The baby's father did not "pay me any mind" although she sent to tell him, and as mentioned before, her mother paid all the bills for the funeral.

Maisie believes that every man and woman should have a child because children are so "helpful"—"look how much I have to help my mother." She thinks girl children are especially good in this respect because even if they are not looked after by their fathers, "if you are into a good job, you wouldn't like to see your father go anyway funny" as it would be carrying down your "prestige, so you would try to help him." She believes childlessness is often due to something "wrong with the womb" and also there are some women "born more on the masculine side."

She thinks a family of 5 children is small, while one of 10 can be considered large, but 7 is a "nice number"—3 boys and 4 girls, as she is partial to girls. She has heard that one can tell how many children a woman is going to have by "the seeds on the afterbirth" but she knows that a woman can stop herself having children by "knotting off her tubes." In her opinion, 3 years is the best spacing between children, so that one can help the other.

Maisie was 11 when she started menstruating and 42 when she stopped. No one explained it to her and when she saw it for the first time at school, she hid it from her mother for 2 days, until the latter discovered it on the bed and told her that it "would have to happen as soon as I reach certain age." She now believes that there is a waste matter in the body that is supposed to pass out and it comes out in that way. Her periods were regular and lasted 5 days.

She used to have a pain in her hip, but it did not affect her normal activities. After she had the baby, she discovered she had a "bad tube" which was removed by a doctor, but at first she thought it was appendicitis.

In those days, mothers did not talk to their children the way they do today, so no one explained sex to her or she might have been "more precautious." She says that a woman can have sexual intercourse before her period but not during menstruation as "that is nastiness ... it's very detrimental to both men and women." One should then wait for 3 days after menstruation "then you get a washout" before having sex. She thinks a woman gets pregnant when "both of you semen get together" but she does not know why it happens at some times and not at others.

Maisie knows that a woman can have her baby "washed out" or take tablets to get rid of it but she does not believe in abortion. On the other hand she thinks family planning is good, so that a woman can stop having children after she has had a certain amount. She feels that to keep on having children is ruinous to the woman's body and health and the children cannot get proper care, and "if the people will take it," it would be very important in the development of the country. In her part of the country she finds that they are very "backward in education."

According to the Bible sex is not good out of wedlock, she says, and it must be very embarrassing for the mother who has, for example, 4 children for 4 different men. She knew of a case where the eldest girl said to her mother, "Mamma, how I name James and Olive name Smith, etc." and Maisie felt it "looks bad."

She admits that sometimes it "works out better" if you live with a man, but "for principle"—appearance's sake—it is better for him to visit. Naturally the union that is most desired is marriage and she seems to have avoided sex as much as possible because of not having been married.

Notes

1. J. H. M. Pinkerton and D. B. Stewart, "Uterine Fibroids," in J. B. Lawson and D. B. Stewart, *Obstetrics and Gynaecology in the Tropics and Developing Countries* (London: The English Language Book Society and Edward Arnold, 1974).
2. For a detailed discussion on this see Sonja A. Sinclair, "A Fertility Analysis of Jamaica: Recent Trends with Reference to the Parish of St. Ann," *Social and Economic Studies* 23, no. 4 (December 1974).

Chapter 12
Conclusions

Modern approaches recognise a wide array of factors influencing the reproductive performance of a society. Its levels of reproduction, reflected in many aspects of fertility, fertility control and mortality, have within recent years come under special scrutiny in developing countries, most of which are now committed to some form of population policy, aimed at containing rates of growth. While the core of such policies takes the form of effecting reductions in levels of fertility, equally prominent are their explicit programmes for improving all aspects of life of the child and the mother. These seek to monitor the health of the pregnant mother and her unborn child, to ensure proper delivery facilities, and, after the birth, to continue to sustain the health of the mother and her newborn child. Integrated into many of these modern policies are provisions for advancing the quality of family life in all sectors of the population. It seems safe to assume that the satisfactory preparation and administering of such policies call for the amassing of a considerable body of relevant information of a social and bio-medical nature. There are many difficulties to be faced in gathering these data. One of the most challenging centers around the frailty of human memory in recalling occurrences and timing of events.[1] At many points in this survey it has been pointed out how these elements introduce gaps into the records. It is still possible to secure substantial bodies of knowledge on which policies can be formulated and evaluated. It is the function of this survey to develop the collection of such material for the island of Jamaica.

This concluding chapter is divided into three parts. In the first place we must bring together the major findings, emphasising the various elements that embrace human reproduction in its wider sense. Secondly, we must consider briefly the implications of these findings. While many frames of reference for outlines of implications can be advanced, for the present purpose it seems best to adopt one in which the focus rests on three separate but closely related phases—the bio-medical, the social and the demographic. Finally, it remains of use to point out fields for future research which seem to be justified in the light of the present findings.

Summary of Findings

While this study is not directly concerned with the important question of the origins of the West Indian family, of necessity it has to take note of some historical features of this institution. Singled out for early discussion is the relationship between religion and prevailing family forms. Of the four religious ceremonies relevant to the family—baptism, confirmation, marriage and burial—the one which seems most important to the emergence of the West Indian family is baptism. It is on this ceremony which missionaries concentrated in such efforts as they made towards the conversion of slaves. Marriage received much less attention; even after the passing of the ameliorating laws during the second decade of the nineteenth century the church made no systematic efforts to promote marriage among slaves.

The seeming absence of change in family forms that emerged after emancipation constitutes another important topic in tracing the history of the West Indian family. Although the society witnessed a number of important developments of a social, economic and political nature, the formation of family unions remains one of the few fields in which there has been no fundamental alteration throughout.

In this very religious society, mothers acknowledge the importance of baptism of their children, but also seem to recognise that without formal marriage neither they nor their children can expect ready acceptance into the church.

Drawing together the experience of Trinidad and Jamaica, we can arrive at patterns of mating in these populations which suggest that, despite slight differences, there is essentially a common scheme linking the two together. The gross mating table shows that the visiting union is slightly more prevalent within Jamaica, whereas formal marriage assumes a more prominent position in Trinidad. The average Jamaican female spends 5.3 years in visiting unions, as compared with 4.1 in the case of Trinidad. The corresponding values for common-law participation are much closer—5.6 years and 5.9 years respectively. The slight advantage in marriage shown by Trinidad women emerges from the fact that the period they spend in formal marriage is 9.6 years as compared with 8.8 for those in Jamaica.

As part of this study, the characteristics of the visiting union have been made the subject of special enquiry. In view of the non-residential nature of this relationship, special significance attaches to the contacts maintained between the partners and between the father and his children. This survey has shown that these contacts are considerable, and that on the average partners spend about 3 hours per day in each other's company. They discuss a variety of topics relevant to the proper functioning of the family, demonstrating that many important decisions are arrived at jointly despite the fact that they do not share a common household. Also to be noted are the effective contacts between the father and his children, which average 4 hours per week.

When use is made of socio-economic indicators based on educational performance, it appears that the highest status is shown by the married, with the visiting coming second and the common-law third. This ranking is in accord with data from the censuses of 1943 and 1960.

Despite evidence of considerable contact and discussion between partners in visiting unions, an examination of the situation of initial visiting types suggests that a strong case can be made out for recognising a sub-category of that type, which is identified in this study as a casual relationship. It is of short duration and usually follows from early sexual contact, which the woman has established. Frequently its only basis for being designated a union is that a pregnancy has occurred and often the discovery of the woman's condition spells the end of the relationship.

Some investigation into menstruation seemed essential, not only because a knowledge of its onset, termination and other characteristics constitute important bio-medical indicators of the population, but also because these may be relevant to the reproductive performance of women and to the general state of their health. Age at menarche for the whole sample is 14.68 years, while the age at menopause for those who have experienced the event stands at 47.86 years. There is convincing evidence of falls in age at menarche from the experience of 3 age cohorts of women, while differentials by educational status show girls born to mothers of advanced levels mature earlier than their counterparts whose mothers enjoy lower educational status.

Those women who have had an artificial menopause amount to 27, which is 21% of all menopausal women. Their age at menarche is slightly lower than it is for those with a natural menopause, while with regard to age at menopause the higher age is shown by those who have not had their reproductive period prematurely terminated. Of considerable interest is the fertility differential between these 2 groups of women. The much lower family size of women with artificial menopause emphasises that this is evidence of a sub-fertile condition to which they were subject long before their medical condition indicated surgery.

Several considerations point to the relevance of knowledge of reproduction and menstruation and these have therefore been introduced into the survey. In the case of knowledge of reproduction, one-third of the women are reported as having no knowledge of the subject, that is reply "don't know," or have failed to state their awareness that sexual intercourse is involved in reproduction. Women who are merely aware that sexual intercourse is involved amount also to about one-third of the sample. At the other end of the scale, there are only 10% who exhibit an adequate knowledge of the subject.

Some interesting relationships between levels of knowledge and degree of information received on sex emerge. The greatest scores are reported for women who received knowledge of the subject from books, although only a small proportion are in this category. Appreciable scores are also recorded for those receiving information on sex from relatives other than mothers and from teachers. It is on the other hand surprising that women who receive such information from their mothers show very low scores of knowledge.

Another finding of the survey is the extent to which ignorance of the menstrual cycle permeates the entire society. The almost total lack of knowledge about it appears from the fact that 82% of the sample have no understanding of it, while only 12% report slight acquaintance with the phases of the cycle. Only 26 women or 5% of the total give answers indicating a satisfactory understanding of the menstrual cycle.

The relationship between levels of knowledge of reproduction and the use of contraception yields some interesting insights into the possible consequence of ignorance of these fundamental topics. In both contexts users of contraception exhibit much higher levels of knowledge than do those who have never made use of such techniques.

The rise in the resort to contraception coincident with the rise in the degree of knowledge of both processes leads us to conclude that the possession of such knowledge is one measure essential to ensure the spread and, possibly, the continued and efficient use of modern contraceptive methods. This argument rests on the premise that an understanding of reproductive processes will prepare users for any changes in their menstrual cycle that may take place; these will be less alarming, as they are expected.

With regard to pregnancy outcome of women in the sample, of the 1,699 pregnancies they report, 1,537 are live births, 35 stillbirths and 127 miscarriages. The majority (63%) of pregnancies are home deliveries and one-half of these are delivered by trained nurses or midwives. The nanas, or untrained attendants at birth, are responsible for 25% of all deliveries and for 41% of all home deliveries.

Probabilities of dying among infants show that, within the early neonatal period (within the first week of life), values are lowest in the case of deliveries made by hospital nurses (11) and greatest in the case of home deliveries made by nurses (19), with the rate for deliveries made by nanas standing midway between these two. This emphasises that nanas have a fairly successful record and do not contribute to high rates of loss among infants in this age range. But at higher ages of infancy the mortality record with regard to births delivered by nanas is less favourable, so that the overall position for the first year of life is as follows. For infants delivered by nurses in hospital the level of mortality is 37 per 1,000, whereas the value for infants delivered in homes by nanas is 67: the probability of dying within the first year of life among infants delivered by nurses at home amounts to 55 per 1,000, which exceeds the comparable value for hospital cases made by nurses.

An important phase of the survey was the examination of effects of deaths of children on the family in general. Virtually all women express some form of grief at the loss of children, and this is at times accompanied by feelings of guilt. The reaction to deaths of young children, in which all members of the family share, was sadness, dismay and general emotional upset. In some cases the mothers showed great distress when being questioned about these deaths.

Losses of more than one child in a family suggest that an approach to infant mortality which relates infant deaths to families rather than to individual births may be rewarding. Rates of mortality based on families may be influenced by 3 factors: size of family, genetic considerations or environmental factors.

The family size aspect is important as all families suffering deaths of children are much larger than those who experience no such loss. The average family size of women who have suffered the loss of one or more children is 6.17, which is 2.6-fold the size of families which have escaped such loss (2.41). Families experiencing a single death show an average size of 5.32 and this moves up fairly regularly with the numbers of deaths to a maximum of 11.3 in the case of those losing 4 children.

There are 26 pairs of twins in this sample and these are born to mothers whose ages range from 18 to 38, with the modal age group being 25 to 29. These 26 pairs are produced by 21 mothers. The majority (17) have only one set, while 3 women have 2 and 1 woman has 3 consecutive sets in 5 years. The 26 pairs consist of 11 all male, 10 all female and 5 male-female sets. When deaths occurring among these twins are examined, it is striking to note that all are female, even in the case where male-female sets are involved.

The great majority of infants in the survey have been breastfed by their mothers; in fact those not breastfed amount to only 4% of the total. Three patterns of breastfeeding are recognised; the most common, at least in the past, extends over 9 months, while 2 others of shorter duration are frequently reported, one of 3 months and the other of 6 to 7 months. Among women of completed fertility, the 9-month pattern is the most common, while only small proportions of their infants are breastfed for 3 months. In terms of type of union, very little separates the general position of women in visiting and common-law unions who are over 45, both of whom show medians of about 10 months. Much lower is the corresponding value for married women of the same age (8.4 months). There is among older women a marked concentration on the 9-month pattern by women in all types of union. Shifts from long to short durations constitute the main aspect of breastfeeding for women under age 45, the reduction in its prevalence being the dominant feature of child care. Marked differentials between women with elementary education and those with post-primary schooling are disclosed, with the former having by far the longer duration.

A prominent phenomenon of the West Indian family is the frequency with which women, especially those not formally married, have their children cared for by relatives or friends. One of the commonest ways in which children are not brought up in their family of procreation is seen when the mother establishes a family while still a resident in her parental home and then later leaves that home to establish one of her own. About 30% of the women in the sample have elected to have some of their children brought up in this manner, and for many of them more than 1 child is involved. Most of the 125 children brought up in these conditions are of low birth order. In the case of males, 57% are first births, while for females there are 34% first-order births. It is to be noted that the overwhelming majority of children being cared for away from their mothers' homes come from visiting-type unions.

It is instructive to examine some of the reasons advanced by mothers for entrusting the maintenance of their children to others. So far as those born to visiting mothers are concerned, economic factors are frequently given, such as the mother having to go to work, or lack of financial support from the father. Another reason that appears often is the grandmother's eagerness to have the child live with her.

In the present context, it is essential to relate children living away from their parents to the latter's family size. For here again there is a substantial proportion of cases in which more than one child from the same family is given out to the care of others; in some cases all the children from a given family are living away from their mother.

It would be expected that a picture in some way complementary to the foregoing would be obtained from the sample in the form of women reporting the presence in their household of children other than their own, for whom they are caring. Both in respect of proportions of children involved and their characteristics there should be some consistency. Unfortunately the sample material on families with children living away is not consistent with data on mothers who have their children in the care of others.

An examination of women with large families, that is more than 10 pregnancies, was undertaken in order to try to identify social and bio-medical elements within them to which their large families might be ascribed. There are 28 such women, or 6% of the total sample, and their reproductive performance means that they are responsible for 18% of total pregnancies recorded for women in the sample. The largest number of pregnancies to any women in the sample is 16. The general educational status of these women is uniformly low. While most of them commence childbearing in a common-law or visiting relationship, by age 45 most of them are married, the aim being to gain a measure of respectability.

The relatively late age at marriage should be viewed in the context of statements made by some to the effect that initially they were "too young" to get married. Also many hold that in visiting unions they retain a measure of freedom, which is denied them in marriage or the common-law state. It is also of interest that many parents prefer their daughters to be engaged in visiting relationships, as "the common-law union is not right."

All these women have been in unions of relatively long duration, while the average number of partners per woman has been 2.6. These 28 women have had in all 316 pregnancies, equivalent to an average of 4.3 per partner, while their rate of infant mortality is 88 per 1,000. There is no indication whatsoever that the large families these women support represent inherited traits. In fact their average family size is much larger than the average of their parents.

There are 70 women in the sample with 3 children or less and their experience has been considered in order to determine whether they reveal any social or bio-medical characteristics which can be firmly identified as associated with their low fertility performance. It is however only from the condition of women with 1 child that satisfactory material on these questions can be gleaned. These para 1 women are for the most part involved in casual relationships and it is within these brief initial unions that their first children are born. In fact even among women who are married their one and only child tends to be the product of the early years of their marriage. Whether interpreting the brief periods they spend in unions as a conscious desire to limit the size of their families is reading too much into the evidence remains at this stage uncertain. But the comparatively brief periods at which they are at risk of childbearing undoubtedly contributes to their low fertility. Further, the substantial number of these women who, either through artificial menopause or reports of medical evidence, experience conditions which impair their fertility constitutes another source making for low fertility.

Medical Implications

Some findings of this survey have implications for the medical interests of the country and it is convenient to open this discussion with the role of the nanas, who have long complemented the official delivery services. Their role is all the more notable because they operate in rural areas where appropriate medical services are much less accessible than in urban centers. With regard to proportions of miscarriages among the deliveries for which they are responsible, their record compares favourably with that of trained nurses. In fact it is only in terms of mortality within the period 1 to 12 months that children they deliver show losses higher than those for children delivered by trained medical personnel. We may conclude that while their competence and knowledge suffice to ensure a level of perinatal wastage which does not depart much from that shown by other infants, they may not be in a position to render to their clients proper advice concerning post-natal care of their newborn infants. Probably steps to upgrade their knowledge in this field may help to contain environmental factors affecting infant mortality.

Another aspect of infant mortality with medical implications appears in the appreciable number of miscarriages and infant deaths reported in respect of deliveries made by doctors. The high level observed here seems to indicate that these result from pregnancies which have been deliberately terminated and which are brought before doctors because of the deterioration in the mothers' condition. To the extent that these conditions are generated by induced abortions performed by untrained operators, they suggest that some reductions in these complications may be effected by the legalising of abortion and providing proper services for its performance.

The steep falls in age at which women wean their infants present both medical and social implications; here it is the former aspects that concern us. It is difficult to envisage any programme, medical or social, which could completely reverse the trend towards the 3-month nursing pattern to which the whole society seems to be moving. Presumably, unless there are compensating innovations in feeding habits, there may be declines in the nutritional status of infants.

The element of the analysis of the menstrual cycle with patent medical implications is the appreciable number of women who experience an artificial menopause. These point to the prevalence of conditions among women which may be responsible for generating sterility and sub-fertility on a substantial scale. These, it will be recalled, have characterised many Caribbean populations in the first 4 decades of the present century, but have fallen appreciably in recent years. A close medical examination of the conditions involved may prove fruitful, as, apart from their possible consequences for fertility, they obviously have adverse effects on the health of women.

Social Implications

Social implications of this study relate largely to characteristics of the family, particularly the visiting type, and it is with certain implications pertaining to the latter that we deal now. That there are close contacts between the partners and that they participate to a considerable degree in joint decision-making for the satisfactory functioning of the family emerges clearly from this study. Many discussions of the family are concerned with whether it performs satisfactorily such functions as the socialisation of the child and the part a non-residential father plays in these processes. While full elucidation of these issues cannot be obtained from this study, the extensive contacts between the father and his children and between him and his partner indicate that current opinion often appreciably understates his role in these important aspects of the family.

Popular views that the visiting union exposes the woman to hardships and that she faces particular difficulty in virtue of the absence of the male from the household do not find much confirmation from the present findings. A careful consideration of views of respondents points definitely to their position that this form of family accords them a degree of freedom and independence which they hold to be greatly to their advantage. Even from the standpoint of the support of their children and the family as a whole, they maintain that the absence of the partner is by no means a disaster. For economically they do not consider their position unduly difficult; such financial assistance as they receive from their partners has not to be spent in partial support of the latter, as would be the case in residential unions. Such funds serve solely for their own support and for the upkeep of their children.

We may recall the argument advanced in the opening chapter that women are fully aware that facilities are available whereby their unions may be endowed with legal sanction, should they desire this. Evidence from the survey does not enable us to say with certainty that the decision to marry is basically theirs. Indeed it appears that they are heavily influenced in this respect by the attitude of parents and the persuasion of friends. Seldom are there references to the part played by their partners in inducing them to marry, although extensive discussions of marriage occupy part of the sessions in which visiting unions involve themselves. In so far as the children play a role here, a factor to be reckoned with is that women may prefer a visiting or common-law union as these ensure fuller control, and even complete custody, of their children, which may be lost in formal marriage. Of course the impressions gained from a female-oriented survey such as this, that it is the woman who is essentially responsible for the conversion of a visiting or common-law union to marriage, may not be confirmed from an analysis in which the situation is explored from the standpoint of the male partner. But certainly the evidence from this study strongly indicates that she is fully cognisant of the advantages and disadvantages of formal marriage and is prepared to enter it only when she is firmly convinced that such a course of action will prove of positive benefit to her and to her children.

The implications of substantial proportions of children living away from their mothers, characteristics of the visiting union mostly, are important, as this further affects the structure of a family form, unique in that the male partner lives away from the mother and her children. The influence of such living arrangements on their families of procreation, on their families of adoption, as well as on the children themselves may be far-reaching. Possibly having to live away from their parents from early life deeply influences the children's relationships to their mothers, as one aspect of the survey illustrates. In many cases the children learn to address their mothers as "Aunt" or some similar term, which though signifying some form of kinship, is in no way the equivalent of "mother." Questions that arise as a consequence of this form of living are many. For instance: How are the socialisation processes of the children affected? Does living away from their mothers in any way affect their educational and health prospects? Are these children at a disadvantage, economically, compared with those living in the homes of their mothers? These remain weighty issues as, according to the survey returns, about 15% of the population under age 15 are involved in such living arrangements.

A further implication which basically seems to have sociological as well as other implications is the very low degree of knowledge of the reproductive processes and of menstruation which seems to permeate the entire society. Apart from the indication these afford of the general tone of knowledge in the society, their chief consequence appears to be with regard to the use of contraceptives which produce disturbances in the menstrual cycle. It seems reasonable to assume that such disturbances may be interpreted as dangerous to their "health" and this of itself may constitute a factor militating against the spread of contraceptives having these side effects. The evidence that levels of knowledge of both reproduction and menstruation associated with users of contraception are much higher than levels associated with non-users implies that women with adequate knowledge of these processes will more readily accept the use of measures of birth control. However this does not rule out the possibility that such advanced knowledge may have been acquired after the commencement of use of the method in question. In either event, it appears that programmes of fertility control may to advantage incorporate campaigns aimed at disseminating appropriate understanding of these fundamental processes.

The growing attention being paid to menstruation in recent studies of female behaviour emphasises the realisation of its significance in every aspect of a woman's life. Her patterns of behaviour, her mobility, her sexual life—these are all synchronised with the phases of the cycle, while underlying beliefs play important roles in ensuring the proper timing of activities in accordance with changes in the cycle. There is nothing unique in the range of opinions about menstruation and the attendant taboos that this survey discloses. The literature emphasises that nearly every society has such beliefs, and the general similarity throughout most of them is remarkable. Respondents' beliefs about aspects of the menstrual cycle, such as the time when sexual intercourse should take place, must of course be distinguished from their actual practice in this respect. The degree to which practice conforms to beliefs was not the subject of enquiry, although its relevance is acknowledgéd.

Demographic Implications

From a sample of only 501 women not much in the way of statistical analysis of fertility can be conducted, but the analysis carried out does yield some useful insights into conditions having effects on fertility and on reproductive processes in general. Detailed histories of women with small and large families point to the existence of bio-medical conditions as playing an important part in the control of fertility. Thus the number of para 1 women who report symptoms indicative of impaired fertility capacity is considerable, whereas among women with more than 10 pregnancies these conditions are rare. Satisfactory treatment of these conditions could conceivably mean an increase in family size for certain sections of the population, with a consequent tendency to decelerate somewhat rates of fertility decline.

The interrelationship between fertility and child mortality is only touched on in this survey, but manifestly suffices to bring out the complexities of the situation. What our analyses demonstrate is the relevance of treating mortality among infants as occurring within families of different sizes. The marked differences in family size between women who experience infant mortality and those who do not, together with the pronounced rise in mortality with increases in size of family, underline the importance of the relationships at work here. Manifestly the substantial reductions in infant mortality that have already taken place are of relevance to discussions of child replacement. For falls in this mortality may induce families to postpone or do without births which, in the presence of higher mortality, might have been essential for the maintenance of the appropriate family size.

Birth spacing represents one of the major elements determining the average family size in all populations; in the present context it therefore remains of considerable relevance, notably in the discussions of fertility levels for women in visiting unions. Lengthy spacing, especially between first and second births, is a prominent feature of what we have called the casual relationships and in so far as this forms part of the overall visiting type, the low fertility of the latter must be due, to an appreciable degree, to the relatively protracted birth spacing up to order 4 or 5. Control over the duration of these casual relationships is effected by the woman (or her partner possibly) ending the initial sexual association at or even before the termination of the initial pregnancy.

As in all populations, mating experience plays a dominant role as a determinant of fertility. The analysis of mating patterns in Chapter 2 demonstrates that women who commence their families in visiting unions subsequently spend appreciable periods in a single state, and we may conclude that the casual relationship contributes substantially to this. The several and sometimes prolonged interruptions of their union history have considerably reduced their period of exposure to the risk of childbearing. By contrast women whose initial unions are of common-law or formal marriage show much shorter periods in the single state, and a corresponding lengthening of the periods during which they are at risk of childbearing. These findings from earlier samples, arrived at by a special technique, are matched by the experience of women in this sample, although the small numbers of the latter preclude rigorous demonstration of this feature. Thus the average period per woman spent in unions of any kind amounts to 26 years in the case of women with 10 or more pregnancies, which appreciably exceeds the corresponding period shown by women with families of 3 or less, which is 19 years.

Future Research

Researchers tend to follow tried approaches which have proved successful in their past work and consequently a degree of impropriety may attach to any proposal that the methodology followed in one project be taken over by future investigators. Still it seems of use to record our satisfaction with the dual method of recording adopted in this study, and to urge consideration of its development in future studies of this nature.

From every standpoint the use of tape recording of interviews has proved rewarding. Not only has it made possible the checking of material recorded on the questionnaire by the interviewer, but the recording conveys the attitudes, feelings and values of the respondent in a way which no other approach could capture. An examination of the form of response to certain questions leads to the conclusion that reliance on questionnaires calling for precoded answers of the Yes/No type are wholly inadequate, and at times misleading, when applied to certain forms of information. Thus questions designed to find out whether the respondent has ever made use of contraception by resort to Yes/No questions leaves much to be desired. Very often in the course of the interview answers such as "yes, occasionally," or "sometimes," are given, from which the interviewer has to decide whether yes or no is the appropriate entry. Either seems inappropriate, and thus without supporting material from a tape recording or information from other questions designed for this purpose, a measure of uncertainty surrounds some answers.

Before listing subjects which, from the present findings, seem to constitute significant aspects for future research, we must re-emphasise that we have in effect presented one face of the coin, so to speak, namely the picture drawn from a female-oriented study. What seems required now is a picture drawn from a male-oriented study, which would form the other face of the coin. This is urged not so much on the ground of uncertainties of responses of women; on the contrary we have every reason to be confident about the reliabilities of their responses. But there are aspects of the formation and the functioning of the family for which information must be supplemented by material obtained from males. This is especially the case in the economic aspects of the family, such as the total income at its disposal, and how the partner makes a living. In other fields as well, answers from the male are needed to supplement others provided by females. Above all, very little is known about the extent to which men in the society father children, how they move from one type of union to another and how frequently they change partners in the course of their lives.

The following are subjects which, from the findings of the present survey, seem to call for further investigation. Some of these may entail an analysis of larger samples for more rigorous quantitative treatment of the data, while others may well call for the study of samples of the size used in this project. Moreover some may be more appropriately derived from a male-oriented study.

1. *Study of Abortion.* It has long been recognised that abortion has been practised on a substantial scale in Jamaica, but no systematic attempt has ever been made to derive reliable estimates of its prevalence. A study aimed at determining these and assessing attitudes towards its performance seems therefore highly necessary.

2. *Study of Living Arrangements of Children.* The effects of these on the mothers and the children involved call for careful study. Issues such as the health of the children, their socialisation, schooling and the effects on their attitudes to parenthood are equally important phases of investigation.

3. *Study of Families.* Both in the analyses of mortality and of living arrangements of children, the relevance of an approach based on the family rather than on the individual has been clearly demonstrated. The further development of such approaches and the application of the family to other fields of enquiry seem fully justified.

4. *Study of Males.* As very few systematic analyses of fertility, mating, reproduction and the family have proceeded in terms of males, very little is known about the direct part they play in these contexts. It is therefore time that a project of this nature be undertaken.

Notes

1. Ranjan Kumar Som, *Recall Lapse in Demographic Enquiries* (Bombay: Asia Publishing House, 1973).

APPENDIX I
Gross Mating Table

Table A Probabilities of Jamaican women in various types of initial unions shifting to second-stage unions

Age interval	Probabilities of women in initial visiting unions shifting to second-stage union as:			Probabilities of women in initial common-law unions shifting to second-stage union as:			Probabilities of women in initial married unions shifting to second-stage union as:		
	Common-law	Married	Single	Visiting	Married	Single	Visiting	Common-law	Single
14–15	0.002	0.001	0.006	–	0.000	0.000	–	–	–
15–20	0.072	0.046	0.066	0.010	0.036	0.015	–	0.005	–
20–25	0.142	0.124	0.101	0.022	0.094	0.039	0.005	–	0.015
25–30	0.116	0.139	0.141	0.005	0.147	0.067	0.008	0.003	0.015
30–35	0.091	0.197	0.144	0.031	0.142	0.077	–	0.003	0.031
35–40	0.107	0.138	0.142	0.012	0.156	0.082	0.005	0.003	0.032
40–45	0.029	0.130	0.203	0.016	0.093	0.137	0.003	0.008	0.070

Table B Probabilities of Jamaican women in various types of second-stage unions shifting to terminal unions

Age interval	Probabilities of women in second-stage unions of visiting type shifting to terminal stage as:			Probabilities of women in second-stage unions of common-law type shifting to terminal stage as:			Probabilities of women in second-stage unions of married type shifting to terminal stage as:			Probabilities of women in second-stage unions as single shifting to terminal stage as:		
	Common-law	Married	Single	Visiting	Married	Single	Visiting	Common-law	Single	Visiting	Common-law	Married
14–15	–	–	–	–	–	–	–	–	–	–	–	–
15–20	0.024	–	–	–	0.010	0.003	–	–	–	0.000	0.001	0.000
20–25	–	–	–	0.005	0.062	0.013	–	–	–	0.009	0.020	0.036
25–30	–	0.024	0.024	0.003	0.111	0.017	–	–	0.008	0.013	0.044	0.047
30–35	–	0.051	–	0.019	0.098	0.062	–	0.002	0.008	0.016	0.037	0.088
35–40	0.081	0.027	0.162	0.020	0.119	0.056	0.008	0.005	0.011	0.017	0.038	0.064
40–45	–	0.037	0.148	0.015	0.118	0.103	0.005	0.002	0.030	0.013	0.022	0.076

Appendix I

GROSS MATING
MOVEMENTS OF COHORT OF 10,000
OF ENTRY INTO INITIAL STAGE
TO SECOND AND
PART

WOMEN ENTERING INITIAL

| Age interval | Women entering initial stage in visiting union | | Outcome of those moving to common-law unions at second stage | | | | |
| | *Total*** | *Remaining in visiting unions** | *Total entering common-law unions at 2nd stage*** | *Remaining in common-law unions** | *Moving to terminal stage as*** | | |
					Visiting	*Married*	*Single*
14–15	623	–	1	–	–	–	–
15–20	2,549	618	229	1	–	2	1
20–25	1,505	2,586	585	227	4	52	13
25–30	559	2,574	337	743	3	119	18
30–35	241	1,932	203	940	26	115	70
35–40	60	1,238	140	932	21	128	60
40–45	39	783	29	863	18	110	101
45–50	–	523	–	663	–	–	–
Total	5,576		1,524		72	526	263

*Remaining in given type up to beginning of stated age interval.
**Moving within stated age interval.

TABLE
WOMEN SUBJECT TO PROBABILITIES
AND PROBABILITIES OF SHIFTING
TERMINAL STAGE

I

STAGE IN VISITING UNION

	Outcome of those marrying at second stage					*Outcome of those becoming single at second stage*				
Total marrying at 2nd stage**	Remaining married*	Moving to terminal stage as**			Total becoming single at 2nd stage**	Remaining single*	Moving to terminal stage as**		
		Visiting	Common-law	Single			Visiting	Common-law	Married
–	–	–	–	–	4	–	–	–	–
145	–	–	–	–	207	4	–	1	1
519	145	–	–	–	413	209	6	14	22
437	664	–	–	9	427	580	13	42	49
422	1,092	–	2	12	310	903	20	44	105
179	1,500	13	8	19	196	1,044	23	49	81
106	1,639	9	3	51	164	1,087	23	30	100
–	1,682	–	–	–	–	1,098	–	–	–
1,808		22	13	91	1,721		85	180	358

GROSS MATING
MOVEMENTS OF COHORT OF 10,000
OF ENTRY INTO INITIAL STAGE
TO SECOND AND
PART

WOMEN ENTERING INITIAL

Age interval	Women entering initial stage in common-law union		Outcome of women moving to visiting unions at second stage				
	Total**	Remaining in common-law unions*	Total entering visiting unions at 2nd stage**	Remaining in visiting unions*	Moving to terminal stage as**		
					Common-law	Married	Single
14–15	279	–	–	–	–	–	–
15–20	937	277	12	–	–	–	–
20–25	567	1,140	38	12	–	–	–
25–30	327	1,469	8	50	–	1	–
30–35	138	1,414	46	57	–	5	–
35–40	26	1,141	14	98	9	3	18
40–45	4	874	14	82	–	3	14
45–50	–	660	–	79	–	–	–
Total	2,278		132		9	12	32

*Remaining in given type up to beginning of stated age interval.
**Moving within stated age interval.

TABLE
WOMEN SUBJECT TO PROBABILITIES
AND PROBABILITIES OF SHIFTING
TERMINAL STAGE
II

STAGE IN COMMON-LAW UNION

	Outcome of those marrying at second stage				Outcome of those becoming single at second stage				
Total marrying at 2nd stage**	Remaining married*	Moving to terminal stage as**			Total becoming single at 2nd stage**	Remaining single*	Moving to terminal stage as**		
		Visiting	Common-law	Single			Visiting	Common-law	Married
1	–	–	–	–	1	–	–	–	–
44	1	–	–	–	18	1	–	–	–
131	45	–	–	–	69	19	1	2	3
256	176	–	–	3	118	82	3	8	10
236	429	–	1	5	129	179	5	11	27
189	659	7	4	9	90	265	7	14	23
85	828	4	1	27	119	311	8	10	34
–	881	–	–	–	–	378	–	–	–
942		11	6	44	544		24	45	97

GROSS MATING
MOVEMENTS OF COHORT OF 10,000
OF ENTRY INTO INITIAL STAGE
TO SECOND AND
PART

WOMEN MARRYING

| Age interval | Women marrying at initial stage within age cohort | | Outcome of women moving to visiting unions at second stage | | | | |
| | Total** | Remaining married * | Total entering visiting union at 2nd stage** | Remaining in visiting unions* | Moving to terminal stage as** | | |
					Common-law	Married	Single
14–15	77	–	–	–	–	–	–
15–20	482	77	–	–	–	–	–
20–25	563	556	5	–	–	–	–
25–30	340	1,098	11	5	–	–	–
30–35	189	1,402	–	16	–	1	–
35–40	86	1,538	9	15	2	1	4
40–45	34	1,560	4	17	–	1	3
45–50	–	1,467	–	17	–	–	–
Total	1,771		29		2	3	7

*Remaining in given type up to beginning of stated age interval.
**Moving within stated age interval.

TABLE
WOMEN SUBJECT TO PROBABILITIES
AND PROBABILITIES OF SHIFTING
TERMINAL STAGE
III

AT INITIAL STAGE

Outcome of women moving to common-law unions at second stage					*Outcome of those becoming single at second stage*				
Total entering common-law unions* at 2nd stage**	*Remaining in common-law unions**	*Moving to terminal stage as***			*Total becoming single at 2nd stage***	*Remaining single**	*Moving to terminal stage as***		
		Visiting	*Married*	*Single*			*Visiting*	*Common-law*	*Married*
—	—	—	—	—	—	—	—	—	—
3	—	—	—	—	—	—	—	—	—
—	3	—	—	—	16	—	—	—	1
4	3	—	1	—	21	15	—	1	2
4	6	—	1	1	49	33	1	3	7
4	8	—	1	1	51	71	2	5	8
13	10	—	3	3	110	107	4	5	17
—	17	—	—	—	—	191	—	—	—
28			6	5	247		7	14	35

APPENDIX II
Survey Questionnaire

Form SCFF

SURVEY OF SOCIO-CULTURAL FACTORS OF FERTILITY
IN JAMAICA, 1975

Identification No.

Parish   Enum. Dist.   Housld No.

□   □□□   □□

1. Did you participate in a similar study in 1971-72?   Yes □□
                                                                No □2□

    If no, why not?   Under age □1□   Not in Area □2□   Refused □3□

2. Respondent No.   □□□□

3. Relationship to Head of Household
    Head □1□   Spouse/Partner □2□   Child of Hd/ Sp □3□   Other Rel □4□   Other □5□

                                        Mth. Year
4. Month and year of Birth   □□   □□

5. Age in completed years   □□

6. Marital status
    Never married □1□   Married □2□   Widowed □3□   Divorced □4□

7. Usual parish of residence ....

8. Parish of Birth ....

9. Number of years lived in this parish   □□

10. Religion ....

11. Educational attainment   Years of primary schooling □
                               Post primary   Yes □1□   No □2□

12. Economic activity. Are you employed now?   Yes □1□   No □2□

13. Socio-Economic group _____
    Agricul.   Profes.   Manag.   Clerical   Per Ser   Skilled   Semi-skilled   Unskilled   Other
    □1□   □2□   □3□   □4□   □5□   □6□   □7□   □8□   □9□

2

PARENTS

14. Were your mother and father married to each other?　Yes ☐[1]　No ☐[2]

15. How many children did your mother have?　☐☐　Exact ☐　Estimate ☐

16. What was your father's socio-economic group? _____

Agricul.	Profes.	Manag.	Clerical	Per Ser	Skilled	Semi-skilled	Unskilled	Other	D/K
[1]	[2]	[3]	[4]	[5]	[6]	[7]	[8]	[9]	[10]

Do you have a husband or partner now or did you have one at age 45?　Yes ☐[1]　No ☐[2]
If yes, complete Questions 17-24.

PARTNER

17. What is your partner's age (completed years)　☐☐　Exact ☐　Estimate ☐

18. What is his religion? ....

19. Educational attainment – Years of primary school ☐☐
　　　　　　　　　　　　Post primary　Yes ☐[1]　No ☐[2]

20. Did he work during the last week?　Yes ☐[1]　No ☐[2]

　If yes, what? ....

21. How many acres of land does your partner cultivate for himself? ....

22. Was his mother married to his father?　Yes ☐[1]　No ☐[2]　Don't know ☐[3]

23. How many children did his mother have?　☐☐　Exact ☐　Estimate ☐

24. What was his father's socio-economic group? _____

Agricul.	Profes.	Manag.	Clerical	Per Ser	Skilled	Semi-skilled	Unskilled	Other	D/K
[1]	[2]	[3]	[4]	[5]	[6]	[7]	[8]	[9]	[10]

Form SCFF   25. PREGNANCY AND MATING HISTORY

RESPONDENT NUMBER ▢▢▢▢

SHEET NUMBER   ▢

					L(ive-birth) S(till-birth) M(is-carriage)	D(octor) N(urse) O(ther)	I(inst.) H(ome) O(ther)	↑BP– High ↓BP– Low } Blood pressure V(omiting) D(iabetes/sugar) O(edema/swelling) A(lbumin)			
(a) Preg-nancy Order	(b) Child's first name	(c) Months preg-nant	(d) Month & year of termina-tion		(e) Out-come	(f) Sex	(g) Attend-ant at birth	(h) Place of delivery	(i) Complications			(j) Mths. of breast feeding
			mth.	yr.					During preg.	At Birth	After Birth	

					M(arried) CL(common- law) V(isiting) S(ingle)					
(k) ontra- ptive ed	(l) Mths. worked while preg.	(m) Partner's			(n) Type of Union	(o) Month and Year				Remarks
		First name	Age at birth of ch.			Started		Ended		
						Mth.	Yr.	Mth.	Yr.	

4

Form SCFF
RESPONDENT NUMBER ☐☐☐☐

SHEET NUMBER ☐

26. PARTICULARS OF CHILDREN UNDER 15 YEARS OF AGE
(including those born alive and who have since died)

Name & livebirth order	Mother's age at birth	Age of child		Cause of death	Cause stated by D(octor) N(urse)	Sex of child	General Health G(ood) F(air) P(oor)	Usual resid-ence A(t home) W(ith father) O(ther fam) E(lse-where)	Under foster care	
		if alive	at death						Yes [1] No [2]	Satis. [1] Dis-satis [2]
(a)	(b)	(c)		(d)	(e)	(f)	(g)	(h)	(i)	

Main activity			If at work:		Child support		Main diet under 2 years of age	Child care – working mothers		REMARKS
					S(elf) F(ather) B(oth) R(elative) O(ther man)	V(olunt-ary) C(ourt order)	E(ggs) M(ilk) B(utter/cheese) V(eg.) M(eat)	R(elative) O(lder child) NE(ighbour) N(ursery)		
Home	Sch.	Work	Age on leaving school	Type of work	By whom	Payment in absence of father		By whom	Satis [1] Dissatis [2]	
	(j)		(k)		(l)		(m)	(n)		REMARKS

5

SCFF   Respondent No. ☐☐☐☐

27. FORMATION OF INITIAL UNION (Type.................................)

Were you friendly with anyone (sexually) before setting up your partnership with ....

Could you tell me something about the conditions which influenced your decision to set up a union with ....

....

....

Probe for:

1.   Role partner..   2.   Affection for partner ....

3.   Pregnancy ....   4.   Mutual support ....

5.   Influence of parent or guardian ....   6.   Financial ....

                                                                               7.   Other ....

      Why this type of union rather than another? ....

      ....

Probe for:

1.   Advantages of this type of union ....

2.   Disadvantages of other types ....

28. CHANGE FROM INITIAL TO SECOND TYPE WITH SAME PARTNER   (Initial ...... Second ....)

Why did you and .... decide to change the type of union?

....

Was this a step you discussed and agreed on? ....

....

Probe whether:

1.   Change in economic status ....

2.   Increase in family ....

3.   Pressure from friends ....

4.   Pressure from relatives ....

5.   Legal considerations ....

6.   Other ....

6

Form SCFF

Respondent No. ☐☐☐☐

29. CHANGE FROM INITIAL TYPE OF UNION TO SECOND TYPE WITH ANOTHER PARTNER

Could you tell me why the relationship between you and ....
came to an end? ....
....

Probe whether:

1. Original partner left because of another woman ....

2. Did you begin to like (fall in love with) someone else? ....

3. Lack of sexual satisfaction ....

4. Economic factors ....

5. Other factors ....

And why this other type of relationship rather than the first?

....
....

Probe whether:

1. New partner required change ....

2. You required change ....

3. Other factors involved ....

[If Second continues up to age 45, no further Questions on Union Status to be asked]

7

Form SCFF   Respondent No. ☐☐☐☐

30. IF TERMINAL DIFFERS FROM SECOND, WITH NO CHANGE IN PARTNER

(Second .... Terminal ....)

Why did you and .... decide to change your type of union?

....

Was this a step that both of you agreed on?

....

If not, who took the initiative?

....

Probe for:

1.   Change in economic status ....

2.   Increase in size of family ....

3.   Factors concerning children ....

4.   Pressure from other relatives ....

5.   Pressure from other sources ....

6.   Legal implications ....

31. IF TERMINAL DIFFERS FROM SECOND, WITH CHANGE IN PARTNER

(Second............ Terminal............)

Why did you and .... your former partner separate?

....

Probe for:

1.   No longer (liked) in love with one another ....

2.   Specify difficulties or problems in order of significance ....

....

3.   Why have you gone into another type of union?..

....

Probe for:

1.   Change in economic status ....

2.   Increase in size of family ....

3.   Factors concerning children ....

4.   Pressure from other relatives ....

5.   Pressure from other sources ....

6.   Legal implications ....

8

Form SCFF

Respondent No. ☐☐☐☐

31a.   PURE TYPE WITH MULTIPLE PARTNERS (Type..........................)

What are the main reasons for your having so many partners?

....

....

....

Probe whether

1.   Partners leave because of other women

2.   Respondent fell in love (came to like) other men

3.   Complaints about lack of sexual satisfaction

4.   Whether economic considerations involved

5.   Responsibility for children

6.   Other elements

Details about partners:

Name of Partner (1)	Woman's age when partnership		Remark (4)
	Begins (2)	Ends (3)	

Note.   Enter the name of the partner in column (1) and woman's age on same line to indicate when partnership begins Column (2) and when it ends, Column (3).

9

32. ROLE OF FIRST CHILD IN ESTABLISHING AND DISSOLVING UNION IN WHICH THE CHILD
WAS BORN (Type of union ....)

(a) Did birth of your first child help you decide to enter this union? If so, how?

....

Probe for:

1. Your desire to set up own home ....
2. Partner desired to set up own home ....
3. Necessity of leaving home of parent or guardian ....
4. Economic considerations ....

How did birth of first child affect your:

(1) sexual relationships ....
(2) other relationships ....

(b) Did birth of this child play part in breaking up your union with ....

....

Probe for:

1. Resulting economic difficulties ....
2. Fundamental changes in attitudes of partner ....
3. Influence of relatives ....
4. Influence of others ....
5. Legal implications ....

(c) Was this pregnancy planned or not?

....

If planned, why?

....

Probe for:

1. Intention to stabilise your union ....
2. Other ....

Also probe for possible distinction between "planned" and "desired.

10

33.   ROLE OF OTHER CHILD IN CHANGING TYPE OF UNION OR DISSOLVING UNION IN WHICH
       THE CHILD WAS BORN (Type.................................... Birth Order ....)

(a)   Did birth of this child help you decide on change or break of union type?

....

Probe for:

1.   Resulting economic difficulties ....

2.   Fundamental changes in attitudes of partner ....

3.   Influence of relatives ....

4.   Influence of others ....

5.   Legal implications ....

(b)   Was this pregnancy planned or not?

....

If planned, why?

....

Probe for:

1.   Intention to stabilise your union ....

2.   Other ....

Also probe for possible distinction between "planned" and "desired."

Did performance of this child in school or other ways influence relationship between you and
your partner?

....

11

Respondent No. ☐☐☐☐

34. WOMAN'S ASSESSMENT OF HER PARTNER

Now I should like to ask you a few questions about your views on your partners.

	Very much			Not so much			Not at all		
	First	Sec.	Term.	First	Sec.	Term.	First	Sec.	Term.
1. Affection for your partner									
2. Economic support given you									
3. Econ. support of children									
4. Sexual partner									
5. Love of children									
6. Ambition for children									

35 WOMAN'S ASSESSMENT OF HER UNION TYPES (for women involved in more than one type of union)

Now I should like to ask you a few questions about the unions in which you have been involved.

	Very much			Not so much			Not at all		
	First	Sec.	Term.	First	Sec.	Term.	First	Sec.	Term.
1. Brought happiness									
2. Affection for your partner									
3. Good for children									
4. Economic wellbeing									
5. Pride in achievement of partner									
6. Pride in achievement of children									
7. Are these unions in accord with your religious beliefs?									
8. Change in status									
9. Despair									

12

35. (a)   RELATIONSHIP BETWEEN YOU AND YOUR PARTNER(S) IN VISITING UNIONS

How frequently do you and your partner meet?...

Do you meet regularly, how many times a week? ....

I want to ask you more about these visits.

SOCIAL OCCASIONS

(a)   Does your partner regularly visit you to take you or the children out to entertainment of any kind? ....

If so, how many times a week? .... And how many hours are involved?

....

(b)   Do you visit his residence regularly? ....

If so, how many times a week? ....And how many hours are involved?

....

(c)   Does he visit your residence regularly? ....

If so, how many times a week? ....

And how many hours are involved? ....

(d)   Has this pattern changed as you have grown older? ....

....

....

....

(e)   Are there any special occasions, such as Church, Cinema, Sports, that you and your partner go to, or to which he takes the children? ....

....

....

GENERAL VISITS

Are there any matters that you meet with your partner to discuss regularly? ....

....

If so, name them...

....

How often do these business visits take place? ....

....

Where are they held? ....

How long do they last? ....

13

SEXUAL VISITS

How often do these take place per week? ....

Where do you meet? ....

Explain ....

How long do they last? ....

Are there any difficulties in arranging these meetings? ....

....

OTHER

On the average how long (hours per week) are you and your partner together ....

....

For any purpose whatsoever (list) ....

....

Do you feel lonely when your partner is not around? ....

How many hours per week do your child(ren) spend with their father? ....

at his home ....

at your home ....

elsewhere ....

36. (a) RELATIONSHIPS BETWEEN YOU AND YOUR PARTNER(S)

Do you expect your partner(s) to be faithful to you? ....

Are you expected to be faithful to them? ....

Do (Did) you enjoy having sex with your partner? ....

On the average how many times per month do (did) you have
    sex with him? ....

(b) COMMUNICATION BETWEEN YOU AND YOUR PARTNER(S)

Did you and your partner discuss questions of
    whether to have children or not? ....

If so, at what stage in the family cycle
    (in terms of parity and union stage)? ....

14

37   WOMEN'S ATTITUDES TOWARDS CHILDBEARING

   1.   How many children do you think make a small family? ....

   2.   How many children do you think make a large family? ....

   3.   Do you think every woman should have a child? ....
....
....

   4.   Do you think every man should have a child? ....
....
....

   5.   Have you ever heard that every woman should have a certain number of children? ....
....

   6.   Have you ever heard how this number can be known? ....
....
....
....

   7.   Do you think that a woman has a choice in the number of children she can have?
....
....

   8.   What is your opinion of a woman who has no children? ....
....
....
....

   9   What do you think are the causes of childlessness? ....
....
....
....

   10.   What do you think is the best spacing between
          (1)   First and Second birth? ....
          (2)   Second and Third birth? ....
          (3)   Third and Fourth birth? ....

   11.   Do you feel better when you are pregnant than when you are not? ....

   12.   If so, why? ....
....

   13.   Do you think that a woman should have a child for each of her partners?
....

15

Form SCFF   Respondent No. ☐☐☐☐

14. How many children do you think a woman should have in her life-time? ....

      (1) Boys ....

      (2) Girls ....

38. **MENSTRUATION**

1. At what age did you have your first menses? ....

2. At what age did you have your last menses? ....

3. (a) Did anyone explain menstruation to you? Yes [1]   No [2]

    (b) If yes, who?

Teacher	Mother	Friend	Older Woman	School-mate	Other
[1]	[2]	[3]	[4]	[5]	[6]

    (c) If no, were you frightened when you saw your period?

      ....

4. Did anyone ever explain sex to you?   Yes [1]   No [2]

    If yes, who? ....

5. (a) Are your periods regular or irregular? ....

    (b) If irregular: (i)   Do you worry? ....

                (ii) Consult a doctor? ....

6   How many days on the average do you menstruate? ....

7. Do you have any problems or complications? ....
    (if yes, please list)

    ....

    ....

    ....

8. Should a woman have sexual intercourse

    (1) Just before menstruation ....

    (2) During menstruation ....

    (3) Just after menstruation ....

9. What does (did) your partner do about sex when you are (were) menstruating?

    ....

    ....

10. What do you think causes menstruation? ....

    ....

11. Do you prefer to be menstruating or to be pregnant? ....

12. Do you find menstruating less of a problem than pregnancy? ....

16

Form SCFF   Respondent No. ☐☐☐☐

13. (a)   Does menstruation affect your normal activities in any way? ....

     (b)   If yes, please explain ....

                  ....

14. What beliefs do you know about menstruation? ....

   ....

   ....

   ....

   ....

15. (a)   How does a woman get pregnant? ....

                  ....

                  ....

                  ....

     (b)   Why at some times and not at others? ....

                  ....

                  ....

16. Have you ever heard of ways or things to get rid of a baby? ....

   What?...

   ....

   ....

   ....

17

Form SCFF   Respondent No. ☐☐☐☐

39. BOND BETWEEN MOTHER AND CHILD

Are there any of your children for whom you have a special feeling? If so, which one?

....

Probe for:

1.   Birth order ....
2.   Sex ....
3.   Complexion of child compared to others ....
4.   School performance ....
5.   Physical characteristics ....
6.   Behaviour in general ....
7.   Was this a wanted or unwanted child? ....
8.   Is this child living with you? ....
9.   If no to 8, under what circumstances would you agree to her living away from you?

      ....

40. HOW CHILD ADDRESSES MOTHER

How did you call your mother? ....
How do your children call you? ....
If term other than mother, mummy, etc., probe why

....

41. CHILDREN NOT LIVING WITH MOTHER

What circumstances made you decide to send them away?

....

Probe for:

1.   Economic considerations
2.   Health factors
3.   Other

What factors determined when they were sent away (at what age)?

....

How long do you think they will be away from you? ....
How did/has their living away from you affected you and the family?

....

....

18

Form SCFF   Respondent No. ☐☐☐☐

42. WOMEN WITH FOSTER CHILDREN

What relationship, if any, is the foster child to you? ....

What are your reasons for taking this child? ....

....

Probe for:

1. Financial gain
2. Companionship
3. Status
4. Genuine love of children
5. Other

How has this addition affected your own family?

....

....

43. REACTIONS TO DEATH OF CHILD

How did you feel about this?

....

Probe for:

1. Whether this made her ill ....
2. Caused emotional disturbance ....
3. Produced feeling of guilt (responsibility) for tragedy ....
4. Was your role as partner affected? ....
5. Was your role as mother affected? ....
6. Was the sexual relationship with your partner affected? ....
7. Was your social relationship affected? ....
8. Did you consider replacing the child? ....

How did the father of the child take this death? ....

....

How were other children of family affected by this death?

....

How did the death of the child affect the family as a whole?

....

19

Form SCFF

Respondent No. ☐☐☐☐

44. (a) What do you think of family planning? ....
....
....

(b) Do you think it is important for the development of the country? ....
....
....

APPENDIX III
Enumeration Districts Comprising the Sample
and Various Statistics on Survey Material

Enumeration Districts Comprising the Sample

Parish	Area	E.D. Nos	No. of women interviewed	No. of documents processed	No. of documents used
Kingston	Rae Town	C. 32	32	21	21
	Prison, North St.	C. 87	31	22	22
St. Andrew	Hagley Park Rd.	E.C. 131	30	30	30
	Swallowfield	N. 68	29	29	28
	Swallowfield	N. 68	30	21	21
	West of Const. Spring Rd.	N. 62	30	23	21
	West of Const. Spring Rd.	N. 62	7	6	6
	Arlene Gardens	N. 76	30	21	21
Portland	Port Antonio	E. 5	30	23	23
	Balcarres	W. 43	26	19	19
St. Mary	Highgate	C. 41	30	25	25
	Claylands	W. 36	6	6	6
St. Ann	St. Ann's Bay	N.E. 11	31	23	23
	Gibraltar	S.E. 56	31	27	27
St. James	Montego Bay	N.W. 71	33	26	26
	Montego Bay Rosemount	N.W. 76	32	27	27
	Salt Spring	N.W. 63	32	25	25
	Salt Spring	N.W. 65	30	28	27
Manchester	Mandeville	C. 12	30	18	18
	Lincoln	N.W. 26	33	29	26
	Lincoln	N.W. 26	25	22	22
St. Elizabeth	Bull Savannah	N.E. 67	20	20	20
	Junction	S.E. 18	18	17	17
Total			626	508	501

Note: These districts are defined in the 1970 Census of Jamaica.

Various Statistics on Survey Material

Interviewers in survey 18

Questionnaires

Received 626
Processed 508
Not processed 84
Incomplete 17
Women over age 65 17
Processed but not worked on 7
Worked on 501
For Kingston & St. Andrew 171
For other parishes 330

Women

Under 45 326
Over 45 175
Single 37
In pure type visiting unions 105
In pure type common-law unions 27
In pure type marriage 65
In three types of unions 60
With partners but no pregnancies 56
With 1 partner 230
With 2 partners 127
With 3+ partners 107

Pregnancies in survey 1700
(no date was given for 1 pregnancy)
Livebirths to women under 45 846
Livebirths to women over 45 692
(no date was given for 1 pregnancy)
Miscarriages 127
Stillbirths 35
Twins 26 sets
(1 has 3 sets; 3 have 2 sets)
Children living away 125
Women caring for children not their own 20
Children for whom they are caring 21
Menopausal women 129
Women in five major religions (Anglican, Moravian,
 Baptist, Roman Catholic & Church of God) 304
Other religions 175
Without religion 22

Case studies

Large families	13
Small families	4
Pure types (visiting)	5
Women with four or more partners	2
Multiple pregnancy wastage	1
Casual relationship	1

APPENDIX IV
Relationship Between Respondents
and Their Partners in Visiting Unions

Visiting Unions
Relationship Between Respondents and Their Partners

Category	Total of the replies	No. of women	Mean value or percent	Comments
Respondent's age	9558.00	270	35.40 years	
Sum of weekly meeting with partner	906.91	267	3.40 days	
Social occasions				
Entertainment:				
No. of times	175.50	128	1.37	
Total hours	488.50	105	4.65 hrs.	
Respondent's visits to partner:				
No. of times	349.25	151	2.31	
Total hours	993.00	120	8.27 hrs.	
Partner's visits to respondent:				
No. of times	849.80	241	3.53	
Total hours	1922.43	219	8.78 hrs.	
Change in pattern of relationship				
Change	84	} 203		% total = 41.38
No change	119			% total = 58.62
Special visits:				
Cinema	87	—	—	
Church	53	—	—	
Clubs, parties etc.	41	—	—	
Sport	39	—	—	
Beach	8	—	—	
Shopping, friends, restaurant	10	—	—	

Category	Total of the replies	No. of women	Mean value or percent	Comments
General visits				
Topics discussed:	—	145	—	The topics discussed
Children	43	—	—	were arranged in
Marriage	34	—	—	23 groups
The future	24	—	—	
Visits				
No. of times	169.83	75	2.26	
Meeting place:				
Her home	102	—	77.86%	
His home	11	—	8.40%	
Both homes	11	—	8.40%	
Elsewhere	7	—	5.34%	
Duration	233.07	102	2.28 hrs.	
Sexual visits				
Times per week	402.83	245	1.64	
Meeting place:				
Her home	168	—	65.37%	
His home	67	—	26.07%	
Both homes	15	—	5.84%	
Elsewhere	7	—	2.72%	
Reasons for choosing above:				
Convenience	24	—	—	Many other reasons
Respondent's own house	13	—	—	given for choice of meeting place
Length of visit	458.92	205	2.24 hrs.	
Difficulties encountered:				
Yes	22	—	8.80%	
No	224	—	89.60%	
Some	4	—	1.60%	
Other visits				
Weekly average of time together	4375.5	193	22.67 hrs.	
Purpose of other visits:				
Sex	19			Many other
To visit children	12	} 48		purposes given
To talk	11			for visits
Whether lonely in absence of partner				
Yes	147	—	61.76%	
No	70	—	29.41%	
Sometimes	21	—	8.82%	

Category	Total of the replies	No. of women	Mean value or percent	Comments
Child(ren)'s time spent with father				
Hours per week	1071.66	74	14.48 hrs.	
Place:				
His home	40	—	54.79%	
Her home	19	—	26.03%	
Both homes	11	—	15.07%	
Elsewhere	3	—	4.11%	
Relationship between partners				
Expectation of partner's faithfulness:				
Yes	257	—	96.62%	
No	7	—	2.63%	
Hopeful	2	—	0.75%	
Expectation of respondent's faithfulness:				
Yes	266	—	99.25%	
No	2	—	0.75%	
Enjoyment of sex:				
Yes	249	—	96.51%	
No	7	—	2.71%	
Other	2	—	0.78%	
Average times of sex per month	1628.00	243	6.70	

APPENDIX V
Statistical Summary of Large Families
and Comparative Statistics for Women With
Large and Small Families

A STATISTICAL SUMMARY OF THE MAJOR FERTILITY

CATEGORIES	1071	2204	2300	2338	2369	4505	6859	6721	6802	6828	6825	6806	6708
										RESPONDENT NUMBER			
Age at menarche	12	14	14	16	15	14	15	11	13	15	14	14	13
Age at menopause	49	49	41	47*	45	54	35*	44*	48*	50	45	51	45*
Biological Years (a) of potential child-bearing	37	35	27	31	30	40	20	33	35	35	31	37	32
Age at termination of 1st pregnancy	19	20	16	17	17	20	18	23	22	18	15	16	21
Age at termination of last pregnancy	41	36	31	36	41	44	35	40	45	43	37	45	40
Actual years of childbearing (b)	22	16	15	19	24	24	17	17	23	25	22	29	19
Years spent in pregnancy (c)	7.5	7	7.2	7.1	7.1	9.0	10	5.7	8.3	7.0	7.3	7.5	10.7
Years spent in breastfeeding (d)	7.5	5.4	3.9	2.3	2.3	7.1	5.5	4.2	8.0	4.3	8.3	13.6	3.2
(c) + (d)	15.0	12.4	11.1	9.4	9.4	16.1	15.5	9.9	16.3	11.3	15.6	21.1	13.9
Rest of period	7	3.6	3.9	9.6	13.6	7.9	1.5	7.1	6.7	13.7	6.4	7.9	5.3
Total Pregnancies	10	10	10	10	9	15	14	10	11	10	12	10	16
(b) as % (a)	59.5	45.7	55.6	61.3	80.0	60.0	85.0	51.5	65.7	71.4	71.0	78.4	59.4
(c) as % (b)	34.1	43.8	48.0	37.4	29.6	37.5	58.8	33.5	36.1	28.0	33.2	25.9	56.6
(d) as % (b)	34.1	33.8	26.0	12.1	9.6	30.0	32.3	24.7	34.8	17.2	37.7	46.9	16.6
(c) + (d) as % (b)	68.2	77.5	74.0	49.5	39.2	67.1	91.2	58.2	70.9	45.2	70.9	72.8	73.2
No. of yrs. per preg. [(b) ÷ by total preg.]	2.2	1.6	1.5	1.9	2.7	1.6	1.2	1.7	2.1	2.5	1.8	2.9	1.2

Note: *indicates women still menstruating.

EVENTS OF THE 28 WOMEN WITH LARGE FAMILIES

6874	7910	7967	7915	8B82	8B83	8C67	8C74	8B62	8B80	4513	2301	6759	2158	6857	Averages
16	19	16	16	17	13	17	16	16	14	14	13	17	15	16	14.82
48	50	41*	42*	50	45*	40*	52*	50	49	48*	38*	40	55	45	48.00
															44.60*
32	31	25	26	33	32	23	36	34	35	34	25	23	40	29	31.46
28	20	24	24	19	19	17	18	20	14	22	16	20	27	24	19.78
42	49	41	42	40	38	39	44	44	36	39	37	42	44	46	40.53
14	29	17	18	21	19	22	26	24	22	17	21	22	17	22	20.75
6.3	11.3	7.3	7.5	9.4	8.7	7.0	9	7.5	9.2	7.5	7.5	6	8.1	7.3	7.89
2.5	12.8	6.7	10.0	7.1	6.0	6.1	9	10	9.0	7.4	8.1	4.4	8.8	4.6	6.71
8.8	24.1	14.0	17.5	16.5	14.7	13.1	18	17.5	18.2	14.9	15.6	10.4	16.9	11.9	14.61
5.2	4.9	3.0	0.5	4.5	4.3	8.9	8	6.5	3.5	2.1	5.4	11.6	0.1	10.1	6.03
9	15	10	10	15	12	10	12	10	13	10	10	8	11	12	11.30
43.8	93.5	68.0	69.2	63.6	59.4	95.6	72.0	70.5	62.9	50.0	84.0	95.6	42.5	75.9	65.95
45.0	36.4	42.6	41.7	44:8	46.0	31.8	34.6	31.2	42.0	44.1	35.7	27.3	47.6	33.2	37.95
17.9	41.3	39.7	55.6	33.8	31.6	27.7	34.6	41.7	40.9	43.5	38.6	20.0	51.8	20.9	32.41
62.9	77.7	82.4	97.2	78.6	77.6	59.5	69.2	72.9	83.0	87.6	74.3	47.3	99.4	54.1	70.34
1.6	1.9	1.7	1.7	1.4	1.6	2.2	2.2	2.4	1.7	1.7	2.1	2.8	1.5	1.8	1.84

Comparative Statistics for Women With Large and Small families

Events	Parity 1		Parity 2		Parity 3		Large families	
	Percentage	Average years	Percentage	Average years	Percentage	Average years	Percentage	Average years
Age		53.38		53.37		52.20		49.57
Primary education		6.92		6.10		7.08		6.10
Religion:								
"established church"	69		74		68		50	
fundamentalist	31		26		32		46	
none	—		—		—		4	
Age at marriage		30.00		30.83		27.89		27.18
Union types:								
married	65.38		57.89		72.00		78.57	
common-law	19.23		57.89		36.00		57.14	
visiting	76.92		63.16		56.00		71.43	
Duration of union:								
most stable		15		16		17		22
total of all		19		22		22		26
total to menopause		15		19		20		25
Years single		16		5.05		5.28		5
Number of partners		(1.8)		(2.2)		(1.8)		(2.6)
Age at menarche		14.58		14.74		14.60		14.82
Age at menopause		45.86		49.25		45.33		48.00
Pregnancies		(1)		(2)		(3)		(11.30)
Age at first pregnancy		22.90		24.32		22.25		19.78
Age at last pregnancy		22.90		29.53		29.03		40.53
Numbers and % married prior to childbearing	23	(6)	26	(5)	32	(8)	18	(5)
Biological potential period of childbearing								
Menopausal		31.18		34.17		31.06		32.50
Non-menopausal		27.75		33.57		40.33		30.43

Note: Figures in parentheses are averages or actual numbers.

APPENDIX VI
Case Studies

Case Studies
Pure-Type Visiting Unions

Respondent 6871

Margaret B. is a Baptist who has lived in the parish of her birth for all of her 62 years. She describes herself as a housewife who is the head of her household although she has never been married nor, by her own choice, lived in a common-law union. Indeed, she says there was no other reason for her breaking off with her 3 partners but that they wanted to live with her and she does not like "sweetheart life." She considers a visiting union better than living together as "you don't in'a no punishment with him." Her father, who did not support her, was an unskilled labourer, who was not married to her mother. The latter died and left Margaret, her only child, at an early age and she then lived with her grandmother until she too died while Margaret was in her early teens. Her grandmother was sick and she had to "wash and cut wood, put on coal, draw it and go to Montego Bay and sell it" to maintain them both, so she says she could not go to school. However she is not entirely illiterate because for about 4 years she would get up in the morning, put on the coal, bathe and go to school for half the day as "the teacher lived near."

After that she lived with "my Grandpa wife" who "raise me" as her mother and grandmother had died and "leave me to her." In fact this lady delivered 7 of her 9 pregnancies as she was a trainee nurse at the hospital—"she never get the diplume [diploma]." When "she got any patient and the patient is a little ticklish, him and the patient go down to hospital" as in those days she was allowed to practise outside the hospital without the benefit of a certificate. All Margaret's children were delivered at home without any complications as she was "hearty, hearty. Go to Montego Bay on Saturday, come back, have baby."

Margaret's 9 pregnancies were for 3 different partners and 4 of the children survive today. The first and third children, whom she had for her first partner, died at 9 and 5 months respectively. She says she "bawl" over them as they were "chubby and looking all right" and she missed them. She does not know what caused the death of the second child but she described in

301

detail how she came home from work and found the first child with fever and she bathed him in bay rum and warm water and "draw some mint tea" and gave him. He drank a little and then threw up. She took him to the doctor the following morning and he gave him medicine and she stayed home from work for about 3 weeks to look after him. She took him to the hospital as well and sometimes she gave him a little "goat milk" but he eventually died. The father of the children "never felt no way different" as he was visiting them and could see that she took good care of them. She breastfed these children up to the time of their deaths, while the second child was breastfed for 9 months.

Two of the 4 children whom she bore for her second partner—her fourth and seventh—were stillborn, and 2 years after having her eighth child for her third partner she suffered a miscarriage when she was 4 months pregnant. She was then 44 years old but said she did not stop menstruating until she was 59. Nevertheless she did not conceive after that, although she did not use any method of contraception.

Margaret was 16 when she had her first child in 1928. She became friendly with the father, of whose age she was entirely ignorant, as "me did want a little help." By that time her grandmother and mother had both died and she had "nobody, as me father never looking after me." She was with her "Grandpa's wife and was battering a work a' cane piece. I work a' cane piece from I was a little girl," so it was a "little hard and I was looking a little help." At the time she cared for him very much but would not live common-law with him, because "me never love the life." In addition she had built a little thatched hut in the yard of her "Grandpa's wife" and lived there, and "my mind never make up to carry a man there because she was living there." She "never live a' house" with any man as "I never have my own place." At the time she used to sell "neeseberry and tobacco and so" for a living, during the pregnancy. After the second child started to walk she found herself pregnant with a third "but when I get fe find out the routine of me mother sickness I leave." We do not know what the respondent meant by this statement but this was the reason given for her breaking off with her first partner before the third child was born—"I leave him off." They had been together for 6 years.

"Nuff time" (4 years) passed between her third and fourth pregnancies during which time she worked on a sugar estate carrying and cutting cane. In fact she was friendly with her second partner about 2 years before her fourth child was delivered stillborn when she was 8 months pregnant. A year later her fifth child was born and 3 years afterwards she had another stillbirth, again when she was 8 months pregnant, when she fell and "the bundle of cane drop on me back." She breastfed her fifth child for 9 months but she "never live a' house neither" with that partner.

After that relationship, which lasted for 8 years, ended, she moved from that district and lived in another area for "nuff years." Her eighth child was born 11 years later for her third partner and delivered by a "Queen midwife" who has since died. She and this partner "never friend no time" (about 2 months)—before she found herself pregnant. She breastfed the child for about a year as she did not have any more "so quick." Two years later, however, she miscarried her ninth and last pregnancy at 4 months and in the same year their friendship came to an end.

She speaks of a fourth partner; she "did dearly love him and he took sick" and died. They were friends for 9 or 10 years but apparently this was not a sexual relationship and they were just good friends.

Margaret declares that she had no special love for any of her partners because "them no care me" and if she hadn't worked for herself she would not be here today. However she seemed to have been very independent and did not encourage any of them to spend too much time when they came to see her: "They have fe go back a dem yard because me na' do nothing fe them." They visited her about once per week and when she found herself pregnant "most of the time me have to consider how, because me never glad fe them to stay, or go up to some merriment nuff nuff time." She says she did not particularly enjoy having sex with them, and as soon as she realised she was pregnant, she refused to have sex with them for the entire pregnancy. Regarding which one was the best sexual partner—"in those days we never consider nothing, we never got no interest in 'a those things." None of her partners took her or the children out for any entertainment and although they visited her home, she never went to theirs. After she had a baby, the baby's father would visit her more often than the usual once per week "though when me have the stomach me never glad fe them." She did not discuss any business matters with them as they were not living with her and she preferred to keep her business to herself. She thought they should have been more faithful to her, as she was to them, but she found them "less care," so that she had to go back to work soon after she had her children. She was solely responsible for schooling her sixth child, a boy, as the father did not give her much help with him as Margaret would not live with him. That same man, however, tried "him very best" with his older daughter who "was along with her grandmother." On the whole she thought her partners did not have any ambition for their children and she had to do most of the "caring."

Margaret had her first menses at 11 and she stopped at 59. She felt that the cause of menstruation was ". . . blood. It is what the Lord limit you to do." No one explained menstruation to her so when she saw her first period she went to her grandmother who was alive at the time. It was a Saturday morning and her grandmother drew out a board box and took out an old sheet and tore it and showed her how to put it on, then she sent to buy 5 yards of brown calico at 3d per yard and she cut out some diapers and gave them to Margaret to hem. Her periods used to be regular and lasted about 5 days. She was told that she should not clean the house as the rubbing was not good while one was menstruating, and also that she should not "look on dead."

No one told her about sex either but she knows that one should not have

sex during menstruation nor up to 8 days afterwards although it is permissible
before the period. As long as a woman "go 'gainst a man" she is likely to get
pregnant, and when she does, "is the time come." She actually preferred
being pregnant to menstruating as she felt no difference and was never sick
but "me no have to menstruate!"

She says it is not every woman who can "birth a child," but if it is possible
every man and woman should have one as he or she may be able "to come up
and help" the mother. "I know if I never have a child I would be sorry."
Nevertheless she continues, "I have to work for myself." She buys "little oil
and two coconut and come and sell it so I can buy any little thing for myself."
One daughter helps her with "a $2 or $3 when she works" but "the balance of
children, they don't know if I eat or if I drink" so philosophically she accepts
that some women have children who help them very much while others do
not get any help from theirs. Despite this, she says she does not love any of
her children more than the other and anything she has she will give to any of
them who need it. Although she does not sound bitter she concludes, "If you
don't have none, it would have even much better, because your energy
wouldn't work out."

Margaret cannot say anything about a childless woman as "is not every
fruit tree that bear . . . that is the Lord affair." Hence it is foolishness to call a
woman a mule. In her case she "never go look for them, get them, never sorry
still." There are some women, she states, who do not want children until they
are ready and when they are ready they cannot have any, while some want
children and do not get them because the Lord says they must not have any.
In these days a woman can control the amount of children she has by using
family planning. Margaret does not find any fault with family planning
because it helps many poor people who cannot help themselves but "children
is borning plenty so I don't see. It good yes, but it don't stop the pickney them
from born to that," because "children born now nuffer" as it is not every
woman taking family planning.

Margaret thinks a family of 1 child can be considered small while 1 or 2
may be large depending on how many children each of those 2 have. One of
her daughters has 7 children and another has 5, one of whom died. However,
she feels that a woman should have 9 children in her lifetime—4 boys and 5
girls. She should not have them for each of her partners, though, because "if
you are a person who runs around" and has 8 partners, by the time you are
50, you "can't have pickney for the 8 of them . . . you no will bruk down."
She tells of her daughter who has the 4 children; "out of the 4 of them there is
not one Saturday morning come, there is one father can hand one a penny
because the father of the two boys is in Kingston—not even a cent—the third
one's father is in Kingston—not even a cent—the little girl's father live nearby
but not even a cent. So suppose there were 6 of those types" or if she,
Margaret, did not help she does not know what would become of them.

Respondent 8B51

Agatha T., aged 51, is an unmarried woman with 2 children. Her mother had 12 children, and it seems as if she has always lived with one or other of her siblings, after she left the parental home. She is now living in the home of one of her older brothers who is "respectably married." The interviewer thinks that it is for this reason she was "holding back" regarding her relationships with her partners who were all in visiting unions. She has lived in the same parish all her life but has recently moved to the area in which she now resides. Agatha had 10 years of primary schooling and is now employed in a job which requires a semiskilled person.

Agatha has not had a partner for many years and although her 2 children are for different men, when asked if a woman should have a child for each of her partners, the reply was a firm "No." She thought a family of 12 children "like what my mother had" is large, while one of 4 is ideal—2 of each sex. At the same time, when discussing family planning, which she considered a good thing, she said "is quite enough" to have 2 children as the population was too large. She thought family planning would "better Jamaica as there are too many children and we have nothing to give them."

No one explained menstruation to her so she was frightened when she started at age 12, and called to one of her sisters to help her. At age 45+ she "was sick in that way and Doctor had to stop me." Her periods were regular and used to last 5 to 6 days but she had pains in her stomach and feet and had to go to bed and sleep. She does not know the causes of either menstruation or pregnancy but does not think a woman should have sex just before, during or just after menstruation. Despite her monthly pains she said she felt better when she was menstruating than when she was pregnant.

One of her sisters has no children and she feels that a woman like her is "not born to have any," while others may take something to prevent themselves having children.

Agatha has a special feeling for her first child "because she is a girl and I am a woman too and she can't stand the hardship of life as the boy." She did not "definitely want" to have her at the time. Her daughter is now an adult living away from home.

Agatha paused for a long while before admitting that she used to have sex with her first boyfriend. Her parents, who were married to each other, were alive then and they "never like to see we live that kind of life without marry." Thus he could not visit her at home and she had to hide to see him (laughter).

Her second relationship began when her sister with whom she was living "did join a church" and the man was a member of the same church. She used to go there with her sister and he would talk to her and tell her he "liked" her but she "was only talking to him then." One night, however, her sister allowed her to sleep at a friend's house and he came up there ... "and we used to talk to each other" but she never considered him "as any friend" but "him try to force himself." After that she used "to get something from him" (money) but she had to hide it from her sister, who did not like him and would not even speak to him, as she was "under my sister care." Agatha was then 24 and her boyfriend was about 5 years older. He was visiting her for a month when she got pregnant and she "never have no business with him after I got the child." Later she says the relationship ended about 3 months before she had the baby. After the baby was born, her sister told him "but up to this moment me and him don't have any argument . . . I never go where him is and I never talk to him because I heard him did have another girl." The baby was delivered in hospital by a doctor and there were no complications.

She met her third partner when she went with others on a trip to the district where he lived. He spoke to them and "him carry us to him home. I never . . . my mother and my father quarrel and said I shouldn't do them things, so for that reason, each of them, is only one time I see the man." This meeting resulted in her second pregnancy but she is a little confused about the dates, as by her calculations she could not have been 9 months pregnant when the baby came. She wrote him about it but he replied "me not to call him name." That child was born $1\frac{1}{2}$ years after the first and was delivered at home by a trained nurse and again there were no complications. She had worked for 4 months at the beginning of the pregnancy but stopped and came home when she realised that she had conceived.

Four years later she initiated a meeting with the same man again, "because I ask him friend for him and him tell me." It was just "one time, and me and him was talking again and him say him going to mind the child but after that I don't see him again." Having not kept his promise to do so, when she found herself pregnant, she realised "that him don't mean no good" and she was so "cross" with herself that she left home and without letting her mother know, she went to a doctor who aborted her in his office. She was then about 3 months pregnant. Perhaps she misunderstood the question asked, later in the interview, if she had ever heard of ways or things to get rid of a baby, because she promptly replied "No."

Agatha says all her partners had other women, and she did not consider any of her unions as "regular." She mentions a male friend she met a week ago but is vague about the relationship.

Respondent 2112

Beatrice R. is an unemployed, 46-year-old woman living in a crowded urban area. She is the head of her household of 3 children and has never been married. She moved to the parish where she now resides 24 years ago and participated in a similar study in 1971–72, at which time she was interviewed by her present interviewer. Her mother had 4 children and was not married to her father, who was a farmer. Beatrice left elementary school at age 14 in 4th Standard after spending 7 years there.

Her present partner is about 52 years old. He is a married man who lives with his wife, but the latter goes to America quite often. Although they have been friends for 3 years, Beatrice does not know his religion nor how many children his mother had but she knows his parents were married to each other and she "thinks" his father was a farmer. She reluctantly admitted the nature of his job perhaps because she did not want him identified. He visits her once or twice per week but more frequently when his wife is away. He takes her out occasionally as well, to the movies or to sports. They have sex once or twice per week at her house as she and her children live in their own home, but she never visits his home.

Her first child was for her first boyfriend. She was 19 years old and he was 26 and the friendship lasted for 2 years when they broke up because "another woman came into the picture." She was living with her mother and had no desire to set up her own home although she says they were in love with each other, and their relationship was good. After it was over he stopped supporting the child and she found things difficult economically. However she says the child played no part in either the formation or dissolving of the union. In fact none of her children has had any influence on her unions—they "just come along as a result of the unions."

Her second child was born 3½ years later for another visiting partner. He was quite a bit older than she, being 48 to her 22. That friendship lasted 3 years but we know very little about it.

Her third partnership also produced a child 5½ years after the second one. She is the only one of the children who spends any time with her father whom she visits at his home. The relationship lasted 10 years, and 5 years after the last child was born she suffered a miscarriage when she was almost 3 months pregnant.

Beatrice started menstruating at 14 and has not stopped yet. She has had an occasional irregular period but it does not happen often enough to worry her or cause her to consult a doctor. Her periods used to last for 6 to 7 days but now they last for only 4 days. She suffers from severe pains in her abdomen and legs as well as nausea and therefore she has to remain in bed for "a little bit" when she is not feeling well. "Irregardless" of these problems, Beatrice preferred menstruation to pregnancy, although she had had no complications with the latter. Her mother had explained menstruation to her before she had had her first period but her idea of the cause of it was "maybe the human body just make it come." The only taboo she had heard about menstruation was that one should not have sex while having it but she does not see anything wrong in having sex just before or just after the period.

Boys told Beatrice about sexual intercourse. She thinks a woman gets pregnant by having sex and "when the both of you discharge at the same time, and the discharge meet" but sometimes the discharge "don't reach" and then she does not conceive. She had heard that a woman can take tablets or go to the doctor and get an injection to get rid of a pregnancy. Sometimes, she says, the doctor may use instruments to induce an abortion.

When she had her third pregnancy, Beatrice was already using the foam tablets as a contraceptive and she now uses them in conjunction with her boyfriend using a condom. She thinks family planning is "a good idea if one keeps up to it and does not get sick by it and so forth ... In my days, if it was as popular as now, probably I would only have one, so I think the most you can do to keep it [the population] down, is better for both you and the children and everybody." She feels that if the population keeps on growing people will not get enough work and "children will suffer both when they are small and when they get big for nowhere to live, food is expensive ... ."

She considers having a child proof that a person is "normal" and gave this as a reason why every man and woman should have one. It also showed that "their organ are functioning right" because when that is not so a woman may be childless; "sometimes the womb is too low or tube problem or something like that."

Despite the fact that she had 3 children for 3 different partners, she did not think it right, "it doesn't look properly, but if you get it and you want to keep it, well ...." She thought 3 children the ideal number to have, however, and considered that would be a small family. She thought a large family was one with 4 or 5 children. She was aware that a woman could choose the number of children she wanted to have by using "preventatives."

Beatrice says she has continued having her partners visit her because none of them has asked her to marry him (the interviewer states that she apparently associates with married men mainly). She finds no advantage in the visiting union and would prefer to be married. She has had 4 partners that we know of because she says she has been trying "to find the right one" and she is bored and lonely when she does not have a boyfriend. These relationships were broken off for varying reasons—because of other women or because she fell in love with someone else, and of course economic considerations have played a part.

Respondent 2127

Sylvia is an unemployed, unmarried woman, aged 59 living in a suburban area. She has always lived with her parents, who were married to each other, and she attended primary school for 13 years. She had 3 children for her only partner in a visiting relationship which lasted almost 20 years. She admits that she "may have desired" to set up her own home during that time but "I didn't have the chance" while her partner, who died at age 38, "was working towards it."

Her father was a farmer and although they were not wealthy, they were not "very poverty" either and as they were "responsible" for her at that time she did not need any financial help from her partner. They had grown up together from childhood and their families "moved together." The birth of the first child when she was 18 influenced her to enter into a serious visiting relationship with him—"We were just young people, we knew each other all the time and then we actually fell in to a trap and had the child"—she adds quickly "not exactly a trap." She says it "could have been" that they were in love and goes on to state definitely that he was in love with her. She "supposes" that they both "neglected" marriage and in fact the question never came up at all. She is noncommittal about the advantages of the visiting relationship but says that marriage has disadvantages as "many marriages are not successful." The common-law union is worst of all in her opinion—"that is not in question at all."

She had 3 children for her partner, each one 8 years apart; when the interviewer commented on this spacing she said "we never live together." Sylvia saw him almost every evening but only occasionally did he stay overnight. They used to go to church together—she is a member of the Church of God, a fundamentalist religion—and sometimes they would go to a fair but there was no cinema nearby for them to attend. She says she cannot remember how often their sexual visits took place and when asked how long these visits lasted, replied "but you couldn't ask me that," but she did say that they took place at her home as it was more convenient. She enjoyed having sex with him and they were both expected to be faithful to each other.

Sylvia had her first child at age 18 and had no complications during her pregnancies. She worked around the house as usual and the first 2 children were delivered at home by a nana. She breastfed them all for about a year. Their father spent most evenings with them as he visited often, as stated before.

Sylvia had her first menses at age 13 and she stopped about age 49. She was a "bit frightened" when she saw it but until now she does not know the cause of it except that it is a natural thing "that is supposed to happen." At the beginning her periods were irregular but afterwards things settled down and they would last for 3 days and did not affect her normal activities in any way. She heard people say that one must not have a cold bath at that time.

No one ever explained sex to Sylvia either but she now knows that a woman gets pregnant by having sexual intercourse and the "germ from the male goes to the female." She is shocked to think that a woman might have sex while menstruating and perhaps having it just before may be dangerous as it might stop it coming. One could have sex just after but she "really does not know about those things." However her partner "did not attempt anything like that" during those times.

On another occasion when she was asked if a woman should have a child for each of her partners she was again shocked by this, "sounds too dreadful," as she thought many women had several partners, and one wouldn't like to know that "they have so many different families."

Sylvia thinks that 2 children in a family is a small amount but no one should have more than 6. In fact she considers 6 the ideal size—3 boys and 3 girls. She feels that if a man can support his children he should have them but every woman should have one as "it is not such a happy life" to work without seeing for whom you are working. At the same time she does not feel that she can hold any opinion about a childless woman because it may not be possible for her to have a child, the reasons for which escape her: "It's too big for me." In these modern days a woman can choose the number of children she wants through family planning but in her day she had never heard of contraceptives. Indeed she says she has never enquired into the methods used in family planning as she is "past the age." Later she said she thought it depended on the individual. If a woman is having too many children and becomes ill her doctor should advise her about it but she is against young unmarried girls "practising these things." It should be for certain people only "mainly the married ones who are having too many children." She admitted that it does help to keep down the population. She says she has never heard of any way of getting rid of a baby and even if it were discussed she would not be listening as she is "definitely against that."

Respondent 8A51

Beulah S. is an unmarried nurse aged 27, living in an urban area. Her partner for whom she had 2 children died 2 years ago and she has been single since then. Their visiting relationship started when she was 16 and he was 41. She was in love with him and he supported her financially. In the first few years of the friendship he used to carry on a business in the town where they both lived, so they met often but when she went to do her training as a nurse, he could only visit her. (The interviewer believes that they were living together but was unable to elicit this from the respondent). After that, they moved from that parish but he had to live near to his business place while she was living further away. Because the business demanded his presence at odd hours he visited her and stayed from time to time but they were not actually living together. He lived with his sister and his children by a previous union. Beulah S. did not get on well with her partner's sister and as he did not "trust to leave her [the sister] alone ... so it was a sort of complicated thing." She says if it had been possible for them to be together "at the last part" they would have done so as they "used to be together before."

She was 23 when she had her first child and sometimes she has a "little more tender feeling for that one" although she stresses that "it doesn't show." "It's a long story ... I don't know if it is because that this person and myself were so much in love that when I finally decide to have a baby, it happened that I was having a little problems, I couldn't get pregnant really, and I tried every possible way . . . I went to the doctor and he was telling me about the safe period affair and then I tried it and it worked, and I was so glad when I got pregnant, I felt so good, and when the baby was born, believe me, I was so happy and loving the man to that extent, I was happy about having a child for him, and the second one it wasn't a matter of preparing for a child, it just happened, so maybe that is why I have a little . . . " Previously she had been using "the pill" as a contraceptive.

She had no problems during the pregnancies and did not work then. The children, born 1 ½ years apart, were both delivered in hospital by a doctor. She did not breastfeed either child. Although she thinks that the best spacing is 2 to 2 ½ years between children depending on the number of children a person plans to have, she would like to have her children quickly and "finish away with it."

She has a helper with whom she leaves the children when she goes to work, and she is now the sole supporter of her family. She is not really satisfied with her helper "as you know what this helper problem is like" but the important thing, she feels, is that somebody is around who can get help from a neighbour if necessary. Her younger son suffers from tonsillitis frequently although at present he is well.

Beulah S. started menstruating at age 12 + and her periods were regular and lasted 3 days. Her grandaunt told her about it "but not intelligently" as she now knows that she did not get "all the facts." However when asked the cause of it, she said, "people were born to menstruate, I think so, and the cause of it is just like you saying why does a person breathe to live—it's just that you were born to breathe." Menstruation does not affect her normal activities and she does not believe in any of the old-time sayings such as "you must not go swimming" at that time.

When they were telling her about menstruation they mentioned sex but she read about it in books and discussed it with her schoolmates. She feels that having sex before, during, and/or after menstruation depends on the preferences of the individual. She feels that there is every likelihood that a woman will get pregnant if she has sexual intercourse without using a contraceptive or not during her safe period.

Beulah says that sometimes circumstances cause women to have children with different partners but for the child's sake as well as the mother's it is best to have them for one man, if that is possible as the woman may keep changing her partners. She believes in family planning but from what she sees around her she cannot agree that it is playing any part in the development of the country as "the people pregnant same way" as they will not practise it. She is aware that although abortion is not legalised one can go to a doctor for a D. and C. if it "mars your health or anything like that." She also mentioned a type of vacuum extraction, which is now available.

She says the cost of living is so high now that she thinks it is best not to have any children at all, and although she considers 3 a large family one has to be satisfied with what one gets. All women and men want to have a child, but whether they should is a different matter. She has heard it said that a woman should "have out her lot," but she can now choose the number of children she wants if any.

Beulah's mother, who has 7 children, is married, but not to her father, whom she did not know, as she was told he died before she was born. She "did not grow" with her mother, so she called her "Miss D" and not "Mamma" as her children call her.

Her biological knowledge is surprisingly limited in view of the fact that she is a trained nurse with 10 years of primary schooling.

Women with Four or More Partners

Respondent 6706

Mildred W. is a 52-year-old unemployed married woman who has lived in the same parish all her life and took part in a similar survey in 1971-72. Her husband, who is 57 years old, and is presently employed as a "houseman," had only 1 year of primary schooling while she had 7. They live in a rural area and are members of the Seventh Day Adventist Church. Both their fathers were cultivators and were not married to their respective mothers. Her mother, whom she called "Mummy," had 3 children while his mother had 9.

Mildred had her only child at age 19 for her first visiting partner who was 24, and although she says they loved each other, she knew he had another girlfriend and he would not give her any financial support. She had an uncomplicated, full-term pregnancy and was delivered at home by a nana. She worked until the day the baby was born and breastfed her but the child died after 1 month from an unstated cause, at which time the relationship with the gentleman ended.

Two years later she had a miscarriage when she was 6 months pregnant for her second partner, aged 23. She did not work during the pregnancy but "I just buck me toe," and she aborted 2 weeks later, before the nana could get to her home. She went back to work about 5 months after the event and was in good health at that time but since she was working in another district, "I just eventually keep away myself and it break off." This relationship, which had started 2 months after the first ended, broke up 6 months after the miscarriage.

She remained single for about 3 years, then had a third visiting partner for about a year. "He was in church and I would like to get married but he didn't so stationary with me for him have his mind on somebody else, so after when I find out that, I just take time and just leave it at that." In addition he "had no manners to his parents so quite likely it would happen to me." Apart from that her affection "was something to think about."

Mildred met her husband 5 years after that and they were married the following year. "After I decide to accept Christ, I just lay low with everything." She did not enter into a common-law union with any of her boyfriends as "I never like that one." During the year he visited her she used to see him at least twice per week and she visited his home about once per week for an hour or two as she was working. They went to church together and to picnics and other activities to do with the church as well and they would discuss the preparation for their wedding. They had sex about 3 times per week and there was never any difficulty in arranging these meetings. She has a great deal of affection for her husband and declares herself happier in marriage. They are both expected to be faithful to each other and she enjoys having sex with him.

Neither of them has any children and when asked about the death of her child who had lived for a month, she said "I was feeling happy ... the maintenance wasn't pretty so I said the child would punish and I would punish also and I would be getting older so fast." She laughed and added, "at that time but it wouldn't be now." They have legally adopted a child who is 4 + now. He was 6-months old when they took him and she was then 48 and her husband 53. The little boy has frequent colds and she takes him to the hospital often for check-ups. For this reason he has not started going to school yet. The interviewer saw her husband bathing the child and looking after him very lovingly. At the end of the questions she anxiously asked the interviewer if she thought it would be "suitable" for her to adopt another child because of her present age.

Mildred thinks a family with 2 children is small, while one with 4 is large. Nevertheless a woman ideally should have 6—3 boys and 3 girls. The reason, she says, every woman should have a child is "it makes the home happy," while for a man "the fruit of his womb is his reward." She believes a childless woman has not found "her match ... they does not find the right partner ... some never born to have ... some too fat." All the same, "she should be happy with those that have." She laughingly said that a woman could tell how many children she was going to have "by the bump at the back of your neck."

Her period started at age 15 and finished at age 49. A friend told her about menstruation before she had it but no one explained sex to her. She used to menstruate for 4 days and her activities were affected as she had to stop working for a day each month. Mildred does not know what causes menstruation which she preferred to pregnancy. She did not feel any difference between the two states: "It [pregnancy] didn't do me anything." She thinks a woman gets pregnant if she has sex immediately "after she see her menses" and without hesitation she declared that a woman should not have sex during her period and not for 5 days immediately before or after. During that time she says her husband "stay away." Mildred did not think a woman should have a child for each of her partners although "them would want you to do it but. . . . " She has heard of ways of getting rid of a pregnancy such as taking tablets but she does not know what kind one can take.

Mildred has never used any method of birth control but she says she wouldn't worry with family planning but would "keep a check on myself" by spacing her children. She had mentioned earlier that the best spacing between the first 4 children should be 3, 5 and 6 years respectively. "It is good to plan your family" and after having one "you wait off and see if you can manage that one before you have another one." She does not say what method she would use to do this. She thought it important for the development of the country as one would have "more chance to school the child the right way."

During the interview one could hear children playing nearby and Mildred was careful to see that they went outside whenever there were any intimate questions asked.

Respondent 1030

June T. is a 54-year-old married dressmaker living in a crowded metropolitan area. She was not included in a similar survey in 1971–72 as she was not then living in the parish. Her father, who was a barber, was married to her mother and June was her only child. She attended primary school for 7 years and says she does not belong to any religion. Her husband, 69, is a pump operator. The relationship which has lasted for 12 years is not going well at present. His parents were also married to each other and his mother had 6 children. He is a Baptist who has had 8 years of primary schooling. His father was an unskilled labourer.

June has had 6 pregnancies for 5 partners—her husband being the father of her last 2 children—yet she states that a woman should not have a child for each of her partners. The truth is she has had many more partners than was stated in the survey, as we shall see from the history given. She was an old primipara, having her first child at age 38. The father of that child was not her first sexual partner. She says she got pregnant many times before she started having these children but at the first signs of conception she always took "aloes and porter and blue" (presumably mixed together) in order to abort as she did not know "who to give them to." She mentioned other methods of abortion such as different kinds of bushes mixed together (in a brew) and quinine tablets. She was not really friendly with the baby's father as he had another girlfriend at that time but he used to take her to his home on Sundays for dinner and give her money when she asked for it and she got pregnant for him. She breastfed the baby for 6 months.

A year later she had her second child for another partner. She suffered from low blood pressure after the birth and breastfed that child for only 2 months.

Eleven months after, her third child for her third partner was stillborn. She was glad about this and it did not trouble her in any way. When asked if she considered replacing the child, she replied, "and me not mad!"

However, only 11 months after the stillbirth she delivered a third son for a fourth visiting partner. Again her blood pressure dropped after the birth but she breastfed the child for 7 months. This man would not support the child and left her and married another woman. June says, "No man don't want me for long. A so it go when you born poor."

Her husband then appeared on the scene. He liked her and said "him sorry how me batter, but every hoe have him stick a bush, so him and me marry." In fact she had her fourth son for him in the visiting union and got married before she had her only daughter. Both these children were breastfed for 2½ months and again she suffered from low blood pressure after the birth of the penultimate child. All her deliveries took place in hospital where she was attended by trained nurses and a doctor for the stillbirth. June has not worked during her pregnancies nor has she used any contraceptives. She said family planning was good, however, and important for the development of the country as it kept down the birth of the criminals and "we get more food."

All the children live at home and are supported by her husband. The fathers who have all visited her for less than a year have not accepted responsibility for the children: "Well like a tell you them only see me pregnant and say is not them for me did have other men." She states that she does not "love" any of them and "all them questions" referring to her assessment of her partners and union types "not for me or the children." The children played no part in establishing or dissolving the unions and, in fact, her opinion of a childless woman is that she is lucky not to have any trouble. However she does not know the reasons for childlessness nor does she think that a woman has any choice in the number of children she can have. June does not believe that every man or woman should have a child but she has heard it said that every woman should have a certain number of children and the number can be known by the "knots on the cord" at childbirth. She says a family of 2 children can be considered small while one with 6 is large. Her ideal number of children in a family is 4—2 boys and 2 girls, and the best spacing is 3 years between the first and second, then 2 and 1 years respectively between the third and fourth. The actual spacing between her children is little more than a year in 1 case and less than that in 2.

No one had explained menstruation to her so she was frightened when she saw her first period at age 12. She is still menstruating and her periods are regular and last for 5 days. They do not affect her normal activities as she has no problems with them, nor does she have any beliefs or superstitions associated with menstruation. June does not know the cause of menstruation but she certainly prefers it to being pregnant as she considers it less of a problem and "you don't have to fret" when you are not pregnant. She does not see any reason why a woman cannot have sexual intercourse before and after menstruation and when asked about sexual relations during menstruation she replied: "I do." She does know a woman gets pregnant by having sex but she does not know why at some times and not at others.

June says neither her partner nor herself is expected to be faithful to each other and she does not enjoy having sex with him and does not know how often this happens anyway. They have never discussed the question of having children. She has no favourites among her children, who all call her "Mamma" just as she called her mother.

Multiple Pregnancy Wastage

Respondent 8C77

Mathilda M., 51 is a married woman who has lived all her life in the same parish, which is situated in the center of the island and is predominantly agricultural. She is a domestic worker who is employed at present and her husband, who is a year younger than she, is a farmer who cultivates half an acre of land for himself. They both had 8 years of primary schooling and belong to the Moravian Church. Neither of their parents was married to each other and their respective fathers were farmers. Her mother had 8 children and his had 4. Apparently she called her mother "Sister Gertie" as "I don't grow with her" and she used to hear her grandaunt call her that.

Her 5 pregnancies have all ended in disaster. The first child died at 1 month and the second, 3 weeks after birth. This was followed by a stillbirth while the fourth miscarried at 2 months. The last baby died at the age of 3 weeks. She could only remember the names of the first and last children but as may be expected she is very confused with her dates and their ages. We are unable to elicit any information which would account for this tragedy, apart from the last child who was premature. Mathilda says, "Until now me wrecked .... When I lose the first two child, I never have that sense to know what is children ... I never have no sense at all because I have them in me young days and I didn't have nobody to explain to me and tell me what is children, but from I lose the three last ones, I can't come to until now, especially the last one." It made her ill "because it made me sort of off me head to know that I have 5 of them and the 5 of them just gone back. When I have the last one I can quite remember ... people have to stay here just to keep me company to just hender me, to see if me can forget it." Her husband was not as affected as she and he took the death "quite good." He went out and he got people to "come and dig grave, make box and everything and get minister to bury it." She considered replacing the children, "all the while I never forget."

She was 9 months pregnant with the first 2 children who were delivered at home, while the stillbirth and the premature baby were delivered in hospital. The miscarriage was taken care of at home. She had no complications except with the last delivery and she was attended by trained nurses. Her blood pressure was high and she had pains during the last pregnancy as well as prolonged labour at birth, going into the hospital from the Tuesday and not delivering until Friday. She was unable to breastfeed this child due to its prematurity. During the pregnancies she did not "work out" but used to "beat oil" at home.

She says the first child was born in 1950 when she would have been 26, but her history indicates that she was much younger. Her grandmother sent her to another district to get her cousin's clothes to wash and when she was coming back, it was night and the young man, whom she said was about 16, led her through a shortcut. She did not want to go but he forced her to do so: "not to say he was me partner . . . . I quite remember say a then is rist him rist [raped] me." However he "didn't own" the child.

Mathilda and her first genuine partner were "together a long time." They used to see each other often as they went to another district together frequently. They liked each other but her grandmother, who reared her, was alive and did not like "the living together" and besides "he was not steady enough" for any other kind of union, but as a visiting friend. He was the father of her second child.

She knew her husband for 10 years before they got married 7 years ago. He visited her for about 7 years and then they lived together in the common-law union for 3 years. In the visiting relationship he used to visit her at her home about twice per week for an hour, but he did not take her out to any form of entertainment. They had sex about twice per week at his home "because the old people didn't like it" at her home. There was no difficulty in arranging these meetings, which lasted for about half an hour. In all they spent about 4 hours per week together and she felt lonely when he was not around.

She got married to him "because we love one another, and we treat one another good, and we never have no quarrel . . . none at all." In reality the thing that precipitated their decision was that the members of their church came and "talk to us and tell me that that life do not suit, so it is best for us to get married." She eventually gave him an ultimatum: "I only get up one day and tell him that if he don't decide to marry, I will have to leave him and live to myself because the life don't suit me." After that, "We decide our mind, just to live a good life."

They are both expected to be faithful to each other but he is "not so faithful," Mathilda says. However she enjoys having sex with him, which is about twice per month now. They did not discuss the question of having children until after the last one died. She had always felt better when she was pregnant because of the hope that she "would live to have one."

Mathilda has never used any method of birth control and she "don't agree with the family planning ... the Lord limit you ... Him know how many children you are to have and I feel to say that taking this family planning and don't have out your lot, it must sick you." In fact she has heard a lot of people complain that "it sick them." She agreed that it would help the development of the country and it is good for Jamaica "but me no like it." Personally she thought it would be better to have a certain number of children then stop for a while "definitely know say that after a time I can be able to have the balance of children," but too many children are born now without a father and "everything just leave on the Government. The Government have it too hard."

She thinks every man and woman should have a child because if her first or second child were alive "they could able to help me now." She says it is "very hard" not to have any children because "just like myself here now, I am here right now and I don't have anybody to give me anything. Me husband not working that amount and I know—me husband not working more than $2 a day—and I know ... if I did have 2 or 3 children out there which would able to help me, things would be more better off." She feels that some women "just don't born to have any children."

In her opinion 2 children constitute a small family while a large one has 12 children. She thinks 4 is an ideal number however—2 boys and 2 girls, and the best spacing between them is 4 years so that "one can help the other." The only way a woman can choose how many children to have is by discussing it with her husband as the choice cannot be hers alone. She does not believe that a woman should have a child for each of her partners.

Mathilda does not know what causes menstruation but she prefers it to being pregnant as she found it less of a problem. No one explained it to her but she was not frightened when she saw her first period at age 17. It was regular and lasted from 3 to 5 days and although she used to "have a lot of pain" in her abdomen, her normal activities were not affected in any way. At the same time she stated that during that time one is not supposed to cook or work and "don't suppose to have sex with no man." She also said that one should not have sex before the period but it was all right to have it immediately after. Her husband did "nothing" during that time. Her menstruation stopped at age 49 when she had an operation for a growth. Nothing about sex was explained to her either but she knows that a woman gets pregnant when she has sex with a man and "the both of them blood hot." She says she has never heard of any methods of abortion.

It seemed sometimes that this lady did not quite understand some of the questions and would answer the interviewer with "yes, nurse" and "no, nurse" without any real meaning. She had not been asked to participate in a similar study conducted in 1971–72.

Large Families

Respondent 4505

Doreen H. is a 55-year-old unemployed married woman who has been separated from her husband for 9 years and seems to have had no partner since. We have no personal data on her husband apart from the fact that he is now 82 years old. Doreen has lived in the same parish for 48 years and did not attend primary school, yet she answers alertly and often volunteers information beyond the scope of the questions asked. Her mother had 9 children and was not married to her father, who was a carpenter. She belongs to the Zion Church, which is a revivalist group, who are against both visiting and common-law unions: "It couldn't work that way, serving God and still living sweetheart life."

She complained that she was "mash up" due to "blood pressure" and "can't retain nothing in my brain again." She found it difficult to give the birth dates and ages of the children without their "age paper" but with some coaxing the interviewer was able to get a comprehensive history from her.

She had 15 pregnancies, 4 of which were miscarriages including male twins, and one child died when she was 6 months old, leaving her with 4 daughters. She had her children very easily, "sometimes just as I cry out I had the baby .... I never go to the hospital with one, because as I feel the pain, if I outside, I just go in'a house and me have me baby." Hence they were all delivered by a nana, and Doreen worked throughout the pregnancies and immediately after delivery was back at work. As an illustration of her good health during her pregnancies she told of an incident when she was having her sixth child: "I climb a breadfruit tree with Agnes—today is Saturday and Tuesday morning I had Agnes." With the last child, however, she was very sick—vomiting during the entire pregnancy and having to see a doctor every week. Just before that, 3 of her 4 miscarriages had taken place, each a year apart. The last child was small and used to choke on the breast so she stopped breastfeeding him immediately but the others were breastfed for 8 to 9 months and the one who died at 6 months was breastfed up to that time. She still sounds most distressed when discussing the latter—her eleventh pregnancy. She sighed, "I did feel it you see." She took him to the doctor who said it was "the water from the teething turn down." After a time she consoled herself that "the Lord give and the Lord take" and when her husband saw her crying he said, "Well Mamma, all you have to do is cry and done, because it's God who do the work." Her neighbours and family were a great source of strength for her.

Doreen has obviously always liked older men, as she was 20 when she had her first child for her common-law partner aged 48. He visited her for about 6 months, until she got pregnant and they started living together as it was hard for him to pay rent for two separate places. She loved him but there were other pressing reasons for her to take up this friendship. She had no parents and she was not working regularly, "only doing a little clothes washing . . . . I couldn't stay hungry, I couldn't walk naked and I want somebody help me, if I sick to take care of me." She didn't like the type of union they were in but by the time her first child was 9 months old, she was 4 months pregnant with twins, which she miscarried when her common-law partner "took sick and died" suddenly. They had been planning to get married, she says, smiling nostalgically. Later, she said that she loved him best of her three partners.

Her second relationship, which lasted about 18 months, was with a visiting partner aged 50. She was then 22, and it began just 3 months after the death of her first partner. They "broke off" shortly after the baby was born because she became interested in her third partner, also aged 50 then, whom she later married. They had had no quarrel whatsoever, she says, but she wrote him a letter saying "everything is closed." She speaks of him with affection, however, and says he still looks after his child very well.

Before they got married, her husband used to visit her about 3 times per week while she would go to his house twice a week and clean it out and tidy it. She hardly ever went out to any entertainment with him but when she was not working she would ask him for some financial assistance to help her to go to market etc. Remarking on how a man changes, for better or worse, in a friendship, she says, "Man a green lizard," meaning they change to suit themselves. Doreen married him when she was about to have his fifth child — as she puts it "with Vincent's stomach," Vincent being her eighth child. She liked being married at the start, "but he is not going on well with me. Tell me lots of bad words and I just can't take it. That's why I leave." He gives her no support at all now and none for the last child who is only 11. The child should have been at school the day this interview took place but she had no lunch money or bus fare to give him. The only help she gets is from her older sons. She had to take the second youngest son out of school early as she could not afford to keep on sending him there. He is now with a cousin learning to be a mechanic—"the boy love trade."

Doreen thinks that a family of 6 or more children can be considered large but she says 6 to 8 is a good number for a woman to have—3 boys and the rest girls. She and her husband preferred having girls, but she has 6 boys and 4 girls alive. Every man and woman "who are born to have" should have a child, as a childless woman has no one to do anything for her and she is "in need of company." She has heard it said that every woman should have a certain number of children but she knows that this is impossible as "who knows God work?" If they plan their families now a woman can choose how many children she wants but this was not available to her when she was having children. In fact she does not sound too enthusiastic about family planning even now as she says it is "all right" for some of the people and it is important for "who it helps." On the average her children are spaced 2 years apart but she thought the best spacing was 5 years.

Doreen had her first period when she was 14 and was 54 years old when she stopped. Her periods were regular and lasted 4 days. Before she started having children, she used to have pains, but they were not bad and she did not go to a doctor. Her mother had told her to expect menstruation before it came but the only reason she can give for it is that it is "ordained." She also has no idea how a woman gets pregnant or why only at certain times. She does say, however, that she prefers menstruating to being pregnant. She does not think it "wise" to have sex before her period, and certainly not during it, but she says that after the period is "even worse." Her partner used to "keep himself quiet" during that time as he was always sorry for her.

She has only contempt for the "foolish gal them, that throw way belly," but she does not know what they use to abort.

With all the disadvantages, Doreen prefers marriage to the other types of unions. She says if you are living a "bad life," however, you will fret regardless of the union.

Statistical summary of pregnancy history

Events		Age	Years	Percentages
Age at menarche		14		
Age at menopause		54		
Biological years of potential childbearing	(a)		40	
Age at termination of 1st pregnancy		20		
Age at termination of last pregnancy		44		
Actual years of childbearing	(b)		24	
Years spent in pregnancy	(c)		9	
Years spent in breastfeeding	(d)		7.1	
(c) + (d)	(e)		16.1	
Rest of period			7.9	

Statistical summary of pregnancy history

Events	Age Years	Percentages
Total pregnancies	15	
(b) as % (a)		60.0
(c) as % (b)		37.5
(d) as % (b)		30.0
(e) as % (b)		67.1
Average number of years per pregnancy 1.6		
(actual years)/(number of pregnancies)		

Respondent 7967

Anita is a 41-year-old married woman who lives in a rural, agricultural area which is backward in many respects—education, housing, etc. She has always lived in that parish. She has had 6 years of primary schooling but her husband, who is 44, has had none. Her parents were married to each other and her mother had 12 children while his mother, who was not married to his father, had 4 children. She is not at present employed but when she works she plaits straw—an occupation which many of the people in the area do, and in which she was employed throughout her pregnancies. Her husband, like both their fathers, is a farmer and cultivates half an acre of land for himself. They both belong to the Anglican Church.

Anita has had only one partner. While he was visiting her she had her first child; 6 more were born in the common-law union and the last 3 since they have been married. The fifth, ninth and tenth are females who are alive and well. She cannot remember any of the dates connected with the changes in her types of union, apart from the year the friendship started, which was 1955, and although she was able to give the years the children were born, she was unable to remember the months for 4 of them. They were all delivered at home by a nana and there were no complications during the pregnancies, at deliveries or after deliveries apart from one which was premature. Anita slipped and fell when she was 6 months pregnant with her sixth child and the baby, born prematurely, lived for only 1 day. The seventh child—male—was born with a hole in the heart. He was hospitalised for most of his short life and died recently at 4 years old. She was very sad at the death of this child and it caused her to have headaches. They had always been a close family and they took it badly but they were able to support each other in this tragedy. Her husband, being stronger than she, did not break down and although she was the same to him, she had no desire to have sex for a long time. However she did not feel in any way responsible for the child's death and did not consider replacing him. The sympathy of the people around made her feel closer to them too.

All the other children are healthy and they were all breastfed for 9 months. The mother gives the 3 youngest children, who are just a year apart in age and not yet going to school, an adequate diet of eggs, milk, butter, vegetables and meat.

She fell in love with her partner J. and because of "nature"—desire for sex—she wanted to start life with him. They were young and had no money or home of their own, so they continued to live with their respective parents, who liked the match. They felt restricted by this type of relationship but they did not live together at that time as they just simply could not afford it.

After the birth of the first child, J. got his own home and she went to live with him. He really wanted to "father" his children and she found that people "took them more seriously" when they lived as man and wife, even though it was in the common-law union. Their relatives approved of this step and in any case her parents' home was becoming too crowded.

About a year after the seventh child was born—and perhaps because of his illness—they both decided that they wanted the children to be "lawful" and there would be more security for the family if her partner died while they were married. In addition they wanted to end the "sweetheart life" and their parents encouraged them to get married. Again they had waited to take this step when they felt they could "afford it."

While they were in the visiting relationship they visited each other's homes daily. They went to sports, fairs, weddings and wakes together—"mostly respectable functions" as often as they took place in the village. They used to spend long periods discussing their future and ways of making enough money to get married when he visited her at her house and that is where they had sex too, about once every 3 weeks. Although she was living with her parents they had no problem in arranging this. Through the years they have been faithful to each other and she enjoys having sex with J. once or twice per month now.

Anita does not think that every man or woman should have a child because "some do not care them." Although this woman was devoted to her family she expressed the opinion that she was sorry for a woman who had no children in some ways, but in others she was lucky as she had no ties or problems and was free. She was probably "not born to have children" or sometimes the couple's blood "don't correspond."

Anita says she will not practise family planning now as she thinks she has stopped childbearing; yet her last child is just a year old and she is still menstruating. Also she thought a woman who had no children for 3 to 4 years would have no more, yet there is a difference of 3 years and 8 months between her second and third children and 4 years and 7 months between her third and fourth children. In fact her idea of the best spacing between the first and second children is 6 years; 9 years between the second and third and 5 years between the third and fourth. Family planning is good for youngsters, she says, as there are too many unwanted children born. She was "unlucky" not to have had it available as she wanted only 2 children—her ideal family being 1 boy and 1 girl. She feels that having fewer children will help in the development of the country as "you can help yourself better." She has heard the expression that a woman should "have out her lot" and that the nana can tell how many you are going to have, but she knows the nana guesses because the one who delivered her told her she would only have 1 more after the sixth child and she has since had 4. She considers that any number of children over 3 makes up a large family.

Anita had her first menses at 16 and was frightened when she saw it as no one had explained menstruation or sex to her. Her periods are regular but last 6 days and the flow is heavy when she works hard. She has no idea what is the cause of menstruation and although she does not believe this entirely, she has been told never to look at the dead at that time as "they say you will never stop bleeding"—a fairly widespread superstition in the country. She thinks a woman can ·have sex immediately before menstruation but not during the time nor up to 2 weeks after. During this time she does not sleep with her husband as they still have the desire for sex but are unable to have it.

Obviously pregnancy is no trouble to her as she feels well and cannot complain "of any bad feelings." Still she prefers to menstruate and finds that even less of a problem than pregnancy. She knows that a woman gets pregnant through having sexual intercourse and the "seed from the man develops" but does not know how or why at some times and not at others. When asked about methods of abortion, she admitted hearing of boiling some kind of bush but stated she had "no idea of those things" and she "never deal in that kind of life."

This lady seemed happy with her partner of 19 years in the 3 types of unions but is most contented in marriage.

Statistical summary of pregnancy history

Events		Age	Years	Percentages
Age at menarche		16		
Age at menopause (still menstruating)		41		
Biological years of potential childbearing	(a)		25	
Age at termination of 1st pregnancy		24		
Age at termination of last pregnancy		41		
Actual years of childbearing	(b)		17	
Years spent in pregnancy	(c)		7.3	
Years spent in breastfeeding	(d)		6.7	
(c) + (d)	(e)		14.0	
Rest of period			3.0	

Statistical summary of pregnancy history

Events	Age	Years	Percentages
Total pregnancies	10		
(b) as % (a)			68.0
(c) as % (b)			42.6
(d) as % (b)			39.7
(e) as % (b)			82.4

Average number of years per pregnancy 1.7
(actual years)/(number of pregnancies)

Respondent 8B82

Gladys M. is a 60-year-old married woman living with her 64-year-old husband in a rural agricultural district. They are still both active—he farms one acre of land for himself and she is at present employed as a worker on a farm. Their fathers were also farmers and were not married to their respective mothers. His mother had 5 children while hers had double that amount—10. She sounds like an outgoing person and it is not apparent in her conversation that she has had only 2 years of primary schooling while her husband was fortunate enough to have had 8. They belong to the Apostolic Church—a fundamentalist religion.

She has had 15 pregnancies of which 4 were miscarriages, 1 a stillbirth and 1 died at 4-months old. Despite a 21-year childbearing span, she states definitely that she feels better when she is not pregnant; and although she has had pregnancies for each of her 3 partners, she says that a woman should not have a child for each of her partners. Another contradiction that exists between her opinions and her life style is in the spacing of the children: she says that 3 to 5 years is best but with only 1 of hers did she have as much as 2½ years difference.

Gladys had her first child when she was 19 years old for a boyfriend she had known for 2 years. He came to the district and they used to work together picking pimento—"I really did like him," but even before the baby came she found "faults" in him, "yet still I have the baby for him. He was a nice looking fellow you know." Sounding nostalgic she says she loved him most of her three partners.

A year later she was in another visiting relationship with a man 29 years older than she. It lasted 2 years and she broke off with him because she had 2 miscarriages, each at 5 months, one after the other, and she "couldn't stand it." She states categorically that he was to blame because "must be something was wrong with him" as she had had no problem with her first child. She was "sick unto the point of death." In retrospect she says she didn't like him at all.

She met her present partner when she went to look for a friend one Sunday and he "start to put up him chats." She never told him "yes" right away but came home and told her parents who later said they would "accept" him. Laughing, Gladys says "him too bad—me did sort of like him." She refers to him always by his surname, sometimes preceding it by Mr. They were friendly for about 6 months before they "knew each other" (had sex) as she "sort of get me 'fraid about that." They seemed to have had sex infrequently until after she had his first child and the relationship was established. However she rates him as her best sexual partner.

Soon after that child was born, they got married—a union which has continued for 27 years. Unfortunately, the baby died when he was 4 months old from an unstated cause. She was very sad about it and she cried a lot but she did not feel any responsibility for his death. The father took it "all right" and although it did not affect their lives deeply she "missed the baby."

All her babies were delivered at home by a nana, but she did see a doctor when she had 3 of the miscarriages. They were breastfed for 9 months, and the child who died at 4 months was breastfed also to the time of his death. She had no problems with her pregnancies, did not use any contraceptives and did not work during any of them. At first she used to have favourites among the children "but not any more." They call her either "Mamma" or "Sister G." as they have heard the villagers call her, while she called her mother the more old fashioned "Mammie."

Gladys feels that a family is small with only 4 children in it, but in these days 8 children constitute a large family—"it's not like my days." Indeed she thinks a woman should have about 8—4 of each sex. She had 6 boys and 4 girls. She knows that it is not every man or woman that is able to have a child, but she feels that those who can should have one or more. She "doesn't carry no feeling against" the childless woman as "she might not be born to have one—the Bible speaks about women like that" but she knows that there are some women who prevent themselves having children.

She did not start menstruating until she was 17, and she stopped when she was 50 years old. When she saw her first menses, she hid it from her mother as she did not know what it was and no one had explained menstruation or sex to her. Her periods were regular and lasted about 7 days with no accompanying problems. All she knows about menstruation is that one should not have sex after one has started or you run the risk of having a baby, but she does not know the cause of it. She knows that a woman gets pregnant by having intercourse and that conception depends on the menstrual cycle but she does not seem too clear about her fertile or safe periods. She is very vague about family planning and says she is "not with it or against it." She believes that a woman should not have sexual intercourse just before, during or up to 9 days after menstruation and she says her partner did not have sex with her during that time.

Gladys says that in marriage you live a better life and you are "stationed one place now" but there are many disadvantages as well because "some of the man dem beat the woman; some of the woman dem bad" and the partners are often unfaithful to each other. "It have plenty failure in it." She realises that the other types of unions have their problems too but she laughingly says that in the visiting union, "you are free to do as you like no disadvantage is in that one." Nevertheless she declares that marriage has brought her the most happiness.

She was not approached to take part in a similar study in 1971–72.

Statistical summary of pregnancy history

Events		Age	Years	Percentages
Age at menarche		17		
Age at menopause		50		
Biological years of potential childbearing	(a)		33	
Age at termination of 1st pregnancy		19		
Age at termination of last pregnancy		40		
Actual years of childbearing	(b)		21	
Years spent in pregnancy	(c)		9.4	
Years spent in breastfeeding	(d)		7.1	
(c) + (d)	(e)		16.5	
Rest of period			4.5	
Total pregnancies		15		
(b) as % (a)				63.6
(c) as % (b)				44.8
(d) as % (b)				33.8
(e) as % (b)				78.6

Average number of years per pregnancy 1.4
(actual years)/(number of pregnancies)

Respondent 7915

Alison B. is a 42-year-old woman living in a common-law union with her 36-year-old partner. They live in a rural agricultural area and she is employed in plaiting straw, while he is a farmer who cultivates 2 acres of land for himself. Her father, also a farmer, was not married to her mother who had 5 children and died before Alison "knew" her. Her partner's mother had 7 children and was also not married to his father. Alison and her common-law "husband" both had 9 years of primary schooling and they belong to the Moravian Church. She has been in the same parish all her life but did not take part in a similar study conducted in 1971–72.

She has 10 children who are all alive and well. Her pregnancies were normal and she worked throughout them. The babies were delivered at home by a trained nurse with the exception of the fifth and sixth who were delivered by a nana. She breastfed each child for a year and has never used any contraceptives. Her last child is less than a year old.

Alison was 19 when she had her first child for a partner a year younger than she. She was living alone at that time and he came to live with her and helped her financially. She would have liked to marry him "but him did have someone else" so marriage was out of the question. She got pregnant for him shortly after the friendship started. The same year that the baby was born, he left for England and never wrote her or sent anything for the baby after that.

Because she had the young baby and no one to help her, she became friendly with another man who was her neighbour, about a year later. He lived with his mother so he only visited her about once or twice per week. She says that neither of them wanted to live together. Again she became pregnant for him almost immediately although she says they had sex only about once per month. This man denied that the child was his and stopped supporting her and moved from the district so she saw him less often. Her relatives agreed that the child was not his but as her friends looked at the baby they said it was his child. He seems to have changed his mind later, however, as he gives his daughter "a little help" now and loves her and during the summer and Christmas holidays, she spends time with him. Any love Alison had for her second partner soon disappeared because of his treatment of her.

Within 9 months of having the second child, the third was born for C., her present partner, with whom she has been living for the past 17 years. She had to "look a help" as she had met with the "same disappointment" twice, and she was hoping to find security in this third relationship, so she allowed him to come and live with her. At the time she was in great financial difficulty as she had 2 babies to support and no help from the fathers. She feels that C. would give her even more support if he could as "him have the mind" but not the money. She laughingly says that she has to say that he is a good sexual partner "since I have so much children." They have both been faithful to each other and she enjoys having sex with him about twice per month. They have discussed the question of having children and decided that they do not want any more. However she has never used any method of family planning and although she says some people have tried it and said it is good, she cannot give any personal opinion of it. She has never heard it said that every woman should have a certain number of children.

Alison does not think that every woman should have a child because "not every woman come in the world to have a child"; some may be sick with such things as having "a growth in the womb." A woman cannot choose how many children she is going to have either. She thinks the best spacing between children is 5 years, although only 1 of hers has been as much as $4\frac{1}{2}$ years apart and 2 have been as close as 9 and 11 months respectively. She thinks that a family can be considered small with only 1 child, while a large one has 12 children. Her ideal family size is 3—1 boy and 2 girls. Her own family consists of 2 boys and 8 girls. They sometimes call her "Mamma" and sometimes "Alison," as they hear other people call her by her Christian name.

Her friends told her about sex but when she had her first period at 16 she was frightened as no one had explained it to her. She still does not know what causes menstruation but she prefers it to being pregnant. Her periods are irregular and she worries about it sometimes but she has never consulted a doctor. The period lasts for 3 days and she has no problems with it, although she complains of a "funny feeling" in her "belly." During that time she does not bathe in cold water, or go swimming, nor can she straighten her hair, or look at the dead.

She thinks a woman can have sex immediately before menstruation, but not during the period or for a few days after it is finished. She knows that a woman gets pregnant by having sex and "an egg leaves from the man to you" but she is not sure that it is only at certain times "that egg comes down or if it is all the time." She has heard that there are certain things one can do to get rid of a baby but does not know what those things are.

Alison thinks the common-law union is better for the children than to have someone visiting, but she says that "the church and the people around have more respect for you when you are married."

Statistical summary of pregnancy history

Events		Age	Years	Percentages
Age at menarche		16		
Age at menopause (still menstruating)		42		
Biological years of potential childbearing	(a)		26	
Age at termination of 1st pregnancy		24		
Age at termination of last pregnancy		42		
Actual years of childbearing	(b)		18	
Years spent in pregnancy	(c)		7.5	
Years spent in breastfeeding	(d)		10.0	
(c) + (d)	(e)		17.5	
Rest of period			0.5	
Total pregnancies		10		
(b) as % (a)				69.2
(c) as % (b)				41.7
(d) as % (b)				55.6
(e) as % (b)				97.2

Average number of years per pregnancy 1.7
(actual years)/(number of pregnancies)

Respondent 6759

Eunice R. is a 57-year-old unemployed woman with 8 years of primary school education. She is an Anglican whose parents were not married to each other, and in fact she never knew her father. Her mother had 3 children while she has had 11 with 5 different partners but at present has no partner. She prefers visiting unions because she doesn't like living with men as she feels they are not worth living with. She did not participate in a similar study in 1971–72 as she was not in the area, although she has lived all her life in the same parish.

Her first union was with L. "He was a nice guy and we loved each other." The union started in 1937 and ended in 1940. Their first and only child was born in September 1938. Although he was giving her financial assistance during the pregnancy, he stopped when the child was born. The birth of this child played no part in her entering into the union, it did not affect her sexual relations with her partner, but did play a part in breaking up the relationship, as he did not want to support the child.

Her second union was with D. and started while she was still seeing L. in 1939. D. would come every day to her house and stay 2 to 3 hours. She occasionally went to his residence but preferred staying at home. They had 3 children together. Eunice was reluctant to discuss her sexual visits. She could not estimate how long they took but there seemed to be no trouble in arranging them. During these visits they would also discuss children, marriage and other plans including getting a house. She estimated that they spent about 28 hours together a week and she did not feel lonely when he was not there. "No sir, I don't feel lonely at all." She did expect her partners to be faithful to her, but "they are not." The union with D. came to an end in 1950 when he died of a stab wound.

Eunice's next 3 unions were very casual. She does not remember the details of them and was not anxious to talk about them. They seem to have brought her no happiness and she summarises her life with her partners in the following way: "The first man didn't treat me good after having the first child. I took a second one and he die. You want some help and I get a next man and he wasn't any good, and none of them were any good. All were the same. It was bad luck for me."

Eunice feels 4 children are a small family and 11 a large one. She feels that every man and woman should have a child but "not too much." She has no feeling about how many children one should have except that now with the price of food so high, you should have fewer children than in the old days when things were cheaper. "The cost of living is so high today you can't manoeuvre." She has no special opinion about women who have had no children and thinks that the cause of childlessness is that "you don't meet good partner, man and woman don't blend. Sometimes you are with a book for years and as you go to the paper you have a child."

Eunice had 8 pregnancies and, of these, 3 consecutive conceptions resulted in live born twins. Two of these twins were for her third partner and one for her fourth. One child of the third set of twins died at one year of age. The pregnancies were normal and there were no complications at or after birth. Except for the first set of twins who were born in the hospital the other children were born at home and delivered by a nurse or nana. Eunice likes all her children but "me have a special love for the second boy." "He's genuine and nice." Her children call her Miss Gerty because everyone else calls her that. At present only 2 children live with her as the others are grown up. She "felt no way" about the child who died. The death doesn't seem to have caused her any physical or mental anguish and she did not feel guilty about it. The other children were not affected by it and "it didn't matter" to the father either.

In assessing her partners, her second partner D. was the one who seemed to be most responsive and satisfactory from the point of view of financial support and affection. It was also the union that lasted the longest. She says of him, "he gave me money but I had to bring them up." The other partners did not give her financial help for the children. She took no part in her partners' achievements and was very categoric on this point. All her partners except D. caused her a great deal of "despair."

Nobody explained sex or menstruation to Eunice. Her menses started at 17 and ended at 40. Her periods were regular and lasted 5 to 6 days. She believes one shouldn't ha\ sex just before, during or after menstruation. When she has her period she "has no business with men." Asked whether she preferred to menstruate or to be pregnant she replied, "me no like none of them." She doesn't know what causes menstruation and finds it less of a problem than pregnancy. She does not know how a woman gets pregnant or why she does at some times and not others. She had heard about ways of getting rid of a baby but was reluctant to say what they were. When pressed on the subject she said she heard of tablets, quinine tablets and "all kinds of different things but me don't remember now."

She doesn't know anything about family planning. When asked how she felt about it she replied, rather logically, that she can't have a feeling about it since she doesn't understand it. It didn't help her so it doesn't interest her.

Statistical summary of pregnancy history

Events		Age	Years	Percentages
Age at menarche		17		
Age at menopause		40		
Biological years of potential childbearing	(a)		23	
Age at termination of 1st pregnancy		20		
Age at termination of last pregnancy		42		

Statistical summary of pregnancy history

Events		Age	Years	Percentages
Actual years of childbearing	(b)		22	
Years spent in pregnancy	(c)		6.0	
Years spent in breastfeeding	(d)		4.4	
(c) + (d)	(e)		10.4	
Rest of period			11.6	
Total pregnancies	8			
(b) as % (a)				95.6
(c) as % (b)				27.3
(d) as % (b)				20.0
(e) as % (b)				47.3

Average number of years per pregnancy 2.8
(actual years)/(number of pregnancies)

Respondent 4513

Jane C. is a 48-year-old woman who had 7 years of primary schooling. She is a Baptist and is presently unemployed. Her father was a farmer and was married to her mother who had 8 children.

Jane married 37-year-old I. in August 1945 at the age of 19, having had no sexual union before her marriage. She was eager to get married, though she never considered the advantages of this type of union as opposed to another and married I. because "I like him, he was loving and kind." She states that they are both expected to be faithful to each other.

Both she and her husband were eager to have a child and their first one was born in July 1949 after a normal pregnancy but died at a young age because he "had water in the head." She describes her reaction to this death of the child as "dismay" and the father's as "disappointment." Both were eager to replace this child.

Her other 9 children were all born at home and delivered by a nana, except for her last one delivered by a nurse. She had no complications or difficulties with her pregnancies except with her last child born in September 1965, when she was 39. During this pregnancy she had "daily illness and low feeling." The first child was breastfed for 8 months and all the others for 9. The children are all healthy and she states that she loves them all equally. Those who are older do not live at home but visit her frequently. At no time during the interview did she indicate that there was any hardship in having 10 children nor did she have any complaints about the children.

The fifth child was born in July 1957. I. had migrated to England in order to improve life for his family. But as she did not hear from him she lost interest in the marriage and started a visiting union with S.

The meetings with S. took place in her house about every 2 days. There seem to have been no difficulties in arranging these visits and though Jane admitted to enjoying sex with S. she was not able to estimate how often and for how long these sexual visits took place. During S.'s visits they discussed business matters whenever possible and "for as long as was necessary." These visits seem to have been pleasant occasions not only for her but also for the children. Two children were born of this union, one in March 1958 and the other in August 1959.

When I. returned from England in January 1961, Jane went back to him as she had the children's interest at heart and according to her it is better to have the children's father living in. She had 3 more children with I. born in October 1961, December 1963 and September 1965. She enjoys having sex with him but cannot estimate the number of occasions.

When asked to make an assessment of her 2 unions and compare her partners as regards affection, support of children etc., it was difficult to obtain clear answers, as in general throughout the interview Jane was very inarticulate. However, S. was judged to be more affectionate but both provided economically for their children. Marriage was more in keeping with her religious beliefs but when asked which union made her more respected in the community she answered "the one that stays with you."

Although she has 10 children she did not discuss the question of having children with either of her partners. Jane never used any method of birth control. She thinks every man and woman should have a child because "it is essential" and every man likes to have a child even to come in and play with. She thinks 8 is a large family and 4 is a small one, 2 girls and 2 boys, and the best spacing is 2 years between each. Jane's opinion of a woman who has no children is "it is very embarrassing" and the causes of childlessness are "medical attention needed." Jane does not know what causes menstruation, she says "it is ordained for women." She thinks a woman can have sex just before menstruation but not during or after. She does not know what her partners did during those times. She has never heard of any method of abortion.

Jane thinks that family planning is good but the methods and means of it are not good. She thinks that with fewer children born the country would have more money for roads and lighting.

Jane's mother had explained menstruation to her. Her menses started at age 14; they last 4 days and she has had no problems with them. She has no special beliefs about menstruation other than that it was ordained for women and that one should not have sex during it. She feels the ideal time for sex is just before the menses.

In answer to the question, how does a woman get pregnant, she replied through sexual intercourse but when asked why at certain times and not others she answered, "because the time came for you to get pregnant when you have sex."

Statistical summary of pregnancy history

Events		Age	Years	Percentages
Age at menarche		14		
Age at menopause (still menstruating)		48		
Biological years of potential childbearing	(a)		34	
Age at termination of 1st pregnancy		22		
Age at termination of last pregnancy		39		
Actual years of childbearing	(b)		17	
Years spent in pregnancy	(c)		7.5	
Years spent in breastfeeding	(d)		7.4	
(c) + (d)	(e)		14.9	
Rest of period			2.1	
Total pregnancies	10			
(b) as % (a)				50.0
(c) as % (b)				44.1
(d) as % (b)				43.5
(e) as % (b)				87.6

Average number of years per pregnancy 1.7
(actual years)/(number of pregnancies)

Respondent 8B83

Sheila A. is a married woman aged 45, living in a remote rural district near the center of the island. She has always lived in that parish and has had little or no schooling. Her mother, who was not married to her father, had 7 children. Although she has been with her partner for 25 years she does not know if his parents were married or how many children his mother had. He now cultivates half an acre of land following in the tradition of both their fathers who were farmers. Presumably there is little else to do in that area. He has had 5 years of primary schooling, somewhat more than she herself has enjoyed. Sheila and her husband both belong to the Apostolic Church which is one of the many fundamentalist religions in the island.

She had 12 liveborn children, 4 of whom died within 9 days of birth. All her children were delivered by her mother, who was untrained and did not deliver anyone else in the village. There is no evidence to suggest that the death of 4 of her children, which from the experience of the survey is very high, is in any way associated with the fact that they were delivered by her mother.

Sheila was 19 when she had her first child who was a month premature and lived for only half an hour. She said she was sick during the pregnancy and had a cold and pains over her body but she did not go to the doctor as she was very young at the time and was "hiding" her condition from her parents. They found out about it only when she was 8 months pregnant. In those days it was different, "not the days of today when we can know what happen to our children." The father of this child, aged 28 at the time the child was born, was her first partner. "She saw him and loved him" and he visited her as that was the type of union most convenient for their age group. When she discovered she was pregnant she broke off the relationship. Even if she had been older at the time she does not think she would have lived with him or married him. The union with her first partner lasted less than a year and she remained single for a very short while.

Her other 11 children were for the man she eventually married and with whom she had a visiting relationship for 10 years prior to her marriage, which took place after the birth of her eighth child. Her second child, born a year after the first, and her fifth child died at 9 and 8 days respectively from fits, while her seventh child, who was born when she was 7 months pregnant, died after 4 days. Unlike her experience with her first child, she had no complications during subsequent pregnancies. She used no contraceptives and breastfed each of her children for 9 months. Her last child was born when she was 38 years old and her husband 41.

She agreed to marry her partner 10 years after the friendship began, as having so many children with him she thought "it would be better than going to another man and having more children." Her mother agreed with their decision. Her husband had taken the initiative as she had not wanted to get married before. She felt that he would change towards her after marriage and she now believes that he was more affectionate in the visiting union and was more thoughtful towards her. She says marriage keeps you "steadier" but there are many disadvantages to it; whether you want to or not you have to obey "by everything" and sometimes it gives you "lots of taking back —regression."

When they were in a visiting relationship she saw him regularly as he would come to her house about 3 times per week and she visited him about once per week. They saw each other at least 5 hours for the week and as the relationship grew he visited more frequently. During these visits to her home they would discuss the needs of the children who, because of their visiting, were able to be with their father 2 to 3 hours per week. They also had sex when he visited her home but as there were difficulties in arranging this, it was not a regular occurrence. Although she and her partner did not go out to any form of entertainment, they went to church together. In comparing her two partners as well as her two types of unions it seems clear that regardless of the disadvantages she mentioned earlier she is happier with her husband in the married union. They have sex about twice per month which she enjoys and she expects that both she and her husband will be faithful to each other.

Sheila feels that every man and woman should have a child: the woman

who has none is not born to have any and "is very poor." She has heard it said
that every woman should have a certain number of children but she has never
heard how this number can be known and her mother who delivered all her
children did not enlighten her about this.

In her opinion the best spacing among the first 4 children is 4, 5 and 6 years
respectively but the greatest space between her own children is $2\frac{1}{2}$ years,
between the ninth and tenth. Although she feels better when she is not
pregnant and her ideal family is 4—2 boys and 2 girls—in 19 years she has had
12 pregnancies. In addition she considers a family of 3 children small while
one of 10 or more large. She thinks the woman has a choice in the number of
children she can have and she should not have a child for each of her
partners. She admits that she and her husband have never discussed the
question of whether or not to have children.

This lady had her first period at 13 and is still menstruating. Her last child,
born when she was 38 years old, is 7 years old. It is not clear whether she is
using any family planning method. She thinks family planning is "all right"
and one does not have to worry while "taking it" and it is important for the
development of the country as one would then have fewer children.

Certainly her knowledge of menstruation—"ordained to be so"—and
conception—"when a man and woman have sex"—is very limited and she has
no idea why one gets pregnant at some times and not at others.

She was frightened when she saw her first period although her mother had
told her about it before it appeared. Her menstruation has been regular and
of 5 days duration and she knows of no beliefs or superstitions connected with
it. She was not told about sex before experiencing it but she feels that a
woman should not have sexual intercourse before, during or up to 4 days after
menstruation. Her partner does not approach her for sex during these times.
She knows of no way of getting rid of a baby.

Despite the number of children she has had, she and her husband were
very sad about those who died. However she did not consider replacing them
nor did she consider herself in any way responsible for their deaths. The other
children were too young to be affected in any way by these events. In this
family of 6 boys and 2 girls, the mother admits to having a special feeling for
the girls and "just loves them." They all call her "Mamma" while she called
her mother the more old fashioned "Mammie."

As can be expected this lady was always busy around her house and could
give the interviewer "no other time." She was cooperative while at the same
time washing her dishes and doing her housework. For some unknown reason
she had not been approached to participate in a similar study in 1971—72.

Statistical summary of pregnancy history

Events		Age	Years	Percentages
Age at menarche		13		
Age at menopause (still menstruating)		45		
Biological years of potential childbearing	(a)		32	
Age at termination of 1st pregnancy		19		
Age at termination of last pregnancy		38		
Actual years of childbearing	(b)		19	
Years spent in pregnancy	(c)		8.7	
Years spent in breastfeeding	(d)		6.0	
(c) + (d)	(e)		14.7	
Rest of period			4.3	
Total pregnancies		12		
(b) as % (a)				59.4
(c) as % (b)				46.0
(d) as % (b)				31.6
(e) as % (b)				77.6

Average number of years per pregnancy 1.6
(actual years)/(number of pregnancies)

APPENDIX VII
Local Terms Used

Local Terms Used

Bruk	Break
Fretration	Worry
Can't lay no treasure	Cannot depend on
Watch ya	Look at
Go to ground	Go to the field
Dead yard	Cemetery
Mauger	Thin, slim
Running belly	Diarrhoea
Nana	Untrained birth attendant
She tan so	She looks so, she is pregnant
When she fall	When she starts having children, becomes pregnant
The very first fast I go fast	First time she had sex she got pregnant
Making a baby	Pregnant
Breeding same way	Still getting pregnant
First pain	First child
Nature	Desire for sex
Germs, juice	Sperm
T'ief a piece	Illicit sex
To dig in	To have sexual intercourse
Too much mix up, mix up, finish the alphabet	Too many surnames
Run the racket	Going with other women
Kill it off	Abortion
Bun-pan	Boiling of different bushes as a drink for the purposes of abortion
See the thing	Menstruation, period
Diaper, pad	Sanitary napkin

Born white	Albino
Lick	To beat, to flog
Never looked so manly	Not mature, unable to settle down
Mule	Woman without or unable to have children

INDEX